T0139867

Evaluation and Management of Dysphagia

Dhyanesh A. Patel • Robert T. Kavitt
Michael F. Vaezi
Editors

Evaluation and Management of Dysphagia

An Evidence-Based Approach

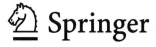 Springer

Editors
Dhyanesh A. Patel
Center for Swallowing and Esophageal
Disorders
Vanderbilt University Medical Center
Nashville, TN
USA

Robert T. Kavitt
Center for Esophageal Diseases
University of Chicago Medical Center
Chicago, IL
USA

Michael F. Vaezi
Center for Swallowing and Esophageal
Disorders
Vanderbilt University Medical Center
Nashville, TN
USA

ISBN 978-3-030-26556-4   ISBN 978-3-030-26554-0   (eBook)
https://doi.org/10.1007/978-3-030-26554-0

This Springer imprint is published by the registered company Springer Nature Switzerland AG
The registered company address is: Gewerbestrasse 11, 6330 Cham, Switzerland

Preface

It is our great pleasure to introduce you to *Evaluation and Management of Dysphagia: An Evidence-Based Approach*.

Dysphagia is a highly prevalent symptom with the most recent national health interview survey in 2012 showing that this symptom affects 4% of the US population (9.44 ± 0.33 million adults), which is approximately 1 in 25 adults annually [1]. It also showed that only 22.7% of adults with dysphagia saw a healthcare professional and, even more staggering, only 36.9% of those that sought care were given a diagnosis. We have also previously shown that adult US inpatients with dysphagia have a longer hospital length of stay, higher inpatient costs, higher likelihood of discharge to a post-acute care facility, and higher inpatient mortality compared to those with similar patient, hospital size, and clinical characteristics without dysphagia [2]. This highlights a critical gap in awareness of the disease and medical providers' ability to provide timely diagnosis and management. The field of esophageal diseases has been transformed over the last decade with the advent of newer diagnostic technologies (high-resolution manometry and EndoFLIP for motility disorders, mucosal impedance device for eosinophilic esophagitis and gastroesophageal reflux disease) and treatment options (per-oral endoscopic myotomy for patients with achalasia) that decrease the latency period for diagnosis and management of these patients.

This book is a comprehensive, state-of-the art review of various esophageal disorders and will serve as a valuable resource for clinicians, surgeons, researchers, and trainees with an interest in the management of patients with dysphagia. The book provides an exhaustive literature review of all the current evidence behind the diagnosis, evaluation, and management of various esophageal disorders and provides the reader with evidence-based algorithms written by prominent clinicians and researchers in the field. When applicable, the writers have graded the recommendations and levels of evidence based on a set criterion:

Level 1A: Large RCTs or systematic reviews/meta-analysis
Level 1B: High-quality cohort study
Level 1C: Moderate-sized RCT or meta-analysis of small trials

Level 1D: At least one RCT
Level 2: One high-quality of non-randomized cohort
Level 3: At least one high-quality case control study
Level 4: High-quality case series
Level 5: Opinions from experts

The chapters are organized so that the reader systematically learns how to recognize and narrow the differential for dysphagia followed by advances in diagnostic tools and includes the most up-to-date information about medical, endoscopic, and surgical options for patients with dysphagia of various etiologies. We are grateful to the contributors and hope that this book provides insight into this commonly encountered symptom and can pave the way for an evidence-based approach to taking care of this patient population.

Nashville, TN, USA   Dhyanesh A. Patel, MD
Chicago, IL, USA   Robert T. Kavitt, MD, MPH
Nashville, TN, USA   Michael F. Vaezi, MD, PhD, MSc (Epi), FACG

References

1. Bhattacharyya N. The prevalence of dysphagia among adults in the United States. Otolaryngol Head Neck Surg. 2014;151:765–9. https://doi.org/10.1177/0194599814549156.
2. Patel DA, et al. Economic and survival burden of dysphagia among inpatients in the United States. Dis Esophagus. 2018;31:1–7. https://doi.org/10.1093/dote/dox131.

Contents

Contributors

Arash Babaei Division of Gastroenterology, Department of Medicine, National Jewish Health, Denver, CO, USA

Jennifer X. Cai Division of Gastroenterology, Hepatology and Endoscopy, Brigham and Women's Hospital, Boston, MA, USA

Harvard Medical School, Boston, MA, USA

Walter W. Chan Division of Gastroenterology, Hepatology and Endoscopy, Brigham and Women's Hospital, Boston, MA, USA

Harvard Medical School, Boston, MA, USA

John O. Clarke Division of Gastroenterology & Hepatology, Stanford University School of Medicine, Redwood City, CA, USA

Ofer Z. Fass Department of Medicine, New York University Langone Health, New York University, New York, NY, USA

Ronnie Fass Case Western Reserve University, Digestive Health Center, Division of Gastroenterology and Hepatology, MetroHealth Medical Center, Cleveland, OH, USA

Nina Gupta Section of Gastroenterology, Hepatology, and Nutrition, University of Chicago, Chicago, IL, USA

C. Prakash Gyawali Division of Gastroenterology, Washington University School of Medicine, St Louis, MO, USA

Afrin N. Kamal Division of Gastroenterology & Hepatology, Stanford University School of Medicine, Redwood City, CA, USA

David A. Katzka The Mayo Clinic, Rochester, MN, USA

Robert T. Kavitt Center for Esophageal Diseases, Section of Gastroenterology, Hepatology, and Nutrition, University of Chicago, Chicago, IL, USA

Betty H. Li Department of Medicine, University of Chicago, Chicago, IL, USA

Kristle L. Lynch Esophageal Physiology Laboratory, The University of Pennsylvania Perelman School of Medicine, Philadelphia, PA, USA

Rishi D. Naik, M.D., M.S.C.I. Section of Gastroenterology, Hepatology, and Nutrition, Center for Swallowing and Esophageal Disorders, Digestive Disease Center, Vanderbilt University Medical Center, Nashville, TN, USA

Kornilia Nikaki Wingate Institute of Neurogastroenterology, Barts and the London School of Medicine and Dentistry, Queen Mary University of London, London, UK

Amit Patel Division of Gastroenterology, Duke University School of Medicine and the Durham Veterans Affairs Medical Center, Durham, NC, USA

Dhyanesh A. Patel, M.D. Section of Gastroenterology, Hepatology, and Nutrition, Center for Swallowing and Esophageal Disorders, Digestive Disease Center, Vanderbilt University Medical Center, Nashville, TN, USA

Joel E. Richter Division of Digestive Diseases and Nutrition, Joy Mccann Culverhouse Center for Swallowing Disorders, Joy Culverhouse Center for Swallowing Disorders, Division of Digestive Diseases and Nutrition, Tampa, FL, USA

Akinari Sawada Wingate Institute of Neurogastroenterology, Barts and the London School of Medicine and Dentistry, Queen Mary University of London, London, UK

Sajiv Sethi University of South Florida Division of Digestive Diseases and Nutrition, Tampa, FL, USA

Daniel Sifrim Wingate Institute of Neurogastroenterology, Barts and the London School of Medicine and Dentistry, Queen Mary University of London, London, UK

Robert M. Siwiec Division of Gastroenterology and Hepatology, Indiana University School of Medicine, Indianapolis, IN, USA

Chapter 1
Dysphagia: How to Recognize and Narrow the Differential

Kristle L. Lynch and David A. Katzka

Introduction

As M.F.K Fisher once wrote, "First we eat, then we do everything else." Though the ability to swallow effortlessly is often taken for granted, dysphagia is a common patient concern with significant impact on quality of life. It can be a challenging symptom to diagnose with causes ranging from benign strictures to chronic allergic disease to widespread malignancy. Narrowing down the differential diagnosis of dysphagia can be difficult by history. This chapter will focus on signs and symptoms that can be used to help pinpoint the underlying cause of dysphagia. Additionally patient-reported outcomes that aid in disease monitoring and treatment will be reviewed.

The word dysphagia stems from Greek terms *dys* (difficulty) and *phagia* (to eat) [1]. This debilitating symptom affects humans across the globe with prevalence rates reported as high as 22% [2]. However, it can be a complex symptom to assess as there is often overlap with other esophageal and pharyngeal symptoms such as globus, heartburn, and regurgitation. Causes of dysphagia vary worldwide. In western nations such as the United States, esophageal adenocarcinoma and eosinophilic esophagitis (EoE) are increasing in incidence. With the introduction and increasing use of proton pump inhibitors, reflux related strictures are decreasing. Contrastingly, eastern nations are noting an increase in squamous cell carcinoma [3].

K. L. Lynch
Esophageal Physiology Laboratory, The University of Pennsylvania Perelman School of Medicine, Philadelphia, PA, USA
e-mail: Kristle.Lynch@uphs.upenn.edu

D. A. Katzka (✉)
The Mayo Clinic, Rochester, MN, USA
e-mail: Katzka.David@mayo.edu

© Springer Nature Switzerland AG 2020
D. A. Patel et al. (eds.), *Evaluation and Management of Dysphagia*,
https://doi.org/10.1007/978-3-030-26554-0_1

Dysphagia Overview

Dysphagia is divided into several main categories, oropharyngeal vs. esophageal and mechanical vs. dysmotility. As apparent in the term, oropharyngeal dysphagia stems from abnormal processes affecting the mouth and pharynx. Patients with oropharyngeal dysphagia have problems transferring liquid or food boluses to the esophagus. Associated symptoms that may help distinguish oropharyngeal dysphagia from esophageal dysphagia include functions related to neuromuscular dysfunction such as drooling, food spillage from the mouth, inability to masticate, piecemeal swallowing, difficulty initiating a swallow, nasal regurgitation, need for repeat swallows, coughing, sialorrhea, xerostomia, dysarthria, dysphonia, or choking [4, 5]. Esophageal dysphagia encompasses all disorders that originate below the upper esophageal sphincter, causing issues with transit to the stomach. Patients classically complain of the sensation of slowed movement of food or liquids boluses in the chest though occasionally may refer symptoms to the neck from a more distal source of obstruction. The onset of symptoms is after the swallow as opposed to during the swallow. These patients do not have respiratory symptoms as the site of obstruction is distal to the airway. Patients with esophageal dysphagia may also tolerate more and/or larger boluses due to the capacious nature of the esophageal body when compared to the pharynx.

Mechanical dysphagia occurs typically though compromise of the lumen diameter. As a result, these patients will note that bolus size and consistency are the most important variables in producing symptoms. As a result, hard, dry, or chunky foods such as meat or rice and also pills cause symptoms in mechanical causes of dysphagia, whereas softer foods and liquids are not problematic unless the narrowing is almost to the point of obstruction. In contrast, motility disorders that cause dysphagia will typically involve both solids and liquids. This is because intact sphincter and esophageal body function are required for passage of all bolus consistencies. Early on in a disease such as achalasia, however, solid dysphagia may dominate with liquids becoming problematic later as lower esophageal sphincter dysfunction worsens. In some esophageal diseases, there may be a combination of dysmotility and mechanical obstruction. For example, a Zenker's diverticulum may form poor upper esophageal sphincter compliance but in turn compress the proximal esophagus.

It is also important to consider the sensory component of dysphagia. Disorders of esophageal hypersensitivity such as functional dysphagia may yield a sense of food sticking or slow transit when in fact motor function is normal and the patient is sensing physiologic passage of the bolus. Conversely, in disorders such as achalasia, where sensory function may be lessened, patients may not be cognizant of bolus impedance until large or multiple boluses have become obstructed.

Oropharyngeal Dysphagia

The most common cause of oropharyngeal dysphagia is neurologic dysfunction in older patients and myopathies, rings, or webs in younger patients [3]. Muscle weakness, drooling, focal weakness, hemiplegia, vision changes, vertigo, tinnitus, fatigability, tremor, ataxia, and trouble speaking are symptoms that may point toward a neurologic deficit, particularly of cranial nerves leading to oropharyngeal dysphagia. Additional attending symptoms with dysphagia are common as a single cranial nerve will typically innervate muscles that contribute to multiple aspects of the swallowing phases as well as speaking. Thus phases such as preparation of the bolus, elevation of the palate, and speaking may all be involved in a single cranial nerve injury. Thus a careful history evaluates all aspects of the swallowing phases. Liquids typically cause more difficulty, particularly with attending respiratory symptoms such as cough. This is because the normal mechanisms that protect the airway are commonly affected in oropharyngeal dysphagia; they are less successful in preventing liquid than solid penetration of the laryngeal vestibule.

If patients present with a known history of neurologic disease such as Parkinson's disease, cerebrovascular accident, multiple sclerosis, or amyotrophic lateral sclerosis, oropharyngeal dysphagia should be suspected. Similarly, patients with striated muscle dysfunction such as with myasthenia gravis or polymyositis commonly have oropharyngeal dysphagia. On the other hand, these and other neuromuscular diseases may present with dysphagia before more evident neurologic symptoms develop [3]. Anatomic abnormalities such as osteophytes may cause oropharyngeal compression but there are no specific differentiating symptoms to raise suspicion for these. A proper oral examination is critical in dysphagia to assess for poor dentition and loss of salivation (often a medication side effect) as probable causes. A full list of potential causes of oropharyngeal dysphagia can be seen in Table 1.1 and a suggested algorithm is seen in Fig. 1.1.

Patients with pharyngeal dysphagia often indicate the sensation of bolus holdup in the cervical esophagus with multiple swallows required to transfer the bolus. However, distal esophageal obstruction can also cause symptoms in the cervical region; this occurred in up to 30% of patients in one study [6]. Thus this is not a specific indicator of location and does not definitively distinguish clinically between oropharyngeal and esophageal dysphagia.

Esophageal Dysphagia

Patients with esophageal dysphagia often indicate food and/or liquids moving slowly or getting stuck in the chest. Classically, dysphagia to solids alone was thought to indicate a structural issue, whereas dysphagia to liquids and solids was

Table 1.1 Differential diagnosis of oropharyngeal dysphagia

Neurologic	*Anatomic*
Cerebrovascular accident	Diverticulum
Parkinson's disease	Malignancy
Multiple sclerosis	Thyromegaly
Central nervous system tumor	Osteophyte
Botulism	Prior head or neck surgery
Supranuclear palsy	Cervical web
Amyotrophic lateral sclerosis	Cricopharyngeal bar
Myotonic dystrophy	*Iatrogenic*
Postpolio syndrome	Medication induced
Tardive dyskinesia	Radiation injury
Acute demyelinating process	Post-surgical
Guillain Barré syndrome	Corrosive
Rabies	
Lead poisoning	
Muscular	*Oral*
Myasthenia gravis	Poor dentition
Polymyositis	Loss of salivation
Pharynx or neck infection	Sjogren's syndrome
Mixed connective tissue disease	
Sarcoidosis	
Myotonic dystrophy	
Upper esophageal sphincter dysfunction	
Paraneoplastic syndromes	

thought to indicate a motility disorder [4]. A recent study reviewed consecutive esophageal manometries in 200 patients with non-obstructive dysphagia and found that achalasia occurred significantly more often in patients with mixed dysphagia than solid food dysphagia [7]. A lack of strong follow-up studies remains. However, clinical application of this teaching may not be unreasonable with the caveat that in any patient with longstanding dysphagia of any type, workup for a motility disorder should eventually be pursued.

There are further clinical clues in dysphagia patients that are often useful. Patients with esophageal dysmotility such as achalasia or Chagas disease often note regurgitation [1, 8]. An associated history of food impaction is classically seen in structural causes such as eosinophilic esophagitis or peptic strictures [3]. In patients who require endoscopic removal of food impaction, it is more likely than not to be from eosinophilic esophagitis in younger patients, with prevalence rates in this subgroup reported to be up to 54%. [9] In older patients, a Schatzki ring is more typical. Dysphagia to solids without food impaction may indicate esophageal webs. Furthermore, it is apparent via clinical observation that patients with mechanical causes of dysphagia tend to feel symptoms at the start of the meal with a single poorly chewed bolus whereas patients with motility disorders feel symptoms later in the meal when several boluses have become compounded in the esophagus. Indeed, some of these patients will describe a stacking effect. Furthermore, patients with mechanical obstruction may regurgitate the single lodged bolus for relief whereas those with motility disorders will regurgitate a

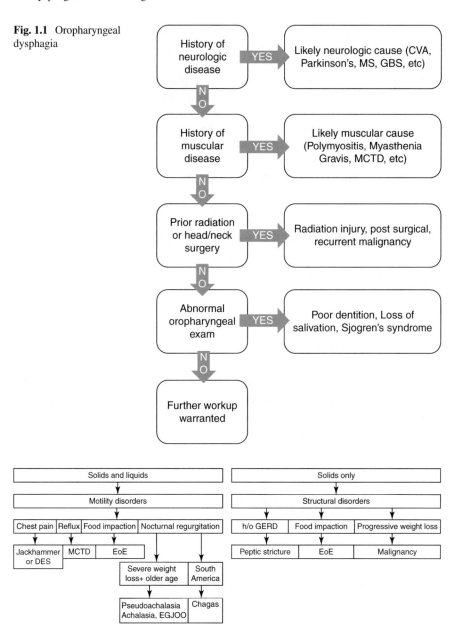

Fig. 1.1 Oropharyngeal dysphagia

Fig. 1.2 Esophageal dysphagia

larger quantity of food and beverage. The absence of regurgitation and vomiting may indicate a patent esophagus such as patients with ineffective esophageal motility, early to moderate scleroderma, or reflux-related esophageal dysmotility. Figure 1.2 notes an algorithm for narrowing the differential diagnosis for esophageal dysphagia based on clinical details.

Regarding structural causes of dysphagia, investigators have used balloon distension techniques to evaluate the accuracy of patient symptom localization. In one study of 139 patients with esophageal strictures, the majority of patients (74%) were able to localize symptoms to within four centimeters of the esophageal lesion as seen on barium esophagram. Patients were significantly more likely to report symptoms from distal lesions being more proximal than vice versa [10]. In another study of 16 distal esophageal rings, only 75% of patients felt any symptom when a marshmallow was impacted at the site. Of these patients, 11 of the 12 reported symptoms more proximal to the implicated area [11]. Further studies reveal similar findings of proximally referred symptoms [12, 13]. Thus patient localization of dysphagia is likely only clinically useful when localized distally, to the substernal area. The broad list of potential causes of esophageal dysphagia is outlined in Table 1.2. Medication lists should be scrutinized as various drugs can lead to oropharyngeal and esophageal dysphagia via both anticholinergic pathways and localized mucosal effects [5, 14] (Table 1.3). For instance, opiates have been described to cause a range of motility disorders from esophagogastric outflow obstruction to type III achalasia [15, 16].

Patient-Reported Outcomes

Patient-reported outcome (PRO) measures are uninfluenced expressions of a patient's experience that are captured in a standardized format to allow assessment of patient-centered outcomes [17]. They can be critical in disease monitoring and treatment response [18]. Thus, PRO measures are used widely in the approval process for medications as well as devices. In fact, most randomized controlled trials funded by the National Institute of Health are required to include PRO measures

Table 1.2 Differential diagnosis of esophageal dysphagia

Motility	Anatomic and structural
Achalasia	Malignancy
Hypertensive esophageal sphincter	Benign tumors
Diffuse esophageal spasm	Esophageal polyp
Jackhammer esophagus	Esophageal rings
Eosinophilic esophagitis	Cervical webs
Ineffective esophageal motility	Eosinophilic esophagitis
Chagas disease	Foreign body
Pseudoachalasia	Strictures
Reflux-related dysmotility	Osteophytes
Scleroderma	Vascular compression
Lupus	Mediastinal or hilar lymphadenopathy
Mixed connective tissue disease	Post-surgical
Medication induced	
Infectious	Other
Candida esophagitis	Functional dysphagia
Viral esophagitis	

Table 1.3 Medications implicated in causing oropharyngeal and esophageal dysphagia [5, 14]	Opioids
	Olanzapine, clozapine
	Amitriptyline
	Botulinum toxin
	Procainamide
	Amiodarone
	Iron
	Potassium
	Non-steroidal anti-inflammatory medications
	Tetracyclines, macrolides
	Bisphosphonates
	Calcium channel blockers
	Nitrates
	Alcohol
	Theophylline
	Cholesterol-lowering medications
	Phenothiazines
	Cytotoxins

[17, 18]. Over the past three decades, there have been over 40 different PROs developed specifically for diseases that cause dysphagia. A recent systematic review of dysphagia-related PROs evaluated the following categories to assess for rigor: conceptual model, content validity, reliability, construct validity, scoring and interpretation, burden, and presentation. Of the 34 studies that met criteria for extraction and analysis, there were 7 studies thought to be of satisfactory analysis. These outcome measures assess mechanical and neuromyogenic oropharyngeal dysphagia, esophageal cancer, achalasia, and eosinophilic esophagitis [18].

General Dysphagia

In 2004 the National Institutes of Health (NIH) launched a patient-reported outcomes initiative to develop publicly available banks to measure patient experience. A gastrointestinal symptom scale was developed by the NIH, and disrupted swallowing was measured via seven questions. This concise questionnaire was not targeted toward any specific esophageal disease but encompassed general dysphagia. It was practical in its ease of availability to the public, the short 7-day recall period, and a reading level that did not exceed that of a sixth grader [19]. The Mayo Dysphagia Questionnaire (MDQ) is another PRO developed for general dysphagia. It was more extensive and consists of 28 items, encompassing dysphagia severity and frequency, presence of allergies, gastroesophageal reflux disease and treatment, and esophageal surgery and dilation history. This takes about 6 minutes to complete and has been used in various clinical trials [20].

Oropharyngeal Dysphagia

Given the high prevalence of oropharyngeal dysphagia in patients over 50 years of age, a quality of life outcomes tool for oropharyngeal dysphagia is definitely justified. Unsurprisingly, numerous PROs have been developed [21]. The first validated dysphagia-specific PRO for patients with head and neck cancer was developed at M.D. Anderson in 2001. The MDADI (M.D. Anderson Dysphagia Inventory) consists of a self-administered questionnaire assessing 20 items that encompass global, emotional, functional, and physical well-being. This has been used in various studies assessing outcomes in head and neck cancer patients [22]. The SWAL-QOL is a quality of care outcomes tool for oropharyngeal dysphagia that assesses ten main categories including symptom frequency, eating duration and desire, fear, mental health, and fatigue. The complementary SWAL-CARE is a medications implicated in causing shorter and more patient-friendly assessment specifically looking into quality of care and patient satisfaction. Brief versions of these PROs can be seen in Table 1.4 [23].

Table 1.4 SWAL-QOL and SWAL-CARE abbreviated versions

Burden	Mental Health
Dealing with my SP is very difficult	My SP depresses me
SP is a major distraction in my life	I get impatient dealing with my SP
	Being so careful when I eat or drink annoys me
Eating Duration	My SP frustrates me
It takes me longer to eat than other people	I've been discouraged by my SP
It takes me forever to eat a meal	
	Social
Eating Desire	I do not go out to eat because of my SP
Most days, I don't care if I eat or not	My SP makes it hard to have a social life
I don't enjoy eating anymore	My usual activities have changed BOM SP
I'm rarely hungry anymore	Social gatherings are not enjoyable BOM SP
	My role with family/friends has changed BOM[a] SP
Symptom Frequency	
Coughing	Fatigue
Choking when you eat food	Feel exhausted
Choking when you take liquids	Feel weak
Having thick saliva or phlegm	Feel tired
Gagging	
Having excess saliva or phlegm	Sleep
Having to clear your throat	Have trouble falling asleep
Drooling	Have trouble staying asleep

Table 1.4 (continued)

Problems chewing	
Food sticking in your throat	*Advice (SWAL-CARE)*
Food sticking in your mouth	Food I should eat
Food/liquid dribbling out your mouth	Foods I should avoid
Food/liquid coming out your nose	Liquids I should drink
Coughing food/liquid out your mouth	Liquids I should avoid
	Techniques to help get food down
Food Selection	Techniques to help me avoid choking
Figuring out what I can eat is a problem for me	When I should contact a swallowing clinician
It is difficult to find foods I both like and can eat	My treatment options
	What to do if I start to choke
Communication	Signs that I am not getting enough to eat or drink
People have a hard time understanding me	Goals of the treatment for my SP
It's been difficult for me to speak clearly	
	Patient Satisfaction (SWAL-CARE)
Fear	Had confidence in your swallowing clinicians
I fear I may start choking when I eat food	Swallowing clinicians explained treatment to you
I worry about getting pneumonia	Swallowing clinicians spent enough time with you
I am afraid of choking when I drink liquids	Swallowing clinicians put your needs first
I never know when I am going to choke	

Reprinted by permission from Springer Nature, McHorney et al. [23]

[a]*BOM* because of my, *SP* swallowing problem. Item content is abbreviated. The SWAL-QOL and SWAL-CARE are available free of charge upon request

Esophageal Cancer

Despite recent advances in neoadjuvant chemotherapy, the mortality rate of esophageal cancer remains dismal. Thus quality of life is a critical consideration for patients when assessing treatment options, and patient-reported outcomes are of utmost value in this disease. Though there have been several PROs developed for esophageal cancer, FACT-E (Functional Assessment of Cancer Therapy Esophageal Cancer subscale) is one of the most comprehensive. FACT-E focuses on physical, social, and emotional well-being as well as esophageal symptom frequency. This PRO has been used in various clinical investigations. [24] The EORTC QLQ-OG25 was developed to assess health-related quality of life in patients with esophageal and stomach cancer. This 25-item questionnaire assesses 6 critical patient outcomes: dysphagia, eating restriction, reflux, odynophagia, pain, and anxiety [25, 26].

Achalasia

Though achalasia treatment response is often evaluated by the well-known Eckardt symptom score, a quality of life assessment has been developed. The MADS (Measure of Achalasia Disease Severity) assessment encompasses food tolerance, behavior modifications, pain, heartburn, distress, lifestyle limitation, and satisfaction [27]. Though it is patient friendly and has shown to be valid and reliable, it has not been widely adapted in achalasia treatment outcomes studies.

Eosinophilic Esophagitis

Eosinophilic esophagitis is a young disease described barely 30 years ago, with an increasing incidence and prevalence. In concordance with this trend, there have been several PROs developed for eosinophilic esophagitis in the recent years. The EoE Activity Index (EEsAI) PRO is a widely used global assessment of EoE that includes seven items that evaluate frequency and duration of dysphagia, severity of dysphagia, and behavioral adaptations to various foods. The recall period is 7 days and 24 hours; completion time is 8 minutes. This is currently being used in clinical trials [28]. Other PRO measures which are not as widely used in EoE include the DSQ which assesses solid food avoidance, dysphagia, and actions to improve dysphagia in a daily electronic diary and the Straumann Dysphagia Index (SDI) which is a non-validated PRO which assesses frequency and intensity of dysphagia events [28, 29].

Summary

Proper oropharyngeal mechanisms and esophageal propagation of food and liquid boluses are essential to daily life. Unfortunately dysphagia is a common patient complaint and can stem from a plethora of causes. A careful review of the patient's history, physical exam, and clinical presentation can often narrow down the differential. It is critical to separate the symptoms into either oropharyngeal dysphagia or esophageal dysphagia, as treatment options differ significantly. Patient-reported outcome measures have been well studied in various esophageal disorders and should be followed to evaluate quality of life in these cumbersome diseases.

References

1. DeVault K. Symptoms of esophageal disease. In: Feldman M, Friedman L, Brandt LS, editors. Fortran's gastrointestinal and liver disease. 9th ed. Philadelphia: Elsevier Inc; 2010.
2. Cho SY, Choung RS, Saito YA, Schleck CD, Zinsmeister AR, Locke GR 3rd, Talley NJ. Prevalence and risk factors for dysphagia: a USA community study. Neurogastroenterol Motil. 2015;27(2):212–9.

3. Malagelada JR, Bazzoli F, Boeckxstaens G, De Looze D, Fried M, Kahrilas P, Lindberg G, Malfertheiner P, Salis G, Sharma P, Sifrim D, Vakil N, Le Mair A. World gastroenterology organisation global guidelines: dysphagia—global guidelines and cascades update September 2014. J Clin Gastroenterol. 2015;49(5):370–8.
4. Abdel Jalil AA, Katzka DA, Castell DO. Approach to the patient with dysphagia. Am J Med. 2015;128(10):1138.e17–23.
5. Philpott H, Garg M, Tomic D, Balasubramanian S, Sweis R. Dysphagia: thinking outside the box. World J Gastroenterol. 2017;23(38):6942–51.
6. Cook IJ, Kahrilas PJ. AGA technical review on management of oropharyngeal dysphagia. Gastroenterology. 1999;116(2):455–78.
7. Chen CL, Orr WC. Comparison of esophageal motility in patients with solid dysphagia and mixed dysphagia. Dysphagia. 2005;20(4):261–5.
8. Newberry C, Vajravelu RK, Pickett-Blakely O, Falk G, Yang YX, Lynch KL. Achalasia patients are at nutritional risk regardless of presenting weight category. Dig Dis Sci. 2018;63(5):1243–9.
9. Furuta GT, Katzka DA. Eosinophilic esophagitis. N Engl J Med. 2015;373(17):1640–8.
10. Wilcox CM, Alexander LN, Clark WS. Localization of an obstructing esophageal lesion. Is the patient accurate? Dig Dis Sci. 1995;40(10):2192–6.
11. Smith DF, Ott DJ, Gelfand DW, Chen MY. Lower esophageal mucosal ring: correlation of referred symptoms with radiographic findings using a marshmallow bolus. AJR Am J Roentgenol. 1998;171(5):1361–5.
12. Roeder BE, Murray JA, Dierkhising RA. Patient localization of esophageal dysphagia. Dig Dis Sci. 2004;49(4):697–701.
13. Zerbib F, Omari T. Oesophageal dysphagia: manifestations and diagnosis. Nat Rev Gastroenterol Hepatol. 2015;12(6):322–31.
14. Antonik S, Shaker R. Disorders causing oropharyngeal dysphagia. In: Richter J, Castell D, editors. The esophagus. 5th ed. Oxford: Blackwell Publishing Ltd. p. 2012.
15. Ravi K, Murray JA, Geno DM, Katzka DA. Achalasia and chronic opiate use: innocent bystanders or associated conditions? Dis Esophagus. 2016;29(1):15–21.
16. Camilleri M, Lembo A, Katzka DA. Opioids in gastroenterology: treating adverse effects and creating therapeutic benefits. Clin Gastroenterol Hepatol. 2017;15(9):1338–49.
17. Ahmed S, Berzon RA, Revicki DA, et al. The use of patient-reported outcomes (PRO) within comparative effectiveness research: implications for clinical practice and health care policy. Med Care. 2012;50:1060–70.
18. Patel DA, Sharda R, Hovis KL, Nichols EE, Sathe N, Penson DF, Feurer ID, McPheeters ML, Vaezi MF, Francis DO. Patient-reported outcome measures in dysphagia: a systematic review of instrument development and validation. Dis Esophagus. 2017;30(5):1–23.
19. Spiegel BM, Hays RD, Bolus R, Melmed GY, Chang L, Whitman C, Khanna PP, Paz SH, Hays T, Reise S, Khanna D. Development of the NIH patient-reported outcomes measurement information system (PROMIS) gastrointestinal symptom scales. Am J Gastroenterol. 2014;109(11):1804–14.
20. Grudell AB, Alexander JA, Enders FB, Pacifico R, Fredericksen M, Wise JL, Locke GR 3rd, Arora A, Zais T, Talley NJ, Romero Y. Validation of the Mayo dysphagia questionnaire. Dis Esophagus. 2007;20(3):202–5.
21. Wallace KL, Middleton S, Cook IJ. Development and validation of a self-report symptom inventory to assess the severity of oral-pharyngeal dysphagia. Gastroenterology. 2000;118(4):678–87.
22. Chen AY, Frankowski R, Bishop-Leone J, Hebert T, Leyk S, Lewin J, Goepfert H. The development and validation of a dysphagia-specific quality-of-life questionnaire for patients with head and neck cancer: the M. D. Anderson dysphagia inventory. Arch Otolaryngol Head Neck Surg. 2001;127(7):870–6.
23. McHorney CA, Robbins J, Lomax K, et al. The SWAL-QOL and SWAL-CARE outcomes tool for oropharyngeal dysphagia in adults: III. Documentation of reliability and validity. Dysphagia. 2002;17:97–114.
24. Darling G, Eton DT, Sulman J, Casson AG, Celia D. Validation of the functional assessment of cancer therapy esophageal cancer subscale. Cancer. 2006;107:854–63.

25. Lagergren P, Fayers P, Conroy T, et al. Clinical and psychometric validation of a questionnaire module, the EORTC QLQOG25, to assess health-related quality of life in patients with cancer of the oesophagus, the oesophago-gastric junction and the stomach. Eur J Cancer. 2007;43:2066–73.
26. Blazeby JM, Conroy T, Hammerlid E, et al. Clinical and psychometric validation of an EORTC questionnaire module, the EORTC QLQ-OES18, to assess quality of life in patients with oesophageal cancer. Eur J Cancer. 2003;39:1384–94.
27. Urbach DR, Tomlinson GA, Harnish JL, Martino R, Diamant NE. A measure of disease-specific health-related quality of life for achalasia. Am J Gastroenterol. 2005;100:1668–76.
28. Schoepfer AM, Straumann A, Panczak R, Coslovsky M, Kuehni CE, Maurer E, Haas NA, Romero Y, Hirano I, Alexander JA, Gonsalves N, Furuta GT, Dellon ES, Leung J, Collins MH, Bussmann C, Netzer P, Gupta SK, Aceves SS, Chehade M, Moawad FJ, Enders FT, Yost KJ, Taft TH, Kern E, Zwahlen M, Safroneeva E, International Eosinophilic Esophagitis Activity Index Study Group. Development and validation of a symptom-based activity index for adults with eosinophilic esophagitis. Gastroenterology. 2014;147(6):1255–66.e21.
29. Dellon ES, Irani AM, Hill MR, Hirano I. Development and field testing of a novel patient-reported outcome measure of dysphagia in patients with eosinophilic esophagitis. Aliment Pharmacol Ther. 2013;38:634–42.

Chapter 2
Advances in Testing for Dysphagia

Afrin N. Kamal and John O. Clarke

Introduction

The act of swallowing relies on a complex series of voluntary and involuntary neuromuscular events to help propel food or liquid bolus past the mouth and along the esophageal lumen into the stomach. Myenteric inhibitory neurons signal relaxation of the lower esophageal sphincter, contraction and shortening of the inner circular and outer longitudinal layers, coordination of peristalsis, and triggering of the swallowing center in the medulla and pons to create a primary peristaltic wave. These functions act together to create what is referred to as a "normal" swallow. Dysphagia, on the other hand, refers to the subjective sensation of difficulty in the swallowing process, estimated to have a prevalence of 6–9% in all age groups, with a rise at age ≥ 50 years. Dysphagia itself remains a broad symptom category, further separated as either oropharyngeal or esophageal in origin. Whereas some patients can experience difficulty with swallow initiation in oropharyngeal dysphagia – with symptoms such as coughing, choking, aspiration, and nasal regurgitation – others can experience a sensation of food "sticking" in the throat or upper chest as seen in esophageal dysphagia.

Etiologies of dysphagia can be the result of structural or neuromuscular dysfunction [1, 2]. Solid food dysphagia often is attributed to structural disorders including inflammatory, fibrotic, or malignant conditions, whereas mixed liquid and solid food dysphagia can reflect underlying dysmotility such as with achalasia and diffuse esophageal spasm [3]. As patients present with symptoms of difficulty swallowing, it is important to choose the appropriate diagnostic modality to help establish the underlying etiology of symptom

A. N. Kamal · J. O. Clarke (✉)

Division of Gastroenterology & Hepatology, Stanford University School of Medicine, Redwood City, CA, USA

e-mail: jclarke2@stanford.edu

© Springer Nature Switzerland AG 2020

D. A. Patel et al. (eds.), *Evaluation and Management of Dysphagia*,

https://doi.org/10.1007/978-3-030-26554-0_2

pathogenesis. This chapter aims to discuss diagnostic tools commonly utilized in dysphagia assessment, reviewing mechanism of action, protocol, and diagnostic yield. Specifically, this chapter will address the role of fluoroscopy, endoscopic evaluation of swallowing, manometry, and the functional lumen imaging probe. Each of these plays an important yet complementary role in the evaluation of dysphagia. While most patients will require only a subset of these tests for optimal evaluation, all have a potential role in evaluation and are part of the armamentarium available to the dysphagia provider. Obtaining a careful history and clinical assessment of the presentation allows one to customize a diagnostic strategy for each individual patient so as to maximize diagnostic yield while simultaneously limiting the number of studies required to achieve a diagnosis.

When considering studies to evaluate dysphagia, it is helpful to separate diagnostic modalities by location. Oropharyngeal dysmotility primarily results from dysfunction of the oropharyngeal musculature and coordination. This is a rapid process and is best evaluated by studies that allow either rapid sequencing or direct visualization. As such, oropharyngeal dysmotility is primarily evaluated by fluoroscopy with rapid sequencing and fiberoptic endoscopic evaluation of swallowing, usually in that order. In contrast, esophageal dysphagia usually results from either structural or motility processes and can be best identified with modalities that do not require rapid sequencing but rather can focus on esophageal mucosa, wall dynamics, and emptying. While endoscopy is often the first study, fluoroscopy (without necessarily rapid sequencing), manometry, and the functional lumen imaging probe all have a complementary and defined role. For the remainder of this chapter, we will address each of these modalities in turn (Table 2.1).

Table 2.1 Summary of the key diagnostic tests available to assess dysphagia with respective advantages and disadvantages of each. (a) focuses on studies available to assess oropharyngeal dysphagia. (b) focuses on studies available to assess esophageal dysphagia

	Advantage	Disadvantage
(a) Oropharyngeal dysphagia		
Videofluoroscopic swallowing study (VFSS)	Visualizes oropharyngeal function Real-time fluoroscopic imaging Less radiation than cineradiography	Lacks visualization of the esophageal lumen and gastroesophageal junction Lack of therapeutic capabilities Requires radiation
Fiberoptic endoscopic evaluation of swallowing (FEES)	Direct visualization of oropharyngeal region Can be utilized using different food consistencies Performed in-office setting without sedation Evaluates aspiration during and after each swallow	Lack of therapeutic capabilities Minimal esophageal lumen structure and/or motility evaluation Can be uncomfortable More invasive than radiography

Table 2.1 (continued)

	Advantage	Disadvantage
(a) Oropharyngeal dysphagia		
High-resolution pharyngeal manometry	Can measure pressure and coordination of oropharyngeal region and upper esophageal sphincter May help define mechanisms of oropharyngeal dysphagia not clear after above	Can be uncomfortable for patients Normative data are limited Analysis is difficult and not supported by current software Clinical significance of many findings remains unclear
(b) Esophageal dysphagia		
Barium esophagram	Assesses structure of the esophagus Can detect gross motility disturbance Can add a 13 mm barium tablet to the protocol for dysphagia Can give information to aid in therapeutic endoscopy	Lack of therapeutic capabilities Requires swallowing oral contrast and radiation May add time and expense if endoscopy is required anyway
Endoscopy	Both diagnostic and therapeutic Ability to biopsy esophagus Only means to diagnose eosinophilic esophagitis	Minimal esophageal motility evaluation Invasive diagnostic tool requiring sedation May miss subtle structural lesions if esophagus not fully insufflated
High-resolution esophageal manometry	Gold standard for assessment of esophageal motility Can provide information for achalasia that can affect prognosis	Patient discomfort can be a factor Only assesses motility Diagnostic only Clinical implications of many manometry diagnoses uncertain
Endoflip	Allows direct measurement of esophageal diameter and wall stiffness Also allows measurement of secondary peristalsis Can guide treatment decisions When combined with endoscopy allows simultaneous assessment of structure and motility	Very limited normative data Not widely available Technical concerns as measurements are based on only one pressure sensor Must be combined with endoscopy Data are more limited as compared to other tests listed

Fluoroscopy

The process of deglutition results in complex muscular coordination, resulting in valvular closure and opening of the upper and lower esophageal sphincters, with in between passage of swallowed material along the upper digestive tract and along the esophageal lumen. The ability to identify abnormalities in deglutition function, therefore, requires examination of two basic processes. First is assessing bolus transport along the upper digestive tract, with safety and airway protection monitoring, followed by measuring bolus passage through the esophagus and into the gastric lumen. As mentioned, dysfunction in these processes can lead to either oropharyngeal or esophageal swallowing dysfunction. Radiographic imaging with ingested barium contrast is a noninvasive contrast-enhanced method enabling visualization of the structural anatomy and function of the gastrointestinal system. Based on anatomical focus, radiographic imaging can range from a focus on the oropharyngeal function with a videofluorographic swallowing study (VFSS), prioritized imaging of the esophagus and gastroesophageal junction (GEJ) via a barium esophagram, or other protocols that may focus on different regions or combine a focus on both oropharyngeal and esophageal function – such as a videopharyngoesophagram [4]. The particular fluoroscopic protocol employed can direct the evaluation as clinically indicated. Specific fluoroscopy protocols are detailed in Table 2.2.

Table 2.2 Summary of common fluoroscopy protocols used in clinical practice, with suggested applications

Study	Summary	Tips and tricks
Esophagram	Barium is swallowed while still images are taken to evaluate esophageal structure and emptying Can add a 13 mm tablet	Reasonable protocol for esophageal dysphagia Tablet can be a very helpful addition in solid dysphagia Can be specific for achalasia but insensitive
Timed barium esophagram	Barium is ingested and then spot images are obtained to assess emptying Minimizes radiation	Helpful for monitoring of achalasia pre/post therapy Limited utility outside of achalasia but can be a validated tool to assess for impaired esophageal emptying
Upper gastrointestinal series (UGI)	Essentially a barium esophagram extended to also look at the stomach and duodenal C-loop	Reasonable to obtain if you are worried about gastric issues in addition to esophageal Probably not necessary if only concerned about dysphagia
Videofluoroscopic swallowing study (VFSS) or Modified barium swallow (MBS)	Rapid sequence images of the oropharynx and upper esophageal sphincter to evaluate oropharyngeal dysphagia or aspiration	Recommended initial diagnostic test for oropharyngeal dysphagia Limited utility at assessing esophageal dysphagia – if not sure based on history whether dysphagia is esophageal or oropharyngeal would ask radiology to extend the study
Videopharyngoesophagram (or cine-esophagram)	Rapid sequence images of the oropharynx and esophagus	Used in some academic centers but probably not necessary in most cases Higher amounts of radiation than the protocols above

In the evaluation of suspected oropharyngeal dysphagia, the videofluorographic swallowing study (VFSS), also referred to as modified barium swallowing examination (MBS), provides a rapid sequence evaluation of oropharyngeal coordination and bolus transit and is often considered the initial instrument of choice for evaluation of oropharyngeal dysmotility. Historically, MBS was also known as the "cookie swallow" technique, reflecting J.A. Lodgeman's protocol instructing patients to swallow 2 cc of radiopaque liquid, 2 cc of paste, and ¼ of a cookie coated with barium. Subsequently, Linden and Siebens et al. from Good Samaritan Hospital and Johns Hopkins University, respectively, created a more individualized approach to videofluorography. In this method, radiopaque food similar to what patients ate on a more ordinary basis was applied, coating foods with barium. Robbins et al. modified this protocol further, adding a cup of 30 cc liquid barium to be swallowed. Authors noted more aspiration events by drinking a higher volume of barium than taking 2 cc boluses, therefore enhancing sensitivity for aspiration detection [5]. Applying these modifications, standard protocols in swallowing content vary from facility to facility but in general consist of a radiopaque material such as barium mixed with liquid and food of diverse consistency and size. As patients are seated upright, real-time fluoroscopic imaging of the swallowing process is obtained, with visualization of the oral cavity, pharynx, larynx, and upper esophagus, following administration of graduated bolus volumes with various radiopaque consistencies. Protocol technique consists of lateral imaging to assess the possibility of aspiration during swallowing and subsequent anterior-posterior views with focus on symmetry and vocal cord function. Due to the required use of fluoroscopy to optimize imaging, optimum duration of fluoroscopy is considered less than 3 minutes in efforts to reduce radiation exposure [6]. Subsequent imaging interpretations are often made collaboratively with radiologists and speech-language pathologists, the latter providing recommendations on diet type and methods to reduce aspiration risks [7].

In contrast to digital cineradiography, which displayed cinematographic recording on tape, VFSS provides the ability to view imaging immediately and with less radiation exposure. On the other hand, acquisition of image frequency by VFSS is less when compared to cineradiography, at 25–30 images/seconds compared to 50–80 images/seconds, respectively, leading to decreased temporal resolution [8]. The application of VFSS has become useful in evaluation of swallowing impairments among patients with neurological deficits, such as in cerebral infarcts (25–50%) [9, 10] and Parkinson's disease (>80%) [11]. By incorporating this form of radiologic study, etiology for oropharyngeal dysphagia symptoms in addition to aspiration risk can be assessed [7, 12].

To measure the interobserver reliability of VFSS, Stoeckli et al. compared assessments of 9 independent observers among 51 patients undergoing videofluoroscopy. As measured by kappa coefficient, parameters for oral and pharyngeal phase, temporal occurrence of penetration, and aspiration, in addition to location of bolus residue, ranged between 0.01 and 0.56. High reliability, as represented by a coefficient of 0.80, was only achieved with defined penetration and aspiration scores. Therefore, the authors concluded that although evaluation of aspiration demonstrated high reliability, this was not as evident among other parameters of oropharyngeal swallow [13].

Furthermore, when assessing accuracy of VFSS, Giraldo-Cadavid et al. performed a systematic review comparing frequencies of positive and negative results among patients with oropharyngeal dysphagia who underwent evaluation via VFSS and fiberoptic endoscopic evaluation of swallowing (FEES). When comparing these two diagnostic techniques, analysis revealed greater sensitivity with FEES for aspiration (0.88 vs. 0.77, $p = 0.03$), penetration (0.97 vs. 0.83; $p = 0.0002$), and laryngopharyngeal residue (0.97 vs. 0.80; $p < 0.0001$), whereas both tests had similar specificity. The authors suggested that FEES offered a slight advantage over VFSS, with the caveat both techniques provided similar specificity in detecting oropharyngeal dysfunction [14].

Whereas VFSS captures dysfunction in bolus transport along the upper digestive tract, barium esophagram is an integral tool to assess for structural and/or motility abnormalities involving the esophageal lumen and gastroesophageal junction. This technique applies radiographic still images with a contrast medium of barium sulfate (45% weight by volume), or less commonly a water-soluble agent such as Gastrografin/diatrizoate, to better characterize the presence of esophageal pathology. Barium sulfate is neither absorbed nor metabolized within a normal gastrointestinal tract and is employed for radiologic imaging for the purposes of improving visualization. Given the radiopaque nature, where barium localizes can visually be seen on X-ray films, generating visual contrasts to allow for identification of the gastrointestinal anatomy. Therefore, interpreting barium esophagram requires recognition of normal anatomy and therefore disruption in anatomy. These abnormalities in anatomy can be seen in the setting of hiatal hernia, esophageal strictures, and achalasia [15, 16].

When performing an esophagram, patients are positioned in a partial lateral decubitus position to displace the esophagus away from the spine during imaging. Patients rapidly drink 100–200 cc of contrast to distend the esophagus. To view more subtle lesions, slight deviations in standard protocol can occur such as mixing water with contrast to reduce thickness or adding effervescent sodium bicarbonate granules immediately prior to swallowed contrast to increase production of air and therefore luminal distension. A barium esophagram is often an initial imaging study performed for dysphagia, having the ability to identify structural lesions such as ulcerations and strictures and benign or malignant neoplasms including fibrovascular polyps and adenocarcinomas, respectively, in addition to gross disruptions in motility such as in achalasia and diffuse esophageal spasm [15].

While barium esophagram focus on the detailed evaluation of the esophagus, the motivation behind timed barium esophagram (TBE) is to concentrate on esophageal emptying while minimizing radiation exposure. By quantifying esophageal emptying, this technique has been applied in the evaluation and monitoring posttherapy of achalasia. Performed similar to barium esophagram, the key modification which occurs is multiple sequential films at pre-defined intervals. To start, patients are advised to complete an overnight fast. At time of the study, patients swallow low-density barium sulfate within 15–20 seconds, followed by three spot left posterior oblique films taken at 1, 2, and 5 minutes to assess esophageal emptying. In the setting of complete esophageal clearance at 2 minutes, many protocols provide an option to omit the 5-minute film [17, 18]. Mechanistically, the degree of esophageal emptying is based on the barium column height, measured from the highest level of luminal contrast to the EGJ, in addition to the esophageal width, measured as the widest part of the barium column. The barium column in most normal subjects empties at 1 minute, whereas at 5 minutes complete barium emptying occurs in all healthy individuals. Therefore, applying these parameters as reference allows readers to differentiate normal emptying from stasis in the esophagus, the latter most notably seen in achalasia. To assess interobserver agreement in this interpretation, de Oliveira et al. applied timed barium swallows among 23 patients with achalasia and measured imaging interpretation among 4 experienced observers. Authors revealed high reliability on height-times-width calculations in addition to qualitative emptying percentage, as represented by a correlation coefficient of 0.87 and 0.93, respectively [19]. Furthermore, TBE has been applied in post-treatment assessment of esophageal emptying [18]. Vaezi et al. assessed pre- and post-dilation barium column heights among 53 patients with achalasia undergoing pneumatic dilation. Authors revealed a significant improvement ($p < 0.001$) in height and symptom relief following dilation [20]. Furthermore, Kostic et al. aimed to quantify similar improvements in esophageal emptying following an esophagomyotomy in patients with achalasia. By comparing pre-myotomy and post-myotomy barium heights and widths relative to surgery, authors demonstrated a postsurgical reduction in column heights at 1, 2, and 5 minutes ($p < 0.001$). Additionally, complete esophageal emptying at 5 minutes was seen in 49% of the measured population. Post-myotomy symptoms of dysphagia and regurgitation, on the other hand, were found to be unrelated to TBE findings, suggesting that although timed barium provides an objective assessment on esophageal emptying following a myotomy, patient symptoms itself may not be as reliable an indicator for assessing postsurgical improvement [21].

Complications to oral contrast are infrequent, mild, and self-limiting, with the most common adverse effect being nausea and vomiting within 30 minutes of swallowing oral contrast. Patients who are dehydrated or diagnosed with cystic fibrosis may experience constipation or intestinal obstruction secondary to colonic impaction, and rarely will patients experience mild allergic reactions. The most serious complications include bronchospasm and laryngeal edema, in addition to contrast aspiration or extravasation into the mediastinum. Safety of barium sulfate during pregnancy is unknown, although radiography itself is contraindicated due to fetal risk, and therefore not generally performed [15, 16]. Please see Fig. 2.1 for examples of fluoroscopic images in patients with dysphagia taken from patients seen in our dysphagia clinic.

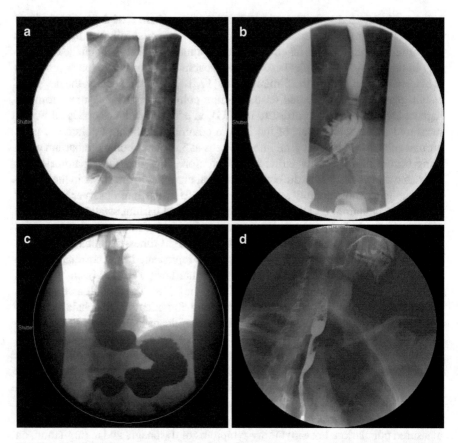

Fig. 2.1 The following images were obtained from patients seen at the Stanford University Dysphagia Clinic. Image (**a**) shows a normal barium esophagram with no signs of structural abnormality. Image (**b**) shows a patient with a large hiatal hernia. Image (**c**) shows a patient with achalasia with a megaesophagus and sigmoidization with a sinktrap deformity. Image (**d**) shows a patient with a cervical esophageal stricture with estimated diameter of 8 mm

Fiberoptic Endoscopic Evaluation of Swallowing

Fiberoptic endoscopic evaluation of swallowing (FEES) provides visualization of the hypopharynx, larynx, and proximal trachea by the use of a flexible fiberoptic rhinopharyngolaryngoscope. The introduction of FEES in 1988 by Langmore et al. [22] opened a new paradigm for swallowing evaluation. The technique applies two endoscopic positions referred as "pre-swallow" and "post-swallow." The former maintains views of the soft palate and tip of the epiglottis, evaluating for premature spillage of a bolus and/or swallowing delay. Patients sound out high-pitched words and cough, allowing the performer to assess for pharyngeal wall approximation and laryngeal adductory tasks. The post-swallow position, on the other hand, concentrates on the inferior larynx and subglottis to assess for the laryngeal penetration and aspiration. This occurs by administering boluses in small amounts, encompassing thin liquids, thick liquids (i.e., nectar), puree, and solids, with evaluation of aspiration events during and after each swallow [23, 24].

Both speech-language pathologists and otolaryngologists can perform FEES with slightly different training practices, the former obtaining 10–14 hours in formal class training and 10–20 FEES observations, whereas the latter group obtaining swallowing physiology through CME courses at workshops or national meetings [1, 2]. The application of FEES in clinical practice, however, has been applied in other medical disciplines. Lee et al. describes an increased frequency of FEES performed by gastroenterologists in South Korea. To characterize the safety and tolerance, the authors evaluated the incidence of laryngospasm, epistaxis, vasovagal syncope, airway compromise, and significant disruption in cardiovascular integrity, in addition to self-reported discomfort. In total, 303 examinations were performed primarily for the evaluation of dysphagia. Gastroenterologist-directed FEES failure occurred in 5 patients and among 128 examinations, only 50.3% and 6.0% reported mild and moderate discomfort, respectively [25].

As mentioned, when comparing FEES to VFSS, Giraldo-Cadavid et al. demonstrated higher sensitivity with FEES in detection of aspiration, penetration, and laryngopharyngeal residue [14]. Langmore et al. aimed to measure similar epidemiologic values when comparing FEES to videofluoroscopy. Among 21 patients with symptoms of oropharyngeal dysphagia, authors calculated a sensitivity of 75% and specificity of 56% for premature spillage, 93% and 50% for pharyngeal residue and, and 100% and 75% for laryngeal penetration, in addition to 88% and 92% for tracheal aspiration, respectively. Furthermore, a positive predictive value (PPV) of 82% in pharyngeal residue and 88% in tracheal aspiration was noted, suggesting FEES adequately predicts "true" findings when compared to videofluoroscopy. Although sample size was relatively low ($n = 21$), the authors concluded FEES was a valuable instrument in evaluating swallowing physiology [26]. Therefore, with the trend in greater supportive data, FEES has often become a benchmark test in the evaluation of swallowing function and oropharyngeal dysphagia [23].

Endoscopy

Esophagogastroduodenoscopy (EGD), often referred to as an upper endoscopy, is an endoscopic procedure enabling direct mucosal visualization of the oral cavity, larynx, and upper gastrointestinal (GI) tract, in addition to tissue acquisition and, when necessary, therapeutic intervention. As endoscopy can be both diagnostic and therapeutic, endoscopy is the most common initial diagnostic tool to evaluate for esophageal dysphagia with an estimated 3000 upper endoscopies performed per 250,000 population annually [27].

Standards for performing upper gastrointestinal endoscopy recommend utilization of a high-definition video endoscopy system. Patients are given intravenous sedation and/or local anesthetic throat spray and positioned in the left lateral decubitus position. Subsequently, the endoscope is passed trans-orally and advanced through the esophagus, stomach, and second portion of the duodenum, with photo-documentation occurring at each anatomical landmark. Applying air insufflation, aspiration, and mucosal cleansing techniques, mucosal inspection occurs at time of upper endoscopy. Moreover, in the presence of a mucosal lesion, placement of biopsy forceps through an instrument channel within the endoscope can facilitate tissue sampling [28, 29].

The underlying principles behind mucosal evaluation and tissue acquisition are to exclude malignant and premalignant conditions, and to assess for underlying etiologies such as a peptic stricture, Schatzki's ring, or eosinophilic esophagitis (EoE). As a chronic, local immune-mediated esophageal disease, EoE is the result of eosinophil-predominant inflammation leading to esophageal dysfunction includ-ing dysphagia, food impaction, and rarely esophageal perforation [3, 30]. With a frequency of 7% of all upper endoscopies in patients with esophageal symptoms, a diagnosis can only be made based on mucosal histology with the presence of ≥ 15 eosinophils per high power field. Therefore in efforts to standardize guidelines for diagnosis, a task force of 21 experts recommended at least six biopsies taken from different locations when suspecting this immune-mediated disease [31]. Furthermore, the American College of Gastroenterology specified biopsies arise from at least two locations (proximal and distal esophagus) [32]. Considering symptoms do not precisely correlate with histology in EoE and patients can often demonstrate normal-appearing mucosa, statement recommendations support esophageal biopsies for mucosal pathology in all patients presenting with esopha-geal dysphagia [33].

Beyond acquisition of tissue for mucosal histology, endoscopic visualization allows for the assessment of structural etiologies for dysphagia. Peptic strictures, a complication of gastroesophageal reflux disease (GERD), accounts for the majority of all benign esophageal strictures. This structural narrowing in the esophagus results from severe esophageal mucosal inflammation, leading to collagen and fibrous tissue deposition. Depending on stricture severity, and therefore effect of esophageal luminal diameter, oral tolerability can vary. A regular diet is tolerated at a diameter of 20 mm, whereas symptoms of dysphagia occur in almost all patients at a diameter of ≤ 13 mm. Between those diameters, symptoms are variable and intermittent. Moreover, stricture diameter facilitates in differentiating between sim-ple and complex strictures. The former characteristically is a short and symmetric stricture, with a diameter of ≥ 12 mm. On the other hand, a complex stricture fre-quently presents as a height of >2 cm, irregular, and a diameter of <12 mm. Understanding the type and size of a stricture often aids in the decision of dilation technique, as complex strictures are associated with more recurrent and dilation-related adverse effects [3].

Esophageal dilation is the act of stretching a narrowed area within the esophagus. Types of esophageal dilators include a wire-guided dilator (Savary-Gillard), weighted push type (Maloney), and balloon dilators (wire-guided and through-the-scope). Savary-Gillard and Maloney bougie dilators depend on tactile perception to feel the degree of resistance with dilator passage. The former consists of polyvinyl with a tapered rigid tip and hollow core to allow guidewire passage, whereas Maloney dilators are passed through the esophagus blindly or under fluoroscopic imaging. On the other hand, polyethylene balloon dilators consist of multiple-size balloons, and are passed either over a guidewire (over-the-wire) or through the upper endoscope (through the scope). Balloon sizes vary from small (6 mm to 20 mm) often applied in sequential dilation with one dilation passage, as utilized in treatment of esophageal strictures, to large (30–40 mm) as seen with pneumatic dilation in treatment of achalasia [3, 34].

Frequently, esophageal pathologies are amenable to dilation, particularly when anatomic change is present as seen with peptic structures, Schatzki rings, and post-radiation strictures. On occasion, however, etiologies for dysphagia will not improve with dilation as seen with esophageal spasm, hypomotility (connective tissue disorders), and extrinsic compression [3]. Considering the process of esophageal dilation encompasses the act of stretching the esophageal lumen, the procedure itself can be linked with an increased risk of complications when compared to a purely diagnostic endoscopy. Esophageal dilation carries an overall risk of 0.4% for all complications, the most common being perforation with an incidence range of 0.1–0.4%. As previously described, complex strictures carry the highest risk for complications with additional risk factors including malignant strictures, prior radiation therapy, caustic ingestion, eosinophilic esophagitis, esophageal pseudodiverticula, surgically altered anatomy with interposition, and chronic steroid use [35]. Suspecting a perforation should be made when visualizing a deep mucosal tear or patient complaint of chest pain and vomiting following dilation. If perforation does occur, management may include stent placement in the esophagus, inhibiting leakage of fluid into the chest [36]. Please see Fig. 2.2 for examples of endoscopic images in patients with dysphagia taken from patients seen in our dysphagia clinic.

Esophageal Manometry

Esophageal manometry is considered to be the gold standard for assessment of esophageal motility. Adapted from conventional water-perfused manometry, high-resolution esophageal pressure topography incorporates the technology of high-resolution manometry (HRM) and esophageal pressure topography as Clouse plots and is an innovative technological advance to assess esophageal motility patterns [37, 38]. HRM translates the measured amplitude contractile events in the esophagus and the upper and lower esophageal sphincter in relationship to time, in addition to pressure that is sensed along the length of a manometry catheter. Whereas conventional line tracing used hydrostatic pressure with limited sensors, HRM advances esophageal evaluation incorporating multiple pressure sensors (up to 36) at 1–2 cm intervals spanning the length from the hypopharynx, through the esophagus, to 3–5 cm within the stomach. Additionally, with the use of a solid catheter that was once not available in conventional manometry, HRM allows for both supine and sitting position measurements [39].

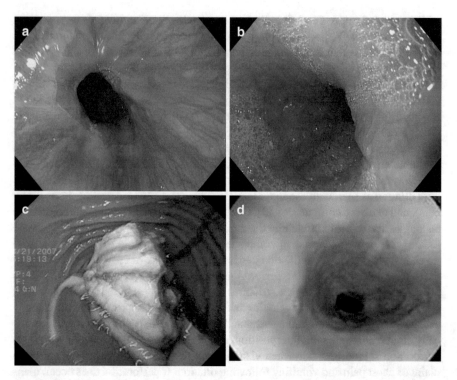

Fig. 2.2 The following images were obtained from patients seen by the authors in clinic for complaints of dysphagia. Image (**a**) shows a relatively unremarkable distal esophagus and gastroesophageal junction. Image (**b**) shows a capacious dilated esophagus with frothy secretions consistent with achalasia, although the diagnosis cannot be established based on the endoscopy alone. Image (**c**) shows food impaction with a piece of chicken in a patient with eosinophilic esophagitis. Image (**d**) shows a cervical esophageal stricture

Pressure topography functions by localizing and tracking focal areas of high pressure, visually allowing a differentiation between sphincters, from adjacent atonic regions, in addition to peristaltic contractions [40]. Applying advanced software algorithm, HRM converts data and allows readers to visualize timing of sphincter relaxation, segmental contraction, in addition to transition zone length between striated and smooth muscle segments – improving methods to assess for esophageal motility disorders [40, 41].

In efforts to standardize definitions of esophageal motility disorders, an international consensus group was created (HRM Working Group) and had their first meeting in San Diego during Digestive Disease Week (DDW) in 2007. Objectives of the group were to adapt data from HRM and pressure topography to clinically meaningful methods to evaluate esophageal motility disorders. This classification scheme coined "The Chicago Classification" was later published in 2009. Over the last several years, two iterations have thus followed with the most recent published in 2015 (version 3) reflecting new developments in the classification system [38, 42, 43].

With esophageal manometry providing an assessment of quantitative and quali-tative measures of peristaltic coordination and pressures, the most common clinical indications to apply HRM has been assessment of nonobstructive dysphagia, local-ization of sphincter landmarks to assist in anti-reflux testing, and evaluation of esophageal motor function prior to anti-reflux surgery [42]. Following catheter cali-bration, the HRM catheter is inserted trans-nasally, initially positioned within the pharynx, and then slid distally with the assistance of the patient swallowing. Correct catheter positioning beyond the EGJ is confirmed with recognition of the pressure inversion point (PIP), a marker of inspiration-associated negative intrathoracic pres-sure inverting with positive intra-abdominal pressure [39, 44].

Following The Chicago Classification (CC) recommendations, a baseline rest-ing pressure of 30 seconds is obtained with the absence of swallows, followed by 10 supine liquid swallows of 5 ml of water. It should be noted that augmentations in this standard protocol have been developed, in efforts to elucidate further abnormalities in esophageal swallowing function. For example, multiple rapid swallows (MRS) function by stimulating neural inhibition, leading to cessation of esophageal body contractions and complete lower esophageal sphincter relax-ation, resulting in subsequent esophageal peristalsis and LES contraction [44]. Fornari et al. aimed to evaluate the yield of MRS to detect disruptions in the normal inhibitory and excitatory functions by applying a protocol of 5 water swallows, 2 ml, separated by 2–3 seconds among 23 healthy subjects and 48 patients with ineffective esophageal motility (IEM). Authors revealed among healthy controls, complete inhibition of esophageal contraction was seen during MRS followed by a strong motor response after MRS completion, whereas only 50% of patients with IEM demonstrated the ability to increase contractile ampli-tudes following MRS. Authors concluded as a complementary test, multiple rapid swallows offers the ability to further evaluate the normal physiological mechanisms within the esophagus among symptomatic patients [45]. As a result, the Chicago Classification v.3.0 published support in using MRS as a supplement test to elucidate peristaltic reserve [43]. Additionally, the incorporation of tex-tured boluses such as thickened liquids or solid foods has been thought to be beneficial in exposing abnormal esophageal motor functions. This application stems from the argument that patient symptoms rarely are triggered by water, let alone at volumes of 5 ml. Therefore, Sweis et al. aimed to measure reference values for both liquid and solid boluses, in efforts to assess for improved sensi-tivity in detection of esophageal dysmotility. Twenty-three asymptomatic volun-teers therefore underwent HRM applying 5 ml water administered with a syringe, in addition to 5 solid swallows of 1 cm bread, completing both in the upright and supine position. Authors revealed a higher integrated relaxation pressure for sol-ids than liquids at both supine and upright (<0.001 both), a significant decrease in contraction front velocity (CFV) for solids versus liquids in upright ($p = 0.01$), although not seen in supine positioning ($p = 0.186$), in addition to a higher distal contractile integral (DCI) for solids than liquids in both upright and supine ($p = 0.001$ and $p < 0.001$, respectively) [46]. Although CC v.3.0 describes HRM based on the analysis in the supine position with liquid swallows, performing in alternate conditions such as upright or following a test meal has been accepted clinically and may be diagnostically helpful in specific situations [43].

Diagnosing esophageal motility patterns applies a hierarchical analytic scheme set by the CC v3.0. Initial evaluation requires interpretation of the integrated relaxation pressure (IRP), a measure of deglutitive relaxation following a swallow. IRP is calculated by measuring 4 seconds of lowest mean axial pressure across the LES during 10 seconds after a swallow, with the median value of all 10 wet swallows signifying the overall IRP. An abnormal value (with the specific level of abnormality dependent on the manometry system employed) indicates abnormal transit across the esophagogastric junction (EGJ), suggestive of an outflow obstruction. Furthermore, in the setting of absent or abnormal peristalsis, suspicion for achalasia occurs. Therefore, IRP is an important metric when evaluating EGJ relaxation and esophageal motility disorders. Furthermore, a focus on contractile function is essential and is based on the distal contractile integral (DCI), distal latency (DL), and peristaltic integrity. The DCI is a sum of pressures within the time/length field between the transition zone to the proximal EGJ, calculated as units of mmHg.s.cm. The CC v.3.0 determined DCI >8000 mmHg.s.cm represented hyper-contractility, whereas values <450 mmHg.s.cm and < 100 mmHg.s.cm signified weak and failed swallows, respectively. The range of normal for DCI is between 450 and 8000 mmHg.s.cm. Additionally, distal latency is an important indicator of esophageal contraction arrival, measuring the start of swallow induced upper esophageal sphincter opening to contractile deceleration. A normal swallow is considered when DL $\geq$4.5, whereas spastic or premature is considered at <4.5 seconds. Lastly, peristaltic integrity is an important aspect of interpreting contractile function, particularly spatial breaks or gaps across the upper esophageal sphincter to the EGJ at 20 mmHg isobaric contour. The CC v.3.0 considers breaks >5 cm as fragmented swallows. The third component on swallowing assessment based on HRM includes interpretation of esophageal pressurization. Manometry provides the advantage of assessing intrabolus pressurization, a defining feature of type II achalasia. Pressurization occurs when swallowed liquid becoming trapped between contracting segments, seen at $\geq$30 mmHg isobaric contour [41]. Identifying these three main components in assessment of swallows and applying definitions based on CC v3.0., major and minor motility disorders can be identified [41].

When applying the Chicago Classification to esophageal manometry, the approach is hierarchical. If deglutitive relaxation, assessed by an abnormal IRP, is abnormal, then the diagnosis is either achalasia (type I, II or III based on the presence or absence of panesophageal pressurization and premature contraction) or EGJ outflow obstruction (if peristalsis is at least intermittently preserved). If deglutitive relaxation is normal, then one looks at the esophageal body to see if there is evidence of hypercontractility (assessed by an elevated DCI), premature contractions (assessed by the DL), or absent contractility. If any of these three esophageal body abnormalities are present, then a major motility disorder is present (Jackhammer esophagus, distal esophageal spasm or absent contractility). If none of these criteria are met, then one looks at peristaltic integrity. If there are significant weak or failed swallows, or large mucosal breaks on at least half of swallows, then a minor motility disorder (ineffective esophageal motility or fragmented peristalsis) is achieved – otherwise the study is considered to be normal.

The addition of impedance to standard esophageal manometry protocols has been added to monitor bolus movement within the esophageal lumen. First described by Silny et al. [47], the concept of impedance is a measurement of the electrical relationship between mounted electrodes on an intraluminal probe and luminal contents surrounding it. High impedance is a reflection of intraluminal air, whereas low impedance is demonstrated by liquid (swallowed or refluxed). Therefore, as impedance rings lay along the length of the esophageal probe, a temporal-spatial pattern can help differentiate swallowed and refluxed liquid, versus air itself [40]. The application of high-resolution impedance manometry therefore is the combination of manometry and impedance, monitoring both pressure and bolus transit simultaneously. Furthermore, to facilitate conductivity 0.3% saline solution is used with each swallows, replacing the standard water protocol [48].

The application of high-resolution impedance manometry has been used to predict incomplete bolus clearance and determine peristaltic integrity. Park et al. measured swallows among 71 patients with esophageal symptoms, classifying each swallow as complete or incomplete bolus clearance based on impedance, where complete bolus clearance was defined as bolus entry and subsequent clearance along all impedance sites and incomplete bolus clearance defined by bolus entry with subsequent failed clearance. Data revealed that small breaks of 3 and 7 cm or less were associated with high bolus clearance (96.8% and 94.7%, respectively). The authors therefore applied impedance to investigate the association between bolus transit and defects in peristalsis [48]. In addition, Liu et al. applied high-resolution impedance manometry among 58 patients with nonobstructive dysphagia, aiming to characterize esophageal motility and transit functions. Among the studied cohort, 28 patients had achalasia, 3 with esophagogastric junction outflow obstruction (EGJOO), 20 with nonspecific esophageal motility disorders, and the rest found to be normal. Applying impedance, incomplete bolus transit was seen in all (100%) of patients with achalasia and 90% with EGJOO, as compared to only 3.5% in the normal cohort. Given traditional HRM does not provide an insight into bolus transit among patients with dysphagia, esophageal impedance enhances the evaluation of esophageal bolus transport and may help characterize underlying pathophysiological mechanisms [49]. However, it should be noted that impedance is most helpful in situations where bolus transit can be intermittent, such as ineffective esophageal motility; impedance may not be as helpful in situations clearly associated with normal or abnormal bolus transit.

Special considerations are made when applying esophageal manometry to measure the proximal esophagus and upper esophageal sphincter (UES) in pharyngeal dysphagia. Since esophageal manometry measures intraluminal pressure and esophageal muscular coordination of pressure activity, this technology has been applied to measure not only esophageal body muscular activity and lower esophageal sphincter (LES) pressure but also further evaluate pharyngeal motor activity and UES relaxation. The UES functions to separate the pharynx from the esophagus, relaxing in response to swallowing followed by coordinated contraction to exclude air from esophageal contents. Abnormalities of the UES have been noted in conjunction with different diseases contributing to symptoms of dysphagia, including Parkinson's disease, globus sensation, scleroderma, and oculopharyngeal muscular dystrophy [50]. Similar to esophageal manometry protocols, UES manometry protocols require proper calibration of the catheter, followed by insertion of the catheter trans-nasally through a lubricated nasal passage while patients are in the sitting or supine position. Catheter positioning will aim to cross along the length of the esophagus, ending with the distal port in the stomach. Following a measurement of basal pressure for 2–5 minutes, patients are instructed to complete multiple swallows, typically 10 with 5 mL of water, in addition to 10 swallows with 1 mL of bread [51]. Unlike esophageal manometry in which the study focuses on esophageal body contraction and LES relaxation, UES manometry aims to assess for UES relaxation – a physiologic inhibition of the cricopharyngeus and simultaneous contraction of the suprahyoid muscles following swallowing. Assessing relaxation, however, is subject to variability between individuals swallows and determining the start and end of relaxation [51].

Normative data of pharyngeal high-resolution manometry values was tested by Jungheim et al., measuring pharyngeal manometry on 29 healthy volunteers in an upright position. Authors revealed normative values of maximum velopharyngeal pressure [mean 269.9, standard deviation (SD) 113.1 mmHg], maximum tongue base pressure (mean 278, SD 93.6 mmHg), maximum UES pressure (mean 205.8, SD 64.0 mmHg), UES resting pressure (mean 42.5, SD 18.7 mmHg), and relaxation UES time (mean 681.6, SD 86.8 ms) [52]. Furthermore, the reliability of pharyngeal manometry was tested by Omari et al., aiming to evaluate intra- and interrater agreement and test-retest reliability among five healthy (mean age 61) patients undergoing pharyngeal high-resolution manometry with impedance measurements. When comparing metrics of contractility, intrabolus pressure, flow timing, and global function, authors demonstrated high intra- and interrater agreement [53]. Similar to esophageal manometry, the application of maneuvers has been tested within pharyngeal manometry. To measure the effects of swallow maneuvers during pharyngeal high-resolution manometry, McCulloch et al. measured manometry among seven subjects during different postural conditions including head turn and chin tuck. Regions of the velopharynx and tongue base were measured for maximal pressure, rate of pressure increase, pressure gradient, and duration of pressure above baseline. Differences in pharyngeal pressures during maneuvers were noted primarily in the UES; however, no changes were observed in the velopharynx or tongue base [54]. Hoffman et al. additionally aimed to assess effects of effortful swallow and Mendelsohn maneuvers during high-resolution pharyngeal manometry, focusing on pressure and timing characteristics. The Mendelsohn maneuver is designed to manage reduced laryngeal excursion and limited cricopharyngeal opening by having a patient hold the larynx up during swallowing. The basis behind this maneuver is to increase extent and duration of laryngeal elevation, and therefore proportionately increasing this extent and duration of cricopharyngeal opening. With the application of these two maneuvers, the authors revealed dependent changes at the velopharynx and UES, critical functions to ensure safe swallowing [55, 56]. Please see Fig. 2.3 for examples of manometric images in patients with dysphagia taken from patients seen in our dysphagia clinic.

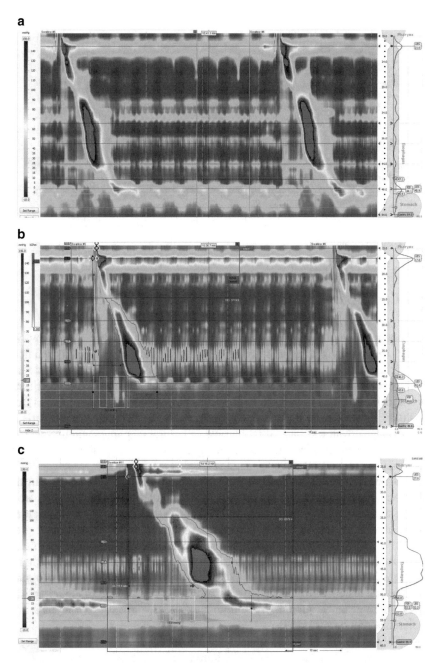

Fig. 2.3 The following images were obtained from patients seen at the Stanford University Dysphagia Clinic. Image (**a**) shows a normal high-resolution esophageal manometry. Image (**b**) shows the addition of impedance (colored in purple) to a normal high-resolution esophageal manometry study. Image (**c**) shows a hypercontractile, or Jackhammer, esophagus. Image (**d**) shows a patient with achalasia, subtyped as type II based on the presence of panesophageal pressurization

d

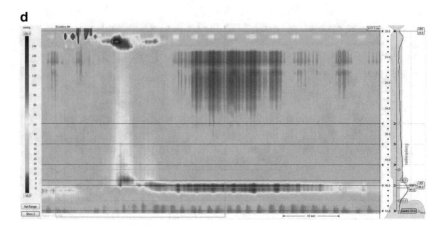

Fig. 2.3 (continued)

Functional Lumen Imaging Probe

The functional lumen imaging probe (FLIP) emerged recently as an innovative method to quantify the radial force of esophagogastric junction (EGJ) sphincter strength measured by the resistance to distension – referred to as distensibility. Sphincters within the gastrointestinal tract, such as the EGJ, create important barriers within the gut. This dynamic function of the EGJ, separating the esophagus from the stomach, relies on both extrinsic and intrinsic factors including gravity, peristalsis, esophageal wall mechanical properties, and crural diaphragmatic muscle tone [57]. As one can imagine, measurement of EGJ competence, therefore, has an important impact on further understanding esophageal diseases.

Traditional methods to measure EGJ sphincter function for the most part has relied on high-resolution manometry (HRM) as the gold standard. Unfortunately, HRM was not created to consider radial force and therefore only provides a measurement of static pressure [57]. Authors have argued, however, sphincter pressure on its own is not a true determinant of sphincter tone [58], and rather distensibility is potentially a more meaningful reflection of sphincter strength. Although barostat and impedance planimetry encompasses this ability to measure luminal distensibility, FLIP offers a more feasible method of adapting principles of impedance planimetry without exposing patients to the pain and intolerance of a barostat [57].

In 2009 an endoluminal functional lumen imaging probe (EndoFlip®, Crospon Ltd., Galway, Ireland) was commercially introduced, marketed as an imaging probe that captured simultaneous measurements of esophageal pressure and luminal diameter. Mechanistically FLIP provides a more accurate measurement of esophageal distensibility by determining resistance to distention, characterized by luminal cross-sectional area (CSA) and intraluminal pressure. Applying high-resolution impedance planimetry electrodes and a balloon filled with conductive saline, as volume-controlled distension occur, measurement of CSA along an axial plane is determined. These measurements are then divided by matched singular pressure levels (CSA/pressure), calculated out to represent luminal distensibility. Therefore, data from FLIP provides an improved assessment of esophageal wall mechanical properties and EGJ opening dynamics – providing different and complementary information to high-resolution manometry [59, 60].

The current FLIP device is made of a 240-mm long, 3-mm outer diameter catheter encompassed with 16 paired impedance planimetry electrodes and a solid-state pressure transducer housed within a distal balloon. Catheter sizes that are commercially available include 8-cm (EF-325) and 16-cm (EF-322) [60]. The FLIP product arrives as either 1.0 or 2.0, the latter converting high-resolution impedance planimetry as a space-time-luminal diameter continuum, or topography, visually displaying esophageal function in response to distension [61].

Variations in FLIP protocol exist among different institutions. At our institution, following sedation the FLIP catheter is placed blinded trans-orally into the esophagus or with direct endoscopic visualization. Although trans-nasal placement in the awake patient can be done, due to patient discomfort, this protocol is not commonly implemented. At a low fill volume (20–30 mL), the esophageal body is identified with a waist identified as the EGJ and allows real-time positioning to set the EGJ as the reference point. Once the catheter is positioned, ideally the tip sitting 2 cm into the stomach, volume-controlled distension of the balloon occurs. Real-time measurements of CSA and pressure is seen with step-wise volumetric distension at 10 ml increments. Measurements for distensibility are taken at all levels but are most validated at balloon distention of 60 ml when using the 16-cm FLIP and at 40 ml when using the 8-cm FLIP [60].

To understand normal thresholds of FLIP distension, Carlson et al. evaluated ten asymptomatic healthy controls (ages 20–49; 6 female) undergoing a 16-cm length FLIP balloon probe placement. Following moderate sedation, the catheter was placed trans-orally, and the distal catheter was positioned 1–3 impedance sensors below the EGJ at a distension volume of 20–30 ml. The majority of healthy controls demonstrated a median and interquartile range (IQR) distension volume of 29 ml (25–35.8), intra-bag pressure of 10.7 mmHg (8.6–15.9), and maximum body diameter of 18.5 mm (17.5–19.6), respectively. Therefore, the authors identified an organized pattern in the esophageal body of healthy controls, providing a characteristic for "healthy" patients. Moreover, the antegrade contractions seen visually on topography were thought to be secondary to sustained volumetric distension, or secondary peristalsis [61]. This normative data has recently been expanded to include an additional 20 healthy subjects.

The clinical utility of FLIP is expanding among various esophageal diseases, with the strongest data in the setting of achalasia. This motility disease is characterized by lower esophageal sphincter dysfunction, leading to failure of LES relaxation and impairment in esophageal peristalsis [62]. Traditionally achalasia was defined by esophageal manometry, a method applying pressure topography and classifying the three types based on pressurization patterns [63]. Treatment is targeted at the EGJ, with aims to improve opening after swallowing. Although high-resolution manometry and timed barium esophagram can facilitate in achalasia diagnosis, Pandolfino et al. aimed to assess if FLIP correlated with symptom severity in achalasia before and after treatment. The authors determined FLIP measurements among 54 patients, separated into two cohorts based on treatment profiles. One cohort received no treatment initially for their achalasia, whereas the second underwent pneumatic dilation ($n = 17$), Heller myotomy with partial fundoplication ($n = 10$), or per-oral esophageal myotomy ($n = 4$). A FLIP protocol using an 8-cm electrode probe was placed at the level of the squamocolumnar junction. EGJ distensibility (CSA/pressure) was a reflection of the narrowest CSA and corresponding pressure. Of those undergoing prior treatment, the authors subsequently categorized patients into either "good" or "poor" treatment response. The data revealed that patients with a successful treatment response correlated with greater EGJ distensibility, compared to those untreated or with poor treatment response ($r = 0.49$; $p < 0.05$). Furthermore, following comparison of EGJ distensibility at 40 mL on FLIP and EGJ function on high-resolution manometry, the authors demonstrated significant correlation for resting EGJ pressure ($r = -0.4$, $p < 0.05$), IRP ($r = -0.51$, $p < 0.001$), and nadir EGJ relaxation pressure ($r = -0.4$, $p > 0.05$). Pandolfino et al. concluded that these study findings suggested FLIP measurement of EGJ distensibility was a feasible tool to apply in achalasia and gauge success to treatment [64].

In addition to measuring EGJ distensibility, FLIP offers a novel method to assess esophageal body contractility through topography. To better define contraction patterns seen on topography, Carlson et al. aimed to compare FLIP topography between patients with achalasia (type I-15, type II-26, type III-10) and ten asymptomatic healthy controls (ages 20–49, 6 female). Applying a 16-cm length FLIP catheter and step-wise distension volumes, topography plots in addition to EGJ distensibility at 50 and 60 mL were recorded. Topography plots were interpreted as propagating or antegrade contractions, with the slope of the line at contraction onset distinguishing the two types. Therefore, propagating direction was determined by a positive slope, whereas a retrograde contraction was a reflection of a negative slope. Additionally, repetitive contractions were defined by ≥ 3 contractions occurring simultaneously. When reviewing topography profiles among healthy controls, the majority (80%) demonstrated repetitive antegrade contractions (RAC) in contrast to achalasia patients, whose contractile patterns were less uniform. Of the 61% exhibiting contractility, 29% were found to be RACs and 35% repetitive retrograde contractions (RRC). When differentiating contractility patterns based on achalasia subtypes, the authors revealed contractility was absent more frequently in type I achalasia compared to type II ($p = 0.017$) or type III ($p < 0.001$). Patients with type II achalasia demonstrated a greater degree of heterogeneity in contractile patterns, with 65% showing some form of contractility whereas type III patients more often demonstrated RRCs than type I ($p = 0.001$) or type II ($p = 0.011$). The fraction of patients with RRCs, however, were all similar among the groups. Carlson et al. therefore concluded FLIP is a useful tool to not only assess EJG distensibility in patients with achalasia but furthermore allowed a qualitative assessment of esophageal contractility [63].

Due to the irreversible degeneration of the nitrogenic neurons of the myenteric Auerbach plexus as seen in achalasia, treatment is often reserved to either medical, endoscopic, or surgical in efforts to improve symptoms. Although classically Heller myotomy with a partial anti-reflux wrap was considered the optimal surgical treatment, more recently the endoscopic alternative per-oral endoscopic myotomy (POEM) has entered into clinical practice [65]. First described in 2007, POEM has gained international attention as an endoscopic therapy that allows selective myotomy of the LES in addition to the esophageal body [66]. Following POEM, therapeutic response is often determined by EGJ appearance on upper endoscopy, esophagram, and esophageal manometry. Familiari et al. therefore aimed to determine if FLIP could be applied prospectively to assess the effects of EGJ distensibility following endoscopic myotomy. Between April 2013 and July 2013, 21 patients underwent FLIP immediately before and following POEM. Using an 8-cm length catheter balloon, pre-procedural mean EGJ diameter and CSA was measured to be 6.3 mm (± 1.8 SD) and 32.9 mm^2 (± 23.1 SD), respectively, with a significant increase to 11.3 mm (± 1.7 SD) and 102.38 mm^2 (± 28.2 SD) following treatment [65]. Additionally, Ngamruengphong et al. aimed to assess FLIP measurements in patients prior to undergoing POEM in efforts to measure correlation between FLIP findings during POEM and postoperative clinical symptoms. In a multicenter study, the authors retrospectively reviewed 63 treated patients, separated by subjective "good" ($n = 50$) and "poor" clinical response ($n = 13$). As one may expect, authors revealed a significantly higher EGJ cross-sectional area among patients with a good clinical response following POEM ($p = 0.01$) and therefore concluded FLIP to be a potential tool in assessing POEM efficacy and outcomes [67].

FLIP has also been employed as a prognostic test in conjunction with Heller myotomy. Teitelbaum et al. applied FLIP intraoperatively for patients undergoing Heller myotomy and POEM. The authors revealed that although both interventions resulted in an overall rise in mean distensibility (LHM- pre 1.4 vs. post 7.6 mm^2/mmHg; $p < 0.001$ and POEM- pre 1.4 vs. post 7.9 mm^2/mmHg; $p < 0.001$), no difference in EGJ distensibility was seen between surgical and endoscopic myotomies [68].

Beyond POEM and Heller myotomy, treatment of achalasia can encompass less invasive techniques including LES botulinum (Botox®) injection and pneumatic dilation. The principle of pneumatic dilation is to weaken the lower esophageal sphincter by tearing muscular fibers through radial force and performed endoscopically using a Rigiflex dilator with fluoroscopic guidance [69]. Currently considered the most effective nonsurgical option in management of achalasia by the American College of Gastroenterology, factors such as personal training, fear of perforation, and exposure to radiation can often hinder the practice of pneumatic dilation [69, 70]. An alternative therefore was the creation of a hydraulic dilation catheter called EsoFlip® (Crospon Ltd., Galway, Ireland). Inferfacing with the EndoFlip® system to visualize the GEJ and shape of the balloon in real-time with dilation, the need for fluoroscopy was removed. Similar to a regular FLIP catheter, one major difference is the type of balloon used. Whereas in FLIP a soft compliant balloon is used with the primary purpose of measuring lumen size, inflated to a pressure of <0.1 bar, a hydraulic balloon dilator applies a high-pressure dilation balloon made of stiffer material, typically inflated to 1.5 bar pressure [71]. The first feasibility study of this form of hydraulic dilation was conducted by Kappelle et al., measuring technical success, clinical success, and complication rates among 10 patients with achalasia. The authors used a probe with a 7-French (Fr) shaft, 2.3 m in length, and consisting of 15 electrodes spaced 5 mm apart located within an 8 cm balloon. At a control rate, diluted saline solution was inserted into the balloon, reaching a maximum diameter of 30 mm. Technical success was defined as visualizing of complete effacement of the balloon at the "waist," or area of EGJ, until the narrowest diameter reached a value greater than ≥ 28 mm. The authors revealed a median increase in EGJ distensibility from 1.1 to 7.0 following dilation (IQR 5.5–17.8, $p = 0.005$), in addition to no major complications or severe adverse effects at follow up [72], therefore introducing hydraulic dilation as a possible and safe means to achalasia treatment.

Gastroesophageal reflux disease occurs following abnormal reflux of gastric contents into the esophagus, resulting in a wide range of typical symptoms including acid regurgitation and heartburn, in addition to atypical symptoms such as dyspepsia, epigastric fullness, and extraesophageal symptoms of chronic cough and hoarseness. The diagnosis of GERD often is made based on clinical symptoms, but diagnostically the use of esophageal pH monitoring has been used to quantify degree of esophageal acid exposure percentage [73, 74]. Considering this rise in acid exposure as a marker for reflux, it was proposed that patients with GERD may have a similar rise in EGJ distensibility seen on FLIP. Studies demonstrate, however, inconsistent findings. As one would expect, authors in a prior study revealed a higher EGJ-DI in patients with symptomatic GERD, compared to healthy controls [59]. On the other hand, when correlating FLIP distensibility measurements with clinical and physiological diagnosis of GERD, Tucker et al. revealed, when comparing to healthy controls, EGJ distensibility at 20 and 30 ml was actually lower in the GERD cohort ($p = 0.001$ and $p = 0.20$, respectively). Upon further comparison between those with and without pathologic esophageal acid exposure (>5.3%) on 48 hour wireless pH monitoring, data exhibited similar EGJ CSA and distensibility measurements ($p = 0.789$ and $p = 0.704$, respectively) [75]. Despite this discrepancy, FLIP has been considered a useful tool following anti-reflux procedures. Patients with severe GERD refractory to medical therapy or looking for an outlook to avoid long-term medication are given an option to pursue a 360° anti-reflux procedure called a Nissen fundoplication [76]. Kwiatek et al. therefore compared patients undergoing fundoplication, this operative technique to replicate normal EGJ distensibility, with healthy controls. Subsequently, a reduction in EGJ distensibility and compliance in patients undergoing a fundoplication was seen, with the least distensible area located at the hiatus [77]. Despite these positive findings, given the degree of inconsistency and reliability on FLIP among patients with GERD, the American Gastroenterology Association (AGA) institute best practice recommended against use of FLIP in routine diagnostic GERD assessment [59].

As described, eosinophilic esophagitis is an atopic pathologic disease characterized by eosinophilic infiltration of the esophageal epithelium, with the potential complication of esophageal fibrosis and luminal narrowing if left untreated. Symptoms can range from esophageal dysfunction and food impaction to those mimicking GERD [78]. Due to this esophageal narrowing, FLIP was studied further in efforts to improve accuracy in identifying esophageal body narrowing beyond pure endoscopic assessment. Chen et al. performed FLIP and upper gastrointestinal endoscopy among 72 adults with EoE, measuring metrics of distensibility slope and plateau compared with the EoE Endoscopic Reference Score (EREFS), a severity degree based on endoscopic presence of rings, furrows, exudates, edema, and strictures. As expected, a Spearman's nonparametric sample correlation coefficient revealed a significant inverse association with ring severity and distensibility plateau ($r_s = -0.46$, $p < 0.0001$), although degree of eosinophilia, severity of exudates, and furrows was not statistically associated with distensibility measurements [79]. Furthermore, Kwiatek et al. aimed to analyze esophageal mechanical properties in patients with EoE applying an 8-cm length FLIP catheter, comparing CSA-pressure response (distensibility) between 35 case patients and 15 healthy controls. Overall esophageal distensibility was found to be significantly reduced in EoE patients, compared to healthy controls ($p = 0.02$). On additional analysis, no significant difference in distensibility was seen between patients with endoscopic visible rings ± furrows (24/33) and structuring disease (9/33), $p = 0.8$ [80]. Nonetheless, as FLIP functions as a unique tool to measure mechanical properties of the esophageal wall, current AGA recommendations in EoE advise against use of FLIP to diagnose the atopic disease, however, support possible use to assess disease severity and therapeutic monitoring [59]. Please see Fig. 2.4 for examples of FLIP images in patients with dysphagia taken from patients seen in our dysphagia clinic.

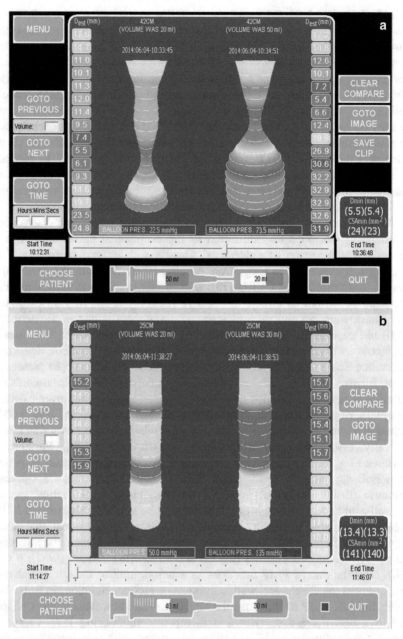

Fig. 2.4 The following FLIP studies were acquired from patients seen by the authors in clinic for complaints of dysphagia. Image (**a**) and (**b**) show static images obtained via the FLIP 1.0 system. Image (**c**) and (**d**) show FLIP topography images obtained via the FLIP 2.0 system. Image (**a**) shows a patient with achalasia, the diagnosis of which had been elusive prior to this study. Image (**b**) shows a patient with eosinophilic esophagitis with dysphagia despite inflammation, but decreased esophageal distensibility on FLIP. Image (**c**) shows normal recurrent antegrade contractions (RACs) consistent with appropriate secondary peristalsis upon balloon distention. Image (**d**) shows the same patient with continued RACs and appropriate EGJ distensibility at a distention volume of 60 cc

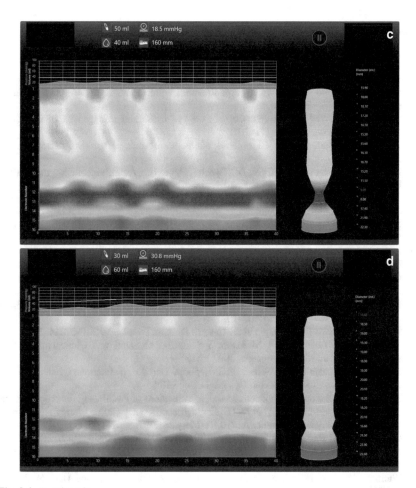

Fig. 2.4 (continued)

Conclusion

Investigation of dysphagia encompasses a range of diagnostic tools and has expanded our assessment of dysphagia, identifying strictures, hiatal hernias, and malignancies in addition to underlying motility disorders. As etiologies for dysphagia can be separated into oropharyngeal and esophageal dysphagia, similar distinctions are seen with each diagnostic tool. Whereas modified barium swallow, fiberoptic endoscopic evaluation of swallowing, and pharyngeal high-resolution manometry are more focused to evaluate an oropharyngeal etiology of symptoms; barium esophagram, endoscopy, high-resolution esophageal manometry, and FLIP are more advantageous in evaluation of esophageal pathology. Diagnostic tools can facilitate in uncovering the underlying etiology for symptoms, with the ultimate goal of shortening time from dysphagia onset to management.

References

1. Kruger D. Assessing esophageal dysphagia. JAAPA. 2014;27:23.
2. Endoscopic findings in patients presenting with dysphagia: analysis of a national endoscopy database. Available at: https://www.ncbi.nlm.nih.gov/pmc/articles/PMC5970000/. Accessed 9th Feb 2019.
3. Pasha SF, et al. The role of endoscopy in the evaluation and management of dysphagia. Gastrointest Endosc. 2014;79:191–201.
4. Dempsey DT. Barium upper GI series in adults: a surgeon's perspective. Abdom Radiol. 2018;43:1323–8.
5. Palmer JB, Kuhlemeier KV, Tippett DC, Lynch C. A protocol for the videofluorographic swallowing study. Dysphagia. 1993;8:209–14.
6. Gramigna GD. How to perform video-fluoroscopic swallowing studies. GI Motil Online. 2006; https://doi.org/10.1038/gimo95.
7. Martin-Harris B, Jones B. The videofluorographic swallowing study. Phys Med Rehabil Clin N Am. 2008;19:769–85.
8. Rugiu M. Role of videofluoroscopy in evaluation of neurologic dysphagia. Acta Otorhinolaryngol Ital. 2007;27:306–16.
9. González-Fernández M, Ottenstein L, Atanelov L, Christian AB. Dysphagia after stroke: an overview. Curr Phys Med Rehabil Rep. 2013;1:187–96.
10. Khoo JB, Buller AS, Wong MC. Modified barium swallow examination in dysphagic stroke patients. Singap Med J. 1996;37:407–10.
11. Suttrup I, Warnecke T. Dysphagia in Parkinson's Disease. Dysphagia. 2016;31:24–32.
12. Martin-Harris B, Logemann JA, McMahon S, Schleicher M, Sandidge J. Clinical utility of the modified barium swallow. Dysphagia. 2000;15:136–41.
13. Stoeckli SJ, Huisman TAGM, Seifert BAGM, Martin–Harris BJW. Interrater reliability of videofluoroscopic swallow evaluation. Dysphagia. 2003;18:53–7.
14. Accuracy of endoscopic and videofluoroscopic evaluations of swallowing for oropharyngeal dysphagia - Giraldo-Cadavid - 2017 - The Laryngoscope - Wiley Online Library. Available at: https://onlinelibrary.wiley.com/doi/full/10.1002/lary.26419. Accessed 9th Feb 2019.
15. Chen A, Tuma F. Barium Swallow. [Updated 2019 Apr 22]. In: StatPearls [Internet]. Treasure Island (FL): StatPearls Publishing; 2019 Jan. Available from: https://www.ncbi.nlm.nih.gov/books/NBK493176/.
16. Widmark JM. Imaging-related medications: a class overview. Proc Bayl Univ Med Cent. 2007;20:408–17.
17. Baker ME, Einstein DM. Barium esophagram: does it have a role in gastroesophageal reflux disease? Gastroenterol Clin N Am. 2014;43:47–68.
18. Neyaz Z, Gupta M, Ghoshal UC. How to perform and interpret timed barium esophagogram. J. Neurogastroenterol. Motil. 2013;19:251–6.
19. de Oliveira JM, et al. Timed barium swallow: a simple technique for evaluating esophageal emptying in patients with achalasia. AJR Am J Roentgenol. 1997;169:473–9.
20. Vaezi MF, Baker ME, Richter JE. Assessment of esophageal emptying post-pneumatic dilation: use of the timed barium esophagram. Am J Gastroenterol. 1999;94:1802–7.
21. Kostic SV, et al. Timed barium esophagogram: a simple physiologic assessment for achalasia. J Thorac Cardiovasc Surg. 2000;120:935–46.
22. Langmore SE, Kenneth SMA, Olsen N. Fiberoptic endoscopic examination of swallowing safety: a new procedure. Dysphagia. 1988;2:216–9.
23. Fiberoptic Endoscopic Evaluation of Swallowing - Hiss - 2003 - The Laryngoscope - Wiley Online Library. Available at: https://onlinelibrary.wiley.com/doi/full/10.1097/00005537-200308000-00023. Accessed 9th Feb 2019.
24. Leder SB, Murray JT. Fiberoptic endoscopic evaluation of swallowing. Phys. Med. Rehabil. Clin. N. Am. 2008;19:787–801, viii–ix.
25. Institute for Digestive Research, Digestive Disease Center, Soonchunhyang University Seoul Hospital, Seoul, Republic of Korea, Lee TH, Lee JS. Safety of flexible endoscopic evaluation

of swallowing examination in gastroenterological practice. Turk J Gastroenterol. 2018; https://doi.org/10.5152/tjg.2018.18279.

26. Schatz K, Langmore SE, Olson N. Endoscopic and videofluoroscopic evaluations of swallowing and aspiration. Ann Otol Rhinol Laryngol. 1991;100:678–81.

27. Beg S, et al. Quality standards in upper gastrointestinal endoscopy: a position statement of the British Society of Gastroenterology (BSG) and Association of Upper Gastrointestinal Surgeons of Great Britain and Ireland (AUGIS). Gut. 2017;66:1886–99.

28. Less patient discomfort by one-man colonoscopy examination - Lee - 2006 - International Journal of Clinical Practice - Wiley Online Library. Available at: https://onlinelibrary.wiley.com/doi/abs/10.1111/j.1368-5031.2006.00891.x. Accessed 9th Feb 2019.

29. Technical skills and training of upper gastrointestinal endoscopy for new beginners. Available at: https://www.ncbi.nlm.nih.gov/pmc/articles/PMC4299329/. Accessed 9th Feb 2019.

30. Gomez Torrijos E, et al. Eosinophilic esophagitis: review and update. Front Med. 2018;5

31. Lucendo AJ, et al. Guidelines on eosinophilic esophagitis: evidence-based statements and recommendations for diagnosis and management in children and adults. United European Gastroenterol J. 2017;5:335–58.

32. Evidenced Based Approach to the Diagnosis and Management of Esophageal Eosinophilia and Eosinophilic Esophagitis (EoE) | American College of Gastroenterology.

33. Liu LWC, et al. Clinical practice guidelines for the assessment of uninvestigated esophageal dysphagia. J Can Assoc Gastroenterol. 2018;1:5–19.

34. Management of benign esophageal strictures. Available at: https://www.ncbi.nlm.nih.gov/pmc/articles/PMC3038317/. Accessed 10th Feb 2019.

35. Kochman ML. Minimization of risks of esophageal dilation. Gastrointest Endosc Clin N Am. 2007;17:47–58.

36. Esophageal perforations. Available at: https://www.ncbi.nlm.nih.gov/pmc/articles/PMC3533215/. Accessed 10th Feb 2019.

37. Soudagar AS, Sayuk GS, Gyawali CP. Learners favour high resolution oesophageal manometry with better diagnostic accuracy over conventional line tracings. Gut. 2012;61:798–803.

38. Bredenoord AJ, et al. Chicago classification criteria of esophageal motility disorders defined in high resolution esophageal pressure topography (EPT). Neurogastroenterol Motil. 2012;24:57–65.

39. Ryu JS, Park D, Kang JY. Application and interpretation of high-resolution manometry for pharyngeal dysphagia. J Neurogastroenterol Motil. 2015;21:283–7.

40. KAHRILAS PJ, SIFRIM D. High-resolution manometry and impedance-pH/manometry: valuable tools in clinical and investigational esophagology. Gastroenterology. 2008;135:756–69.

41. Yadlapati R. High-resolution esophageal manometry: interpretation in clinical practice. Curr Opin Gastroenterol. 2017;33:301–9.

42. Roman S, Gyawali CP, Xiao Y, Pandolfino JE, Kahrilas PJ. The Chicago classification of motility disorders: an update. Gastrointest Endosc Clin N Am. 2014;24:545–61.

43. Kahrilas PJ, et al. The Chicago Classification of esophageal motility disorders, v3.0. Neurogastroenterol Motil. 2015;27:160–74.

44. Carlson DA, Pandolfino JE. High-resolution manometry in clinical practice. Gastroenterol Hepatol. 2015;11:374–84.

45. Fornari F, Bravi I, Penagini R, Tack J, Sifrim D. Multiple rapid swallowing: a complementary test during standard oesophageal manometry. Neurogastroenterol Motil. 2009;21:718–e41.

46. Sweis R, et al. Normative values and inter-observer agreement for liquid and solid bolus swallows in upright and supine positions as assessed by esophageal high-resolution manometry. Neurogastroenterol Motil. 2011;23:509–e198.

47. Intraluminal Multiple Electric Impedance Procedure for Measurement of Gastrointestinal Motility - Silny - 1991 - Neurogastroenterology Motility - Wiley Online Library. Available at: https://onlinelibrary.wiley.com/doi/abs/10.1111/j.1365-2982.1991.tb00061.x. Accessed 25th Jan 2019.

48. Eui Ju Park JSL, Kim J-O. High-resolution impedance manometry criteria in the sitting position indicative of incomplete bolus clearance. J. Neurogastroenterol. Motil. 2014;20:491–6.

49. Liu Z, et al. Assessment of esophageal high-resolution impedance manometry in patients with nonobstructive dysphagia. Gastroenterol Res Pract. 2018;2018:1.

50. Hila A, Castell JA, Castell DO. Pharyngeal and upper esophageal sphincter manometry in the evaluation of dysphagia. J Clin Gastroenterol. 2001;33:355–61.
51. Bhatia SJ, Shah C. How to perform and interpret upper esophageal sphincter manometry. J. Neurogastroenterol. Motil. 2013;19:99–103.
52. Jungheim M, Schubert C, Miller S, Ptok M. Normative data of pharyngeal and upper esophageal sphincter high resolution manometry. Laryngorhinootologie. 2015;94:601–8.
53. Omari TI, et al. The reliability of pharyngeal high resolution manometry with impedance for derivation of measures of swallowing function in healthy volunteers. Int J Otolaryngol. 2016;2016:1. https://doi.org/10.1155/2016/2718482.
54. McCulloch TM, Hoffman MR, Ciucci MR. High resolution manometry of pharyngeal swallow pressure events associated with head turn and chin tuck. Ann Otol Rhinol Laryngol. 2010;119:369–76.
55. Hoffman MR, et al. High-resolution manometry of pharyngeal swallow pressure events associated with effortful swallow and the Mendelsohn maneuver. Dysphagia. 2012;27:418–26.
56. Inamoto Y, et al. The Mendelsohn maneuver and its effects on swallowing: kinematic analysis in three dimensions using dynamic area detector CT. Dysphagia. 2018;33:419–30.
57. Ata-Lawenko RM, Lee YY. Emerging roles of the endolumenal functional lumen imaging probe in gastrointestinal motility disorders. J. Neurogastroenterol. Motil. 2017;23:164–70.
58. Harris LD, Pope CE. 'SQUEEZE' VS RESISTANCE: AN EVALUATION OF THE MECHANISM OF SPHINCTER COMPETENCE. J Clin Invest. 1964;43:2272–8.
59. Functional lumen imaging probe for the management of esophageal disorders: expert review from the clinical practice updates Committee of the AGA Institute. Available at: https://www.ncbi.nlm.nih.gov/pmc/articles/PMC5757507/. Accessed 4th Jan 2019.
60. Carlson DA. Functional lumen imaging probe: the FLIP side of esophageal disease. Curr Opin Gastroenterol. 2016;32:310–8.
61. Carlson D, et al. Utilizing functional lumen imaging probe (FLIP) topography to evaluate esophageal contractility during volumetric distention: a pilot study. Neurogastroenterol Motil. 2015;27:981–9.
62. Park W, Vaezi MF. Etiology and pathogenesis of achalasia: the current understanding. Am J Gastroenterol. 2005;100:1404–14.
63. Carlson DA, et al. The functional lumen imaging probe detects esophageal contractility not observed with manometry in patients with achalasia. Gastroenterology. 2015;149:1742–51.
64. Pandolfino JE, et al. Distensibility of the esophagogastric junction assessed with the functional lumen imaging probe (FLIP™) in achalasia patients. Neurogastroenterol Motil. 2013;25:496–501.
65. Familiari P, et al. EndoFLIP system for the intraoperative evaluation of peroral endoscopic myotomy. United Eur Gastroenterol J. 2014;2:77–83.
66. Peroral endoscopic myotomy (POEM) vs laparoscopic Heller myotomy (LHM) for the treatment of Type III achalasia in 75 patients: a multicenter comparative study. Available at: https://www.ncbi.nlm.nih.gov/pmc/articles/PMC4486039/. Accessed 16th Jan 2019.
67. Ngamruengphong S, et al. Intraoperative measurement of esophagogastric junction cross-sectional area by impedance planimetry correlates with clinical outcomes of peroral endoscopic myotomy for achalasia: a multicenter study. Surg Endosc. 2016;30:2886–94.
68. Comparison of esophagogastric junction distensibility changes during POEM and Heller myotomy using intraoperative FLIP. - PubMed - NCBI. Available at: https://www.ncbi.nlm.nih.gov/pubmed/24043641. Accessed 16th Jan 2019.
69. Chuah S-K, Wu K-L, Hu T-H, Tai W-C, Changchien C-S. Endoscope-guided pneumatic dilation for treatment of esophageal achalasia. World J. Gastroenterol. 2010;16:411–7.
70. Diagnosis and Management of Achalasia | American College of Gastroenterology.
71. O'Dea J, Siersema PD. Esophageal dilation with integrated balloon imaging: initial evaluation in a porcine model. Ther Adv Gastroenterol. 2013;6:109–14.
72. Kappelle WFW, Bogte A, Siersema PD. Hydraulic dilation with a shape-measuring balloon in idiopathic achalasia: a feasibility study. Endoscopy. 2015;47:1028–34.

73. Badillo R, Francis D. Diagnosis and treatment of gastroesophageal reflux disease. World J Gastrointest Pharmacol Ther. 2014;5:105–12.
74. Gyawali CP, et al. Modern diagnosis of GERD: the lyon consensus. Gut. 2018;67:1351–62.
75. Tucker E, et al. Measurement of esophago-gastric junction cross-sectional area and distensibility by an endolumenal functional lumen imaging probe for the diagnosis of gastro-esophageal reflux disease. Neurogastroenterol Motil. 2013;25:904–10.
76. Frazzoni M, Piccoli M, Conigliaro R, Frazzoni L, Melotti G. Laparoscopic fundoplication for gastroesophageal reflux disease. World J Gastroenterol. 2014;20:14272–9.
77. Kwiatek MA, et al. Esophagogastric junction distensibility after fundoplication assessed with a novel functional luminal imaging probe. J Gastrointest Surg. 2010;14:268–76.
78. Cianferoni A, Spergel J. Eosinophilic esophagitis: a comprehensive review. Clin Rev Allergy Immunol. 2016;50:159–74.
79. Chen JW, et al. Severity of endoscopically identified esophageal rings correlates with reduced esophageal distensibility in eosinophilic esophagitis. Endoscopy. 2016;48:794–801.
80. Kwiatek MA, et al. Mechanical properties of the esophagus in eosinophilic esophagitis. Gastroenterology. 2011;140:82–90.

Chapter 3
Oropharyngeal Dysphagia

Robert M. Siwiec and Arash Babaei

Introduction

The clinical approach to dysphagia commonly begins with an objective determination of the anatomic level of dysphagia. Oropharyngeal dysphagia (OD) is defined as dysfunction in bolus movement from the oral cavity to the upper esophageal sphincter (UES) [1], and esophageal dysphagia (ED) is generally attributed to difficulty in transporting the bolus from the UES to the gastric cavity. Deglutition is controlled through complex interactions between brainstem nuclei and feedback loops between both oropharyngeal and esophagus phases of swallowing. Although each phase of swallowing can affect the other, predominant disruption in one phase usually plays a more critical role in a patient's clinical presentation. For example, nearly half of patients with esophageal achalasia (a prototype disorder of ED) may present with unsuspected pharyngeal manifestations [2], while poor dentition may unmask an otherwise subclinical patent distal esophageal ring due to impaired mastication and suboptimal bolus formation.

Dysphagia must be differentiated from globus sensation [3]. Globus is commonly described as a lump in the throat, though a persistent or intermittent non-painful sensation of tightness, fullness, or foreign body sensation in the throat is commonly described by patients. Patients with globus sensation do not present with weight loss and usually have no difficulties during swallowing [4]. Globus sensation and associated nuisance symptoms are generally more noticeable in between meals

R. M. Siwiec
Division of Gastroenterology and Hepatology, Indiana University School of Medicine, Indianapolis, IN, USA

A. Babaei (✉)
Division of Gastroenterology, Department of Medicine, National Jewish Health, Denver, CO, USA
e-mail: Babaeia@njhealth.org

© Springer Nature Switzerland AG 2020
D. A. Patel et al. (eds.), *Evaluation and Management of Dysphagia*,
https://doi.org/10.1007/978-3-030-26554-0_3

Table 3.1 Symptoms of oropharyngeal dysphagia

Food spillage from the lips
Drooling
Hesitation or inability to initiate the swallow
Nasal regurgitation
Food sticking in the throat
Repetitive swallowing
Coughing and choking – before, during, or after swallowing
Posture changes during eating
Frequent throat clearing
Voice hoarseness
Weight loss
Recurrent pneumonia
Prolonged meal duration
Exclusion of certain food consistencies
Nasal speech and dysarthria
Avoidance of social dining

[4]. Although a distinct etiology remains elusive, globus sensation can be seen in patients with underlying esophageal disorders including hiatal hernia, GERD [4], or esophageal dysmotility [5].

OD arises from disorders affecting the oral preparatory phase and/or the pharyngeal phase of swallowing. Given the wide array of clinical manifestations and presentations, the diagnosis of OD requires a high index of suspicion. Some patients may be completely asymptomatic and present with pneumonia whereas others may complain of weight loss, coughing, prolonged meal duration, frequent throat clearing, repetitive swallowing, and hoarseness (Table 3.1). OD must be distinguished from ED as the causes of oropharyngeal pathology are often much different from those of ED. A multidisciplinary approach is considered essential given the diverse etiologies of OD. Managing patients with OD requires healthcare providers to coordinate care between gastroenterologists, radiologists, speech pathologists, otolaryngologists, neurologists, dietitians, geriatricians, and home caregivers.

Patients may point to areas where they sense difficulties and/or obstruction; however, the clinical diagnosis of OD is not equivalent to a patient's perceived level of dysphagia. Dysphagia sensation in the cervical region often times (30–60%) can be attributed to pathology in the distal esophagus (e.g., Schatzki ring with intermittent transient food stasis) [6, 7]. Studies have repeatedly shown that determination of the level of dysphagia by patients is clinically unreliable [8–10]. Furthermore, elderly patients or patients with neurologic disorders are frequently unaware of their swallowing dysfunction [11]. Therefore, OD is not synonymous with cervical dysphagia as a symptom.

OD can affect individuals of all ages, stemming from a diverse range of structural and neuromuscular etiologies. Children and adolescents can experience oral dysphagia caused by congenital cleft lip/palate [12] or cerebral palsy [13]. Poor dentition [14, 15] and xerostomia [16, 17] in older adults are common yet unrecognized etiologies of dysphagia [18]. The term OD is often erroneously used to mean a distinct disease, while it usually represents as a manifestation of a diverse range of etiologies. There are many causes of oropharyngeal dysphagia including neuromuscular, neurological, structural, myogenic, and iatrogenic. OD can be mechanistically divided into voluntary oral and reflexive pharyngeal causes of dysphagia. The focus of this concise review will be the involuntary reflexive pharyngeal phase of swallowing in the adult population.

Epidemiology

Although reliable epidemiological data with a uniform definition of OD are not available, based on screening questionnaires, it is estimated that 11–22% of independently living older adults are affected by OD [19–22]. The prevalence of OD in institutionalized elderly approaches 32–51% of patients based on bedside clinical swallow assessment [15, 19]. OD is associated with aging-related neurological impairments and neurodegenerative processes [23]. In patients with frontotemporal dementia [24], Parkinson's [25], and Alzheimer's disease [26], the prevalence of OD reaches an alarming rate of 57–84%. Impaired cognitive factors and reduced functional capacity due to frailty can significantly contribute to severity and prevalence of OD in the elderly [27, 28].

Physiology

Swallowing consists of three phases: oral preparatory, pharyngeal, and esophageal. Humans swallow upwards of 900 times a day with each swallow involving more than 30 pairs of striated muscles [12] and bolus transfer into the esophagus taking less than a second [1]. Thus, precise timing and muscle coordination during the oral preparatory and pharyngeal phases are essential for normal human swallowing [12].

The pharynx is comprised of three distinct compartments: nasopharynx, oropharynx, and laryngopharynx (Fig. 3.1). The nasopharynx extends from the base of the skull to the distal edge of the soft palate, communicating through the pharyngeal isthmus with the oropharynx. The oropharynx extends from the soft palate to the base of the tongue. Lastly, the laryngopharynx extends from the valleculae to the inferior margin of the cricoid cartilage. The laryngopharynx is a complex anatomic chamber that is 99% of the time part of the respiratory tract [29]. Only during swallowing (<1% of time) does the laryngopharynx morph into an essential component of the digestive tract for less than a second [1].

Successful food ingestion depends on the coordination between oral and pharyngeal function. The oral preparatory phase is mostly under voluntary control and involves cranial nerves V (trigeminal), VII (facial), and XII (hypoglossal) [12].

Fig. 3.1 Pharyngeal
anatomic compartments

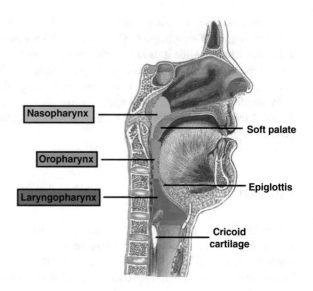

The autonomic nervous system is involved in salivary secretion to assist with both oral breakdown of materials and bolus lubrication [16]. During the oral preparatory phase, the bolus remains in the oral cavity, being processed by mastication and altered chemically by mixing with saliva. This produces a bolus with suitable size, shape, and consistency for safe transit through the pharynx and esophagus [30]. Within the oral cavity, the lips, teeth, hard and soft palates, mandible, mouth floor, and tongue help to break down solid food and form a "swallowable material" [31]. Liquid bolus requires volitional containment mainly with control of the tongue and palatal assistance before propulsion into the pharynx [12]. Propulsion of a liquid bolus involves rapid sequence of positioning of the bolus on the superior surface of the tongue and tongue movement to place the tip against the hard palate, and lingual oral-aboral sequential contraction then propels the bolus beyond the palatine arches into the hypopharyngeal conduit and esophagus [12]. Elevation of the posterior portion of the tongue by the mylohyoid muscles elevates the soft palate, sealing the nasopharynx and preventing nasopharyngeal regurgitation [32]. Conventional semi-solid and solid food, however, is a gradual process of cyclical accumulation of small aliquots of triturated bolus on the pharyngeal surface of the tongue progressing toward the vallecular space until lingual and pharyngeal peristalsis propels the bolus into the hypopharynx and esophagus [31].

The pharyngeal phase, unlike the oral preparatory phase, is mostly under reflexive control and involves cranial nerves V (trigeminal), IX (glossopharyngeus), X (vagus), and XII (hypoglossal) [12]. During this phase, the tongue seals the oropharynx, while the soft palate and proximal pharyngeal wall seal off the nasopharynx. The vocal cords and arytenoids close off the laryngeal openings, and the epiglottis covers the laryngeal vestibule, leading to a transiently closed airway [33]. Simultaneously, the larynx and hyoid are pulled upward and forward by several centimeters allowing the bolus to pass over the larynx without aspiration and causing relaxation of the cricopharyngeus, the predominant muscle of the upper esophageal sphincter (UES) [34]. These events allow for successful bolus transfer through the UES and into the esophagus, with pharyngeal peristalsis velocities 7–17 cm/seconds [35]. During this time, respiration is reflexively inhibited [36, 37].

Swallowing depends on a central pattern generator (CPG) located in the medulla oblongata, which involves several brainstem motor nuclei (V, VII, IX, X, XII) and two main groups of interneurons: a dorsal swallowing group in the nucleus tractus solitarius (NTS) and a ventral swallowing group located in the ventrolateral medulla above the nucleus ambiguous [36, 38]. Within the CPG, neurons in the dorsal swallowing group play the leading role in generating the swallow pattern, while neurons in the ventral swallowing group act as switching neurons, distributing the swallowing drive to the various motor neuron pools [39–41]. The cerebral cortex also contributes substantially to the control of swallowing [42]. During both volitional [43, 44] and reflexive [45, 46] swallowing, a number of brain regions have been shown to be activated including the cingulate cortex, insula, prefrontal cortex, primary sensorimotor, and premotor cortex. While the discrete role of cortical regions in orchestration of swallow components remain unknown, recent studies have started to decipher potential contribution of individual cortical regions. Postcentral somatosensory activity occurs 1–2 seconds before the pharyngeal phase of swallowing, and the precentral motor activation ensues 10–16 seconds after swallowing indicating sequential involvement of cortical regions [47]. Airway protective maneuvers resulted in higher posterior insular activity [48], and gustatory/olfactory stimulation increased prefrontal [49], cingulate [49], and sensorimotor [49, 50] cortical activity indicating their distinctive coordination and sensory role, respectively.

Pathophysiology

Traditionally, the underlying etiologies of OD are classified into structural, neuromuscular, and iatrogenic groups (Table 3.2). Weakness of the tongue and other oral cavity muscles or loss of oral sensation can impair oral preparatory and propulsive stages resulting in premature spillage of food from the mouth, improper bolus formation, or inadequate bolus positioning [12]. Mechanistically, pharyngeal dysphagia could be classified into three core categories: (1) pharyngeal peristalsis dysfunction (i.e., pump problem), (2) reduced pharyngeal lumen compliance (i.e., pipe problem), and (3) airway compromise. These mechanisms may present independently or in combination. For example, a patient with a history of head and neck cancer and chemoradiation therapy may suffer from all three mechanistic elements of OD. Airway compromise (penetration or aspiration) may occur in isolation due to impaired airway protective mechanisms but usually is a consequence and manifestation of pharyngeal peristalsis dysfunction and reduced pharyngeal lumen compliance. Airway compromise therefore may occur before, during or after act of swallowing depending on the underlying pathophysiology. Patients with OD

Table 3.2 Common causes of oropharyngeal dysphagia

Structural	Posterior pharyngeal diverticulum (Zenker's)	
	Cricopharyngeal bar	
	Oropharyngeal tumors (benign and malignant)	
	Thyroid enlargement or tumor	
	Esophageal tumors (benign and malignant)	
	Foreign bodies	
	Dental pathology	
	Skeletal abnormalities (cervical stenosis, osteophytes)	
	Esophageal strictures or webs	
Neurological	Cerebrovascular accident	
	Parkinson's disease	
	CNS tumors	
	Dementia	
	Cerebral palsy	
	Amyotrophic lateral sclerosis	
	Tabes dorsalis	
Iatrogenic	Medications	
	Radiation to head and neck	
	Postsurgical effects	
Myogenic	Oculopharyngeal muscular dystrophy	
	Myasthenia gravis	
	Inflammatory myopathies	
	Polymyositis/dermatomyositis	
	Scleroderma	
	Inclusion body myositis	
	Paraneoplastic syndromes	
	Critical illness and sepsis	

experience difficulties in swallow often with resultant symptoms of choking and/or a sensation of incomplete pharyngeal bolus clearance.

Pharyngeal peristalsis dysfunction most commonly occurs as a result of either neurological or muscular disease. Weakness or incoordination of pharyngeal muscles can result in slowed bolus transit or retained food residue in the oropharynx, significantly increasing the risk of aspiration [51, 52]. Oropharyngeal muscle weakness can result in inadequate pharyngeal bolus propulsion [53]. Muscle weakness and incoordination can often prevent the pharynx from successfully transitioning from an organ of respiration to one of digestion, with incomplete closure of the laryngeal vestibule resulting in aspiration.

Stroke also known as cerebrovascular accident (CVA) produces dysphagia symptoms in approximately 50–60% of patients, and up to 20% of patients develop aspiration pneumonia which can contribute significantly to patient mortality [54–56].

Dysfunction in pharyngeal peristalsis predisposes individual to upper airway compromise. Various mechanisms have been found to contribute to aspiration pneumonia in patients with stroke: absence or delay in triggering a swallow, reduced lingual control, weakened laryngopharyngeal musculature, and sensorimotor impairments. The location of the stroke can influence the type of dysphagia which is likely to occur. Cortical infarcts can cause both oral and pharyngeal dysphagia [57]; however, their effect on the oral phase of swallowing arises from loss of cortical modulation of the oral swallow. This results in problems ranging from the inability to retain food within the mouth to tongue incoordination [56, 57]. Conversely, brainstem infarcts result mostly in pharyngeal dysphagia due to injury involving the NTS, CPG, swallowing interneurons, and/or efferent motor neurons. Translational studies utilizing transcranial magnetic stimulation (TMS) have demonstrated that individuals have a dominant and nondominant cerebral hemisphere with respect to swallowing. OD and risk of aspiration pneumonia are more likely to occur in individuals with CVA involving the dominant hemisphere [58].

Parkinson's disease (PD) is a common, progressive disease of the central nervous system involving loss of dopaminergic neurons of the substantia nigra. Studies have shown that the presence of OD in PD can be as high as 82%; however, only 15–20% of patients with PD report swallowing difficulties [25, 59]. Delayed swallow response coupled with a weak pharyngeal contraction can result in vallecular and pyriform sinus residue. Dystonia has been shown to cause impaired relaxation of the UES which can also contribute to increased pharyngeal residue thereby increasing the risk of aspiration [59].

Amyotrophic lateral sclerosis (ALS) is a neurodegenerative disease characterized by a progressive loss of upper and lower motor neurons resulting in paralysis and death within 2–5 years from the time of diagnosis. Generally, death occurs because of respiratory failure, aspiration pneumonia, malnutrition, and dehydration [60]. Approximately 1 in 3 patients with ALS at the time of diagnosis have dysphagia. Eventually, more than 80% of patients will have dysphagia during the advanced phases of the disease [61]. OD is related to tongue atrophy, dysfunction in the closure of the soft palate and larynx, and diaphragm dysfunction. Prompt assessment of swallow function is crucial in order to organize proper interventions and prevent rapid clinical deterioration [61]. The decline in swallowing function nevertheless is progressive and predictable, invariably leading to gastrostomy feeding.

Oculopharyngeal muscular dystrophy (OPMD) is an autosomal dominant late-onset progressive muscle disorder typically characterized by ptosis, dysphagia, and proximal limb weakness. OPMD is caused by an abnormal increase in the number of repeats of the alanine encoding trinucleotide in the *PABPN1* gene located on chromosome 14 [62]. The highest prevalence of OPMD has been reported in Bukhara Jews (1:600) and French Canadians (1:1000) [63]. Weak or absent pharyngeal contractions result in hypopharyngeal stasis, predisposing to aspiration pneumonia and asphyxia.

Various classes of pharmacological agents can result in OD. Antipsychotics medications act on cortical dopaminergic neurons that help regulate motor neurons supplying motor and pharyngeal muscles [64]. Clinical studies have shown that both typical (e.g., haloperidol, chlorpromazine) and atypical (e.g., olanzapine, risperidone) antipsychotics cause OD and increase aspiration risk [65, 66]. Sedatives like benzodiazepines and opiate medications can alter an individuals' level of consciousness which can then impair the initial voluntary phase of swallowing [67, 68]. As a result, essential swallowing events including mastication, bolus formation, and adequate positioning of the bolus prior to transfer to the pharynx are negatively impacted, increasing the risk of OD and aspiration. Moreover, opioid receptors are ubiquitously present in the esophagus [69, 70] and result in impaired deglutitive LES relaxation and disrupted peristaltic sequence [71, 72]. Recent opioid exposure and chronic daily opioid intake are clinically associated with dysmotility [73] and dysphagia [74]. Relationship between opioids and OD, specifically pharyngeal striated muscle and UES function, requires further investigation.

Reduced pharyngeal luminal compliance may be secondary to pathology in the muscle layer (e.g., cricopharyngeal bar), mucosal layer (e.g., cancer), or the surrounding soft tissue (e.g., radiation-related soft tissue remodeling). Cricopharyngeal (CP) bars are common radiographic findings that can be incidentally found on radiologic examinations of elderly patients with no complaints. A CP bar is seen as a posterior indentation of the esophageal lumen between cervical vertebrae 3 and 6, resulting in reduced UES diameter during opening and resulting in dysphagia [75, 76]. Radiographic presence of CP impression is not evidence of upper esophageal sphincter or pharyngeal dysfunction [77]. Reduced compliance by fibrosis is thought to be the etiology for pathophysiologic CP bars and pharyngeal diverticulum [78, 79]. UES dysfunction (impaired relaxation) can obstruct bolus passage from the pharynx to the esophagus [80]. Reduced UES compliance can result from scarring or fibrosis as well as from vagal nerve lesions and resultant-impaired relaxation [1]. Suprahyoid muscle weakness can also result in ineffective UES opening [53]. High-resolution impedance manometric studies show an increase in hypopharyngeal intrabolus pressures that represents the resistance to flow across the UES [81].

Zenker's diverticulum (ZD) is defined as a pseudo diverticulum given that it contains only some of the layers of the esophageal wall with diagnosis being confirmed by radiographic contrast swallowing examinations (Fig. 3.2). ZD emerges

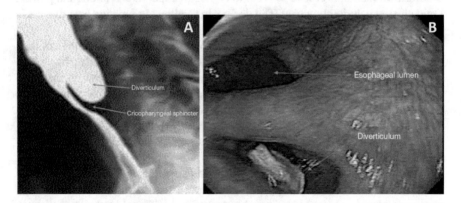

Fig. 3.2 Zenker's diverticulum. (**A**) Luminal outpouching posteriorly above the cricopharyngeal muscle. (**B**) Occasionally residual food particles are noted endoscopically

from a hypopharyngeal muscular wall defect in Killian's triangle above the cricopharyngeal muscle, a natural area of weakness. The borders of Killian's triangle are formed by the oblique fibers of the inferior pharyngeal constrictor muscle and the cricopharyngeus. Chronic increased pressure on Killian's triangle and resultant esophageal evagination can arise from various factors including abnormal esophageal motility, UES dysfunction, impaired bolus passage resulting in increased intrabolus pressures, hiatal hernia, and gastroesophageal reflux disease [79, 82–84]. For unclear reasons, men are two to three times more likely to have a ZD compared to women. Patients present later in life with the majority of ZD found above the age of 75. Symptoms range from OD to halitosis to pulmonary aspiration to regurgitation. Mucosal abnormalities arising within the diverticulum include ulcerations and bleeding from retained medications and in rare cases squamous cell carcinoma [85].

Clinical Evaluation

A comprehensive history and physical examination are essential when evaluating patients with OD symptoms [86]. A general timeline should be obtained as to when symptoms began and whether they have become progressive and associated with nutritional deficiencies. Associated symptoms of dysphagia may include weight loss, anemia, nasopharyngeal regurgitation, choking sensation, coughing spell, and other respiratory symptoms.

Medication history should be obtained with particular attention to anticholinergic medications, opiate medications, and benzodiazepines. A history of head and neck surgery or radiation may provide valuable insight into potential etiologies for OD. Dentition, symmetry, and presence or absence of saliva should be evaluated during inspection of the oropharynx. Careful examination of the eyes, skin, and joints may provide insight into underlying systemic disorders. A neurological exam with particular attention to cranial nerves V, VII, IX, and XII is critical. Neck palpation may reveal masses that could be impacting UES opening. Laboratory testing, although not required for OD evaluation, may be needed if systemic symptoms suggest an underlying myopathy, connective tissue disorder, or drug toxicity.

Aspiration risk is often the key driver for pursuing clinical investigations of oropharyngeal dysphagia. A timely diagnosis requires the assistance from various specialties including gastroenterology, radiology, speech and language pathology, otolaryngology, and neurology. Screening tools allow clinicians to identify patients at increased risk and triage those who necessitate further assessment. Various screening methods have been proposed for select populations and clinical settings; however, only a few screening tools were shown to have modest evaluation metrics (sensitivity >70%, specificity >60%, and reliability $\kappa > 0.7$) [87]: Toronto Bedside Swallowing Screening Test [88]; Volume-Viscosity Sallow Test [89]; Standard Swallow Assessment [90]; and Gugging Swallowing Screen [91]). Screening tools however provide no information regarding dysphagia severity, etiology, or optimal treatment.

Videofluoroscopic swallow studies, modified barium swallow (MBS), provide dynamic and continuous anatomical and physiological assessment of the oral cavity, pharynx, and UES. Lateral and frontal views provide comprehensive information on oropharyngeal mechanics while a patient swallows different consistencies containing barium. Abnormalities involving the oral phase, pharyngeal phase, transport function, and UES can be well characterized (Table 3.3). If disordered swallowing is identified, various postural maneuvers and therapeutic interventions can be tried to assess their effects on swallow function. Clinical radiologic swallow studies have limitations including the need for radiation exposure and the qualitative nature of the information obtained. Furthermore, the interrater reliability of radiologic swallow studies has been shown to be highly variable, often times

Table 3.3 Oropharyngeal dysphagia therapies	
	Dietary modification
	NPO
	Increase bolus texture
	Reduce bolus volume
	Flavor enhancement
	Bolus temperature
	Compensatory maneuvers
	Chin tuck
	Head rotation
	Effortful swallow
	Supraglottic swallow
	Rehabilitation
	Jaw exercises
	Tongue exercises
	Mendelsohn laryngeal excursion
	Masako tongue hold
	Shaker head lift
	Expiratory muscle and voice treatment
	Investigational
	Biofeedback
	Pharyngeal electrical stimulation
	Transcutaneous neuromuscular stimulation
	Transcranial direct current cortical stimulation
	Transcranial magnetic cerebral and cerebellar stimulation
	Operative and endoscopic interventions
	Cricopharyngeal dilation
	Cricopharyngeal botulinum toxin injection
	Cricopharyngeal myotomy
	Zenker's repair
	Gastrostomy
	Vocal fold medialization
	Laryngeal suspension

dependent not only on the analytical method utilized by speech pathology and radiology but also other study factors [92]. Enormous research efforts have been directed to standardize and transform the MBS protocol into a more quantitatively driven diagnostic instrument [93].

Fiberoptic endoscopic evaluation of swallowing (FEES) allows for the direct visualization of pharyngeal and laryngeal structures before, during, and after swallowing [94]. This technique is generally well-tolerated and does not involve any radiation exposure. Given its portability, FEES can be performed at the patient's bedside. During the test, the device is introduced transnasally and advanced to enable visualization of the tongue base, pharynx, and larynx. During the examination, the patient swallows a variety of foods and liquids mixed with a colored contrast agent to maximize visualization of the bolus. The procedure provides valuable information regarding morphology, timing of swallow onset and bolus clearance, presence or absence of residue, and presence or absence of aspiration and penetration [95].

High-resolution manometry (HRM) measures contractile activity of the pharynx, UES, esophageal body, and lower esophageal sphincter (LES) during swallowing. Extensive research efforts have characterized muscular function of the pharynx and UES in health and disease; however, the use of HRM in clinical practice for patients with OD is limited by the lack of normative values, no classification system for UES motility disorders, and no reliable link to predicting a patient's aspiration risk. The addition of impedance measurement to HRM allows for computation of pressure flow dynamics. Pressure flow analysis (PFA) derives and integrates several swallow function variables resulting in a more complete understanding of the pressure-flow structure of the swallow [96]. PFA has high intra-rater and inter-rater reproducibility [97]. Aspiration risk can be easily predicted using PFA of four pharyngeal pressure-flow parameters [98].

Functional lumen imaging probe (FLIP) is a technique that has been developed to test the distensibility properties of a lumen. Sphincter geometry can be reconstructed using multiple estimated cross-sectional area measurements. FLIP was originally designed to evaluate esophagogastric junction compliance; however, it has since been used to evaluate the sphincter of Oddi, esophageal lumen, pylorus, and anorectal canal. UES function has been explored using FLIP in healthy subjects, post-laryngectomy patients, and patients with dysphagia, with studies showing good patient tolerability and no significant major adverse events [99, 100].

Clinical Management

The majority of patients with suspected OD are evaluated by speech pathologists in the US [101]. Swallow evaluation is often performed using either videofluoroscopy or fiberoptic endoscopic evaluation of swallowing (FEES). Timely comprehensive assessment provides the opportunity for early implementation of mechanism-specific OD deficit-directed treatments and prevent pulmonary and nutritional complications [102]. Nonetheless, in the absence of high-level evidence, uniform dietary modifications and/or general compensatory maneuvers are recommended to most patients with OD. Various swallowing maneuvers and exercises have been shown to improve specific dysphagia mechanisms (Table 3.3), but robust randomized trials are lacking. Unfortunately, despite the extraordinary efforts in the field of dysphagia to prove the efficacy of commonly implemented interventions on meaningful patient-oriented clinical outcomes, high-level of evidence is still difficult to find [102].

One of the most common strategies employed in dysphagia management is dietary modifications. There is a broad spectrum of dietary recommendations ranging from elimination of oral intake (NPO and institution of alternative routes of nutritional support) and food texture modification to minor bolus modifications. Aspiration of oropharyngeal contents into the respiratory tract is universally considered a worrisome occurrence [103], being associated with a risk of aspiration pneumonia [104], respiratory failure, and even death [105, 106]. However, NPO recommendations in patients with radiographic evidence of aspiration have not proven to be effective in reducing pulmonary events or improving survival [107]. Modifying food texture to a thickened consistency is a commonly used intervention in OD management. Mild and moderate thickening of liquids (i.e., honey and nectar consistency, respectively) has been shown to significantly reduce radiographic aspiration [108]. This clinical benefit, however, was hampered by an increased risk of dehydration and urinary tract infection [109].

Reducing the bolus volume to an optimal size and preventing premature spillage is a common sense approach [110] with an underlying mechanistic rationale – to prepare a safer swallowing condition in patient with dysphagia [111–113]. Modifying bolus features to enhance oropharyngeal stimulation using sour flavor [114] and cold temperature [115] have been associated with improved swallowing parameters in both neurogenic dysphagia and head and neck cancer patients [114, 116, 117].

Similar to bolus modifications, the clinical use of postural maneuvers such as chin tuck [118] and head rotation [119] are based on improvement in certain aspects of the swallowing mechanism. In a randomized controlled trial, chin tuck was less effective than thickened liquids in reducing radiographic aspiration [108], but the incidence of clinically important pneumonia in both groups was similar, and patients preferred the postural maneuver to food texture modification [109]. Head rotation may offer clinical benefits in patients with unilateral pharyngeal weakness [120]. Supraglottic and effortful swallow are maneuvers designed to facilitate pharyngeal bolus propulsion and efficient airway protection [121–123]. They have been used in cancer-related and neurogenic OD [124]. Combined application of dietary modification and compensatory maneuvers together significantly reduced aspiration pneumonia and death/hospitalization after acute stroke [125].

Swallowing rehabilitation is based on behavioral exercises that offer lasting improvements in neuromuscular function of the oropharyngeal swallowing apparatus. Unlike dietary modifications and postural maneuvers that inherently require adherence with each meal and every swallow to be effective, these behavioral exercises can be applied with or without meals at different times. Improved neuromuscular function with tongue exercises [126], Mendelsohn laryngeal excursion maneuver [127], Masako tongue-holding [128], and Shaker head lift exercise [129] are related to increased muscle strength and restoration of premorbid muscular function in patients with OD. Expiratory muscle strength training (EMST) increases submental muscle force generation and improves deglutitive hyolaryngeal movement along with augmented cough strength [122]. In a randomized controlled study, daily EMST in Parkinsonism improved swallowing safety by reducing airway compromise and enhancing swallow-related quality of life [130]. Behavioral therapies theoretically offer additional benefit of long-term neural adaptations that are rooted in principles of neuroplasticity [131].

Employing all of the above treatment strategies in a randomized clinical trial setting has undoubtedly supported their collective clinical value [125]. In an acute stroke study, implementation of a vigorous daily swallowing therapy for a month significantly correlated with eating a general diet after 6 months [125]. The clinical benefits of rehabilitative measures in progressive neurodegenerative disorders remains less certain [132].

Biofeedback along with peripheral and central neuromuscular stimulation are investigational novel techniques based on a sound foundation but are not yet considered mainstream dysphagia therapies in the clinical practice. Several uncontrolled small trials have shown benefit of videoendoscopic [133], electromyographic [134], and manometric [135] biofeedback in OD therapy but require further clinical validation. Although pharyngeal electrical stimulation [136], transcutaneous neuromuscular electrical stimulation [137], transcranial electrical direct current stimulation [138], magnetic cortical [139, 140] and cerebellar [141] stimulation, or a combination of peripheral and central techniques [142] are promising, their concrete clinical benefit remains far from certain [143, 144].

Obstructive CP bars and Zenker's diverticulum are considered as the continuum of the same poorly compliant UES disorders [79, 145]. UES ablative therapies such as botulinum toxin injection, CP dilatation, and CP myotomy have all shown significant clinical efficacy and improvement in patient symptoms [146]. The best therapeutic option for symptomatic Zenker's and CP bars is cricopharyngeal myotomy with 84% success and less than a 2% complication rate [146]. CP myotomy is indicated when there is a limitation in UES opening but only if the pharyngeal pressure is sufficient to propel a bolus through an open UES [147]. CP myotomy helps to normalize the UES opening and may improve pharyngeal contraction [148]. Transcervical operative techniques have gradually been replaced by their less invasive endoscopic counterparts with similar efficacy [149–152]. Despite common utilization in clinical practice, comparative randomized controlled investigations of various UES ablative techniques are still lacking.

References

1. Cook IJ, Kahrilas PJ. AGA technical review on management of oropharyngeal dysphagia. Gastroenterology. 1999;116:455–78.
2. Jones B, Donner MW, Rubesin SE, et al. Pharyngeal findings in 21 patients with achalasia of the esophagus. Dysphagia. 1987;2:87–92.
3. Purcell J. A Treatise of Vapours, or, Hysterick Fits. Containing an analytical proof of its causes... Together with its cure, etc. London: Edward Place; 1703.
4. Malcomson KG. Radiological findings in globus hystericus. Br J Radiol. 1966;39:583–6.
5. Moser G, Vacariu-Granser GV, Schneider C, et al. High incidence of esophageal motor disorders in consecutive patients with globus sensation. Gastroenterology. 1991;101:1512–21.
6. Smith DF, Ott DJ, Gelfand DW, et al. Lower esophageal mucosal ring: correlation of referred symptoms with radiographic findings using a marshmallow bolus. AJR Am J Roentgenol. 1998;171:1361–5.
7. Edwards D. History and symptoms of esophageal disease of the esophagus. In: Vantrappen G, Hellemans J, editors. Diseases of the esophagus. New York: Springer; 1974.
8. Ashraf HH, Palmer J, Dalton HR, et al. Can patients determine the level of their dysphagia? World J Gastroenterol. 2017;23:1038–43.
9. Jones B, Ravich WJ, Donner MW, et al. Pharyngoesophageal interrelationships: observations and working concepts. Gastrointest Radiol. 1985;10:225–33.
10. Roeder BE, Murray JA, Dierkhising RA. Patient localization of esophageal dysphagia. Dig Dis Sci. 2004;49:697–701.
11. Ortega O, Martin A, Clave P. Diagnosis and management of oropharyngeal dysphagia among older persons, state of the art. J Am Med Dir Assoc. 2017;18:576–82.
12. Matsuo K, Palmer JB. Anatomy and physiology of feeding and swallowing: normal and abnormal. Phys Med Rehabil Clin N Am. 2008;19:691–707. vii
13. Calis EA, Veugelers R, Sheppard JJ, et al. Dysphagia in children with severe generalized cerebral palsy and intellectual disability. Dev Med Child Neurol. 2008;50:625–30.
14. Furuta M, Komiya-Nonaka M, Akifusa S, et al. Interrelationship of oral health status, swallowing function, nutritional status, and cognitive ability with activities of daily living in Japanese elderly people receiving home care services due to physical disabilities. Community Dent Oral Epidemiol. 2013;41:173–81.
15. Siebens H, Trupe E, Siebens A, et al. Correlates and consequences of eating dependency in institutionalized elderly. J Am Geriatr Soc. 1986;34:192–8.
16. Stuchell RN, Mandel ID. Salivary gland dysfunction and swallowing disorders. Otolaryngol Clin N Am. 1988;21:649–61.
17. Guggenheimer J, Moore PA. Xerostomia: etiology, recognition and treatment. J Am Dent Assoc. 2003;134:61–9; quiz 118-9.
18. Ortega O, Parra C, Zarcero S, et al. Oral health in older patients with oropharyngeal dysphagia. Age Ageing. 2014;43:132–7.
19. Cabre M, Serra-Prat M, Palomera E, et al. Prevalence and prognostic implications of dysphagia in elderly patients with pneumonia. Age Ageing. 2010;39:39–45.
20. Bloem BR, Lagaay AM, van Beek W, et al. Prevalence of subjective dysphagia in community residents aged over 87. BMJ. 1990;300:721–2.
21. Lindgren S, Janzon L. Prevalence of swallowing complaints and clinical findings among 50-79-year-old men and women in an urban population. Dysphagia. 1991;6:187–92.
22. Holland G, Jayasekeran V, Pendleton N, et al. Prevalence and symptom profiling of oropharyngeal dysphagia in a community dwelling of an elderly population: a self-reporting questionnaire survey. Dis Esophagus. 2011;24:476–80.
23. Ney DM, Weiss JM, Kind AJ, et al. Senescent swallowing: impact, strategies, and interventions. Nutr Clin Pract. 2009;24:395–413.
24. Langmore SE, Olney RK, Lomen-Hoerth C, et al. Dysphagia in patients with frontotemporal lobar dementia. Arch Neurol. 2007;64:58–62.

25. Kalf JG, de Swart BJ, Bloem BR, et al. Prevalence of oropharyngeal dysphagia in Parkinson's disease: a meta-analysis. Parkinsonism Relat Disord. 2012;18:311–5.
26. Horner J, Alberts MJ, Dawson DV, et al. Swallowing in Alzheimer's disease. Alzheimer Dis Assoc Disord. 1994;8:177–89.
27. Clave P, Rofes L, Carrion S, et al. Pathophysiology, relevance and natural history of oropharyngeal dysphagia among older people. Nestle Nutr Inst Workshop Ser. 2012;72:57–66.
28. Rofes L, Arreola V, Romea M, et al. Pathophysiology of oropharyngeal dysphagia in the frail elderly. Neurogastroenterol Motil. 2010;22:851–8, e230.
29. Rudney JD, Ji Z, Larson CJ. The prediction of saliva swallowing frequency in humans from estimates of salivary flow rate and the volume of saliva swallowed. Arch Oral Biol. 1995;40:507–12.
30. Ardran GM, Kemp FH. A radiographic study of movements of the tongue in swallowing. Dent Pract. 1955;5:252–61.
31. Hiiemae KM, Palmer JB. Food transport and bolus formation during complete feeding sequences on foods of different initial consistency. Dysphagia. 1999;14:31–42.
32. Dantas RO, Dodds WJ, Massey BT, et al. Manometric characteristics of glossopalatal sphincter. Dig Dis Sci. 1990;35:161–6.
33. Shaker R, Dodds WJ, Dantas RO, et al. Coordination of deglutitive glottic closure with oropharyngeal swallowing. Gastroenterology. 1990;98:1478–84.
34. Kahrilas PJ, Dodds WJ, Dent J, et al. Upper esophageal sphincter function during deglutition. Gastroenterology. 1988;95:52–62.
35. Matsubara K, Kumai Y, Samejima Y, et al. Propagation curve and velocity of swallowing pressure in healthy young adults. Dysphagia. 2015;30:674–9.
36. Jean A. Brainstem organization of the swallowing network. Brain Behav Evol. 1984;25:109–16.
37. Sumi T. The activity of brain-stem respiratory neurons and spinal respiratory motoneurons during swallowing. J Neurophysiol. 1963;26:466–77.
38. Jean A. Brain stem control of swallowing: neuronal network and cellular mechanisms. Physiol Rev. 2001;81:929–69.
39. Kessler JP, Jean A. Identification of the medullary swallowing regions in the rat. Exp Brain Res. 1985;57:256–63.
40. Saito Y, Ezure K, Tanaka I. Swallowing-related activities of respiratory and non-respiratory neurons in the nucleus of solitary tract in the rat. J Physiol. 2002;540:1047–60.
41. Chiao GZ, Larson CR, Yajima Y, et al. Neuronal activity in nucleus ambiguous during deglutition and vocalization in conscious monkeys. Exp Brain Res. 1994;100:29–38.
42. Martin RE, Sessle BJ. The role of the cerebral cortex in swallowing. Dysphagia. 1993;8:195–202.
43. Babaei A, Ward BD, Ahmad S, et al. Reproducibility of swallow-induced cortical BOLD positive and negative fMRI activity. Am J Physiol Gastrointest Liver Physiol. 2012;303: G600–9.
44. Hamdy S, Mikulis DJ, Crawley A, et al. Cortical activation during human volitional swallowing: an event-related fMRI study. Am J Phys. 1999;277:G219–25.
45. Toogood JA, Barr AM, Stevens TK, et al. Discrete functional contributions of cerebral cortical foci in voluntary swallowing: a functional magnetic resonance imaging (fMRI) "Go, No-Go" study. Exp Brain Res. 2005;161:81–90.
46. Hamdy S, Aziz Q, Rothwell JC, et al. The cortical topography of human swallowing musculature in health and disease. Nat Med. 1996;2:1217–24.
47. Kamarunas E, Mulheren R, Palmore K, et al. Timing of cortical activation during spontaneous swallowing. Exp Brain Res. 2018;236:475–84.
48. Malandraki GA, Sutton BP, Perlman AL, et al. Neural activation of swallowing and swallowing-related tasks in healthy young adults: an attempt to separate the components of deglutition. Hum Brain Mapp. 2009;30:3209–26.
49. Babaei A, Kern M, Antonik S, et al. Enhancing effects of flavored nutritive stimuli on cortical swallowing network activity. Am J Physiol Gastrointest Liver Physiol. 2010;299:G422–9.

50. Mulheren RW, Kamarunas E, Ludlow CL. Sour taste increases swallowing and prolongs hemodynamic responses in the cortical swallowing network. J Neurophysiol. 2016;116:2033–42.
51. Pearson WG Jr, Molfenter SM, Smith ZM, et al. Image-based measurement of post-swallow residue: the normalized residue ratio scale. Dysphagia. 2013;28:167–77.
52. Molfenter SM, Steele CM. The relationship between residue and aspiration on the subsequent swallow: an application of the normalized residue ratio scale. Dysphagia. 2013;28:494–500.
53. Williams RB, Wallace KL, Ali GN, et al. Biomechanics of failed deglutitive upper esophageal sphincter relaxation in neurogenic dysphagia. Am J Physiol Gastrointest Liver Physiol. 2002;283:G16–26.
54. Scmidt EV, Smirnov VE, Ryabova VS. Results of the seven-year prospective study of stroke patients. Stroke. 1988;19:942–9.
55. Gresham SL. Clinical assessment and management of swallowing difficulties after stroke. Med J Aust. 1990;153:397–9.
56. Smithard DG, O'Neill PA, England RE, et al. The natural history of dysphagia following a stroke. Dysphagia. 1997;12:188–93.
57. Han DS, Chang YC, Lu CH, et al. Comparison of disordered swallowing patterns in patients with recurrent cortical/subcortical stroke and first-time brainstem stroke. J Rehabil Med. 2005;37:189–91.
58. Singh S, Hamdy S. Dysphagia in stroke patients. Postgrad Med J. 2006;82:383–91.
59. Ali GN, Wallace KL, Schwartz R, et al. Mechanisms of oral-pharyngeal dysphagia in patients with Parkinson's disease. Gastroenterology. 1996;110:383–92.
60. Kiernan MC, Vucic S, Cheah BC, et al. Amyotrophic lateral sclerosis. Lancet. 2011;377:942–55.
61. Kuhnlein P, Gdynia HJ, Sperfeld AD, et al. Diagnosis and treatment of bulbar symptoms in amyotrophic lateral sclerosis. Nat Clin Pract Neurol. 2008;4:366–74.
62. Richard P, Trollet C, Stojkovic T, et al. Correlation between PABPN1 genotype and disease severity in oculopharyngeal muscular dystrophy. Neurology. 2017;88:359–65.
63. Blumen SC, Nisipeanu P, Sadeh M, et al. Epidemiology and inheritance of oculopharyngeal muscular dystrophy in Israel. Neuromuscul Disord. 1997;7(Suppl 1):S38–40.
64. Dziewas R, Warnecke T, Schnabel M, et al. Neuroleptic-induced dysphagia: case report and literature review. Dysphagia. 2007;22:63–7.
65. Stewart JT. Dysphagia associated with risperidone therapy. Dysphagia. 2003;18:274–5.
66. Trifiro G. Antipsychotic drug use and community-acquired pneumonia. Curr Infect Dis Rep. 2011;13:262–8.
67. Dantas RO, Nobre Souza MA. Dysphagia induced by chronic ingestion of benzodiazepine. Am J Gastroenterol. 1997;92:1194–6.
68. Hardemark Cedborg AI, Sundman E, Boden K, et al. Effects of morphine and midazolam on pharyngeal function, airway protection, and coordination of breathing and swallowing in healthy adults. Anesthesiology. 2015;122:1253–67.
69. Rattan S, Goyal RK. Identification and localization of opioid receptors in the opossum lower esophageal sphincter. J Pharmacol Exp Ther. 1983;224:391–7.
70. Storr M, Geisler F, Neuhuber WL, et al. Endomorphin-1 and -2, endogenous ligands for the mu-opioid receptor, inhibit striated and smooth muscle contraction in the rat oesophagus. Neurogastroenterol Motil. 2000;12:441–8.
71. Dowlatshahi K, Evander A, Walther B, et al. Influence of morphine on the distal oesophagus and the lower oesophageal sphincter--a manometric study. Gut. 1985;26:802–6.
72. Penagini R, Picone A, Bianchi PA. Effect of morphine and naloxone on motor response of the human esophagus to swallowing and distension. Am J Phys. 1996;271:G675–80.
73. Ratuapli SK, Crowell MD, DiBaise JK, et al. Opioid-induced esophageal dysfunction (OIED) in patients on chronic opioids. Am J Gastroenterol. 2015;110:979–84.
74. Babaei A, Szabo A, Shad S, et al. Chronic daily opioid exposure is associated with dysphagia, esophageal outflow obstruction, and disordered peristalsis. Neurogastroenterol Motil. 2019:e13601.

75. Leonard R, Kendall K, McKenzie S. UES opening and cricopharyngeal bar in nondysphagic elderly and nonelderly adults. Dysphagia. 2004;19:182–91.
76. Leaper M, Zhang M, Dawes PJ. An anatomical protrusion exists on the posterior hypopharyngeal wall in some elderly cadavers. Dysphagia. 2005;20:8–14.
77. Dantas RO, Cook IJ, Dodds WJ, et al. Biomechanics of cricopharyngeal bars. Gastroenterology. 1990;99:1269–74.
78. Cook IJ, Blumbergs P, Cash K, et al. Structural abnormalities of the cricopharyngeus muscle in patients with pharyngeal (Zenker's) diverticulum. J Gastroenterol Hepatol. 1992;7: 556–62.
79. Cook IJ, Gabb M, Panagopoulos V, et al. Pharyngeal (Zenker's) diverticulum is a disorder of upper esophageal sphincter opening. Gastroenterology. 1992;103:1229–35.
80. Cook IJ, Dodds WJ, Dantas RO, et al. Opening mechanisms of the human upper esophageal sphincter. Am J Phys. 1989;257:G748–59.
81. Pal A, Williams RB, Cook IJ, et al. Intrabolus pressure gradient identifies pathological constriction in the upper esophageal sphincter during flow. Am J Physiol Gastrointest Liver Physiol. 2003;285:G1037–48.
82. Anagiotos A, Preuss SF, Koebke J. Morphometric and anthropometric analysis of Killian's triangle. Laryngoscope. 2010;120:1082–8.
83. Fulp SR, Castell DO. Manometric aspects of Zenker's diverticulum. Hepato-Gastroenterology. 1992;39:123–6.
84. Sasaki CT, Ross DA, Hundal J. Association between Zenker diverticulum and gastroesophageal reflux disease: development of a working hypothesis. Am J Med. 2003;115(Suppl 3A):169S–71S.
85. Herbella FA, Dubecz A, Patti MG. Esophageal diverticula and cancer. Dis Esophagus. 2012;25:153–8.
86. Castell DO, Donner MW. Evaluation of dysphagia: a careful history is crucial. Dysphagia. 1987;2:65–71.
87. Kertscher B, Speyer R, Palmieri M, et al. Bedside screening to detect oropharyngeal dysphagia in patients with neurological disorders: an updated systematic review. Dysphagia. 2014;29:204–12.
88. Martino R, Silver F, Teasell R, et al. The Toronto Bedside Swallowing Screening Test (TOR-BSST): development and validation of a dysphagia screening tool for patients with stroke. Stroke. 2009;40:555–61.
89. Clave P, Arreola V, Romea M, et al. Accuracy of the volume-viscosity swallow test for clinical screening of oropharyngeal dysphagia and aspiration. Clin Nutr. 2008;27:806–15.
90. Perry L. Screening swallowing function of patients with acute stroke. Part one: identification, implementation and initial evaluation of a screening tool for use by nurses. J Clin Nurs. 2001;10:463–73.
91. Trapl M, Enderle P, Nowotny M, et al. Dysphagia bedside screening for acute-stroke patients: the gugging swallowing screen. Stroke. 2007;38:2948–52.
92. Baijens L, Barikroo A, Pilz W. Intrarater and interrater reliability for measurements in videofluoroscopy of swallowing. Eur J Radiol. 2013;82:1683–95.
93. Gullung JL, Hill EG, Castell DO, et al. Oropharyngeal and esophageal swallowing impairments: their association and the predictive value of the modified barium swallow impairment profile and combined multichannel intraluminal impedance-esophageal manometry. Ann Otol Rhinol Laryngol. 2012;121:738–45.
94. Hiss SG, Postma GN. Fiberoptic endoscopic evaluation of swallowing. Laryngoscope. 2003;113:1386–93.
95. Langmore SE, Schatz K, Olsen N. Fiberoptic endoscopic examination of swallowing safety: a new procedure. Dysphagia. 1988;2:216–9.
96. Cock C, Omari T. Diagnosis of swallowing disorders: how we interpret pharyngeal manometry. Curr Gastroenterol Rep. 2017;19:11.

97. Omari TI, Papathanasopoulos A, Dejaeger E, et al. Reproducibility and agreement of pharyngeal automated impedance manometry with videofluoroscopy. Clin Gastroenterol Hepatol. 2011;9:862–7.

98. Omari TI, Dejaeger E, van Beckevoort D, et al. A method to objectively assess swallow function in adults with suspected aspiration. Gastroenterology. 2011;140:1454–63.

99. Regan J, Walshe M, Rommel N, et al. New measures of upper esophageal sphincter distensibility and opening patterns during swallowing in healthy subjects using EndoFLIP(R). Neurogastroenterol Motil. 2013;25:e25–34.

100. Regan J, Walshe M, Timon C, et al. Endoflip(R) evaluation of pharyngo-oesophageal segment tone and swallowing in a clinical population: a total laryngectomy case series. Clin Otolaryngol. 2015;40:121–9.

101. Watts S, Gaziano J, Jacobs J, et al. Improving the diagnostic capability of the modified barium swallow study through standardization of an esophageal sweep protocol. Dysphagia. 2019;34:34–42.

102. Martino R, McCulloch T. Therapeutic intervention in oropharyngeal dysphagia. Nat Rev Gastroenterol Hepatol. 2016;13:665–79.

103. Rosenbek JC, Robbins JA, Roecker EB, et al. A penetration-aspiration scale. Dysphagia. 1996;11:93–8.

104. Almirall J, Rofes L, Serra-Prat M, et al. Oropharyngeal dysphagia is a risk factor for community-acquired pneumonia in the elderly. Eur Respir J. 2013;41:923–8.

105. McClave SA, DeMeo MT, DeLegge MH, et al. North American summit on aspiration in the critically ill patient: consensus statement. JPEN J Parenter Enteral Nutr. 2002;26:S80–5.

106. Ickenstein GW, Riecker A, Hohlig C, et al. Pneumonia and in-hospital mortality in the context of neurogenic oropharyngeal dysphagia (NOD) in stroke and a new NOD step-wise concept. J Neurol. 2010;257:1492–9.

107. Bock JM, Varadarajan V, Brawley MC, et al. Evaluation of the natural history of patients who aspirate. Laryngoscope. 2017;127(Suppl 8):S1–S10.

108. Logemann JA, Gensler G, Robbins J, et al. A randomized study of three interventions for aspiration of thin liquids in patients with dementia or Parkinson's disease. J Speech Lang Hear Res. 2008;51:173–83.

109. Robbins J, Gensler G, Hind J, et al. Comparison of 2 interventions for liquid aspiration on pneumonia incidence: a randomized trial. Ann Intern Med. 2008;148:509–18.

110. Logemann JA. Approaches to management of disordered swallowing. Baillieres Clin Gastroenterol. 1991;5:269–80.

111. Wintzen AR, Badrising UA, Roos RA, et al. Influence of bolus volume on hyoid movements in normal individuals and patients with Parkinson's disease. Can J Neurol Sci. 1994;21:57–9.

112. Lazarus CL, Logemann JA, Rademaker AW, et al. Effects of bolus volume, viscosity, and repeated swallows in nonstroke subjects and stroke patients. Arch Phys Med Rehabil. 1993;74:1066–70.

113. Butler SG, Stuart A, Case LD, et al. Effects of liquid type, delivery method, and bolus volume on penetration-aspiration scores in healthy older adults during flexible endoscopic evaluation of swallowing. Ann Otol Rhinol Laryngol. 2011;120:288–95.

114. Logemann JA, Pauloski BR, Colangelo L, et al. Effects of a sour bolus on oropharyngeal swallowing measures in patients with neurogenic dysphagia. J Speech Hear Res. 1995;38:556–63.

115. Cola PC, Gatto AR, Silva RG, et al. The influence of sour taste and cold temperature in pharyngeal transit duration in patients with stroke. Arq Gastroenterol. 2010;47:18–21.

116. Pauloski BR, Logemann JA, Rademaker AW, et al. Effects of enhanced bolus flavors on oropharyngeal swallow in patients treated for head and neck cancer. Head Neck. 2013;35:1124–31.

117. Bisch EM, Logemann JA, Rademaker AW, et al. Pharyngeal effects of bolus volume, viscosity, and temperature in patients with dysphagia resulting from neurologic impairment and in normal subjects. J Speech Hear Res. 1994;37:1041–59.

118. Castell JA, Castell DO, Schultz AR, et al. Effect of head position on the dynamics of the upper esophageal sphincter and pharynx. Dysphagia. 1993;8:1–6.

119. Ohmae Y, Ogura M, Kitahara S, et al. Effects of head rotation on pharyngeal function during normal swallow. Ann Otol Rhinol Laryngol. 1998;107:344–8.
120. Logemann JA, Kahrilas PJ, Kobara M, et al. The benefit of head rotation on pharyngoesophageal dysphagia. Arch Phys Med Rehabil. 1989;70:767–71.
121. Hoffman MR, Mielens JD, Ciucci MR, et al. High-resolution manometry of pharyngeal swallow pressure events associated with effortful swallow and the Mendelsohn maneuver. Dysphagia. 2012;27:418–26.
122. Wheeler-Hegland KM, Rosenbek JC, Sapienza CM. Submental sEMG and hyoid movement during Mendelsohn maneuver, effortful swallow, and expiratory muscle strength training. J Speech Lang Hear Res. 2008;51:1072–87.
123. Bulow M, Olsson R, Ekberg O. Videomanometric analysis of supraglottic swallow, effortful swallow, and chin tuck in healthy volunteers. Dysphagia. 1999;14:67–72.
124. Jensen CB, Evans DL. Swallowing problems in patients with head and neck cancer. Occup Ther Health Care. 1986;3:49–62.
125. Carnaby G, Hankey GJ, Pizzi J. Behavioural intervention for dysphagia in acute stroke: a randomised controlled trial. Lancet Neurol. 2006;5:31–7.
126. Robbins J, Kays SA, Gangnon RE, et al. The effects of lingual exercise in stroke patients with dysphagia. Arch Phys Med Rehabil. 2007;88:150–8.
127. Kahrilas PJ, Logemann JA, Krugler C, et al. Volitional augmentation of upper esophageal sphincter opening during swallowing. Am J Phys. 1991;260:G450–6.
128. Lazarus C, Logemann JA, Song CW, et al. Effects of voluntary maneuvers on tongue base function for swallowing. Folia Phoniatr Logop. 2002;54:171–6.
129. Shaker R, Easterling C, Kern M, et al. Rehabilitation of swallowing by exercise in tube-fed patients with pharyngeal dysphagia secondary to abnormal UES opening. Gastroenterology. 2002;122:1314–21.
130. Troche MS, Okun MS, Rosenbek JC, et al. Aspiration and swallowing in Parkinson disease and rehabilitation with EMST: a randomized trial. Neurology. 2010;75:1912–9.
131. Robbins J, Butler SG, Daniels SK, et al. Swallowing and dysphagia rehabilitation: translating principles of neural plasticity into clinically oriented evidence. J Speech Lang Hear Res. 2008;51:S276–300.
132. Guttman M, Slaughter PM, Theriault ME, et al. Parkinsonism in Ontario: comorbidity associated with hospitalization in a large cohort. Mov Disord. 2004;19:49–53.
133. Denk DM, Kaider A. Videoendoscopic biofeedback: a simple method to improve the efficacy of swallowing rehabilitation of patients after head and neck surgery. ORL J Otorhinolaryngol Relat Spec. 1997;59:100–5.
134. Crary MA, Carnaby Mann GD, Groher ME, et al. Functional benefits of dysphagia therapy using adjunctive sEMG biofeedback. Dysphagia. 2004;19:160–4.
135. O'Rourke A, Humphries K. The use of high-resolution pharyngeal manometry as biofeedback in dysphagia therapy. Ear Nose Throat J. 2017;96:56–8.
136. Jayasekeran V, Singh S, Tyrrell P, et al. Adjunctive functional pharyngeal electrical stimulation reverses swallowing disability after brain lesions. Gastroenterology. 2010;138:1737–46.
137. Shaw GY, Sechtem PR, Searl J, et al. Transcutaneous neuromuscular electrical stimulation (VitalStim) curative therapy for severe dysphagia: myth or reality? Ann Otol Rhinol Laryngol. 2007;116:36–44.
138. Yang EJ, Baek SR, Shin J, et al. Effects of transcranial direct current stimulation (tDCS) on post-stroke dysphagia. Restor Neurol Neurosci. 2012;30:303–11.
139. Khedr EM, Abo-Elfetoh N, Rothwell JC. Treatment of post-stroke dysphagia with repetitive transcranial magnetic stimulation. Acta Neurol Scand. 2009;119:155–61.
140. Verin E, Leroi AM. Poststroke dysphagia rehabilitation by repetitive transcranial magnetic stimulation: a noncontrolled pilot study. Dysphagia. 2009;24:204–10.
141. Vasant DH, Sasegbon A, Michou E, et al. Rapid improvement in brain and swallowing behavior induced by cerebellar repetitive transcranial magnetic stimulation in poststroke dysphagia: a single patient case-controlled study. Neurogastroenterol Motil. 2019:e13609.

142. Michou E, Mistry S, Rothwell J, et al. Priming pharyngeal motor cortex by repeated paired associative stimulation: implications for dysphagia neurorehabilitation. Neurorehabil Neural Repair. 2013;27:355–62.
143. Bath PM, Scutt P, Love J, et al. Pharyngeal electrical stimulation for treatment of dysphagia in subacute stroke: a randomized controlled trial. Stroke. 2016;47:1562–70.
144. Pingue V, Priori A, Malovini A, et al. Dual transcranial direct current stimulation for poststroke dysphagia: a randomized controlled trial. Neurorehabil Neural Repair. 2018;32:635–44.
145. Belafsky PC, Rees CJ, Allen J, et al. Pharyngeal dilation in cricopharyngeus muscle dysfunction and Zenker diverticulum. Laryngoscope. 2010;120:889–94.
146. Kocdor P, Siegel ER, Tulunay-Ugur OE. Cricopharyngeal dysfunction: a systematic review comparing outcomes of dilatation, botulinum toxin injection, and myotomy. Laryngoscope. 2016;126:135–41.
147. Kelly JH. Management of upper esophageal sphincter disorders: indications and complications of myotomy. Am J Med. 2000;108(Suppl 4a):43S–6S.
148. Allen J, White CJ, Leonard R, et al. Effect of cricopharyngeus muscle surgery on the pharynx. Laryngoscope. 2010;120:1498–503.
149. Hernandez Mondragon OV, Solorzano Pineda MO, Blancas Valencia JM. Zenker's diverticulum: submucosal tunneling endoscopic septum division (Z-POEM). Dig Endosc. 2018;30:124.
150. Pang M, Koop A, Brahmbhatt B, et al. Comparison of flexible endoscopic cricopharyngeal myectomy and myotomy approaches for Zenker diverticulum repair. Gastrointest Endosc. 2019;89:880–6.
151. Johnson CM, Postma GN. Zenker diverticulum--which surgical approach is superior? JAMA Otolaryngol Head Neck Surg. 2016;142:401–3.
152. Bonavina L, Aiolfi A, Scolari F, et al. Long-term outcome and quality of life after transoral stapling for Zenker diverticulum. World J Gastroenterol. 2015;21:1167–72.

Chapter 4
Gastroesophageal Reflux Disease

Amit Patel and C. Prakash Gyawali

Introduction

Gastroesophageal reflux disease (GERD) is exceedingly common, with prevalence estimates of 18–28% in North America, and increasing over recent decades [1]. GERD accounts for an estimated 5.5–7 million ambulatory visits in the United States each year [2, 3] and annual direct costs to the United States healthcare system totaling over 9 billion dollars [4].

The most frequent mechanism for reflux, transient lower esophageal sphincter (LES) relaxation, is inherent in all individuals as the belch reflex from gastric distension. Gastroesophageal reflux becomes pathologic when the retrograde movement of gastric contents into the esophagus leads to bothersome symptoms and/or esophageal mucosal injury [5]. This modern-day GERD definition from the Montreal consensus recognizes heartburn and regurgitation as typical symptoms [5]. Atypical symptoms can include chest pain, cough, or even dysphagia. Esophageal complications from GERD can manifest as reflux esophagitis, reflux-mediated (peptic) esophageal strictures, Barrett's esophagus (BE; intestinal metaplasia), or esophageal adenocarcinoma (EAC).

In the setting of suspected GERD, dysphagia is an alarm symptom that indicates a need for further invasive evaluation to evaluate for complications of GERD and/or alternate diagnoses [6, 7]. This is mainly because esophageal mucosal injury from GERD, luminal restriction from peptic strictures, or EAC can all generate

A. Patel
Division of Gastroenterology, Duke University School of Medicine and the Durham Veterans Affairs Medical Center, Durham, NC, USA

C. P. Gyawali (✉)
Division of Gastroenterology, Washington University School of Medicine,
St Louis, MO, USA
e-mail: cprakash@dom.wustl.edu

© Springer Nature Switzerland AG 2020
D. A. Patel et al. (eds.), *Evaluation and Management of Dysphagia*,
https://doi.org/10.1007/978-3-030-26554-0_4

Table 4.1 Mechanisms of dysphagia in gastroesophageal reflux disease (GERD)

Dysphagia directly related to GERD
Erosive esophagitis
Reflux-induced peptic stricture
Esophageal adenocarcinoma from Barrett's esophagus
Dysphagia indirectly related to GERD
Hiatus hernia
Esophageal hypomotility
Post-fundoplication dysphagia
Dysphagia following radiofrequency ablation of Barrett's esophagus
Dysphagia from disorders mimicking GERD
Pill esophagitis
Eosinophilic esophagitis
Achalasia and esophageal outflow obstruction
Infectious esophagitis
Lichen planus
Acute esophageal necrosis (black esophagus)
Caustic esophagitis

dysphagia. Alternatively, conditions that mimic GERD, including eosinophilic esophagitis (EoE) and achalasia, can also result in dysphagia [8]. Consequently, upper endoscopy is a common investigative procedure performed in the setting of alarm symptoms. Further testing can include esophageal function testing, barium radiography, and endoscopic functional lumen imaging probe (endo-FLIP), all of which can provide complementary information in further evaluation of dysphagia.

In the context of GERD, dysphagia can either be directly related to GERD (i.e., a GERD complication), indirectly related to GERD, or part of a disorder mimicking GERD (Table 4.1).

Dysphagia Directly Related to Gastroesophageal Reflux Disease

Although not a common primary symptom of uncomplicated GERD, dysphagia can manifest as part of the symptomatic reflux spectrum either as a stand-alone symptom or more often in conjunction with other typical or atypical GERD symptoms. According to the ROME IV definitions of functional esophageal disorders, GERD must be ruled out before a diagnosis of functional dysphagia can be made [9], since solid food dysphagia can coexist in patients with longstanding heartburn and GERD [10].

One of the common mechanisms of dysphagia in GERD is erosive esophagitis. Dysphagia was reported in over one-third of a cohort of 12,000 patients with reflux esophagitis enrolled in 5 clinical trials, despite the absence of strictures, BE, or malignancy [11]. Invasive evaluation of dysphagia with endoscopy allows inspec-

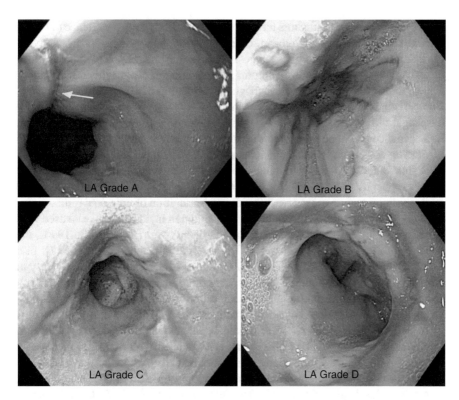

Fig. 4.1 Los Angeles (LA) grades of reflux esophagitis. Grade A: mucosal breaks <5 mm in length, not extending across mucosal folds; Grade B: mucosal breaks >5 mm in length, not extending across mucosal folds; Grade C: mucosal breaks extending across mucosal folds, occupying <75% of esophageal circumference; Grade D: mucosal breaks occupying >75% of the esophageal circumference

tion of the esophageal mucosa for esophageal mucosal injury, which is described as breaks in the distal esophageal mucosa. The Los Angeles (LA) Classification is the most frequently used descriptive classification of esophagitis and grades the severity of reflux esophagitis into the following four grades (Fig. 4.1) [12, 13]:

1. Grade A: mucosal breaks <5 mm in length but not extending between the tops of two mucosal folds
2. Grade B: mucosal breaks >5 mm in length but not extending across the tops of two mucosal folds
3. Grade C: mucosal breaks continuous between tops of at least 2 mucosal folds but not involving <75% of esophageal circumference
4. Grade D: mucosal breaks involving >75% of the esophageal circumference [12, 13]

Using this classification scheme, patients with advanced grades of esophagitis (LA Grades C or D) were more likely to have dysphagia at baseline (43%), in contrast to milder grades (LA Grades A or B, 36%, $p < 0.001$ compared to advanced grades) [11]. Other investigators have reported a similarly high prevalence (47%) of intermittent dysphagia symptoms in severe reflux esophagitis unresponsive to medical therapy [14]. These findings suggest that distal esophageal acid exposure may be associated with dysphagia symptoms in the setting of esophagitis. The relationship of motor abnormalities to dysphagia in the setting of GERD remains unclear. Comparison of esophageal body motor function in GERD patients with and without dysphagia did not reveal differences during stationary manometry, but provocative testing in the upright position or during meal times demonstrated a lower likelihood of simultaneous contractions in patients without dysphagia [15].

Reflux-induced (peptic) strictures occur at the squamocolumnar junction or the distal esophagus and can result in mechanical dysphagia [6]. Peptic strictures are more common among older patients with longer duration of untreated reflux symptoms, as well as in those with hiatus hernias, although incidence has decreased with increasing PPI use in recent decades. In a British cohort from the late 1990s, the incidence of esophageal stricture was 1.1 per 10,000 person-years [16, 17]. In a US study of over 280,000 endoscopic procedures, Caucasians were more likely to have peptic strictures, though Hispanics were more likely to have esophagitis [18]. Evaluation for reflux strictures is another reason for endoscopic evaluation of dysphagia, since strictures can be managed with esophageal dilation during endoscopy.

In 5–15% of patients with chronic esophageal acid exposure, reflux can lead to intestinal metaplasia, or BE [19–21]. BE is associated with a 10-fold increase in risk for EAC [22], though as many as 40% of EAC cases may not have a history of chronic GERD symptoms [23]. Luminal compromise from EAC can result in mechanical dysphagia, which can be a presenting symptom in EAC. Guidelines recommend targeted screening for BE in patients with multiple risk factors for BE and EAC, including male gender, Caucasian race, age > 50 years, longstanding GERD, central obesity, smoking history, and/or a family history of EAC [24, 25]. Early identification of advanced dysplasia in BE and EAC can lead to better management outcomes, which is yet another reason for esophageal endoscopic evaluation in dysphagia.

Dysphagia Indirectly Related to GERD

Anatomic separation of the LES from the diaphragmatic crura defines a hiatus hernia, which can be seen in the setting of GERD. Hiatus hernias can be associated with abnormal esophageal reflux burden and GERD, which can lead to dysphagia. Hiatus hernias can be obstructing, particularly paraesophageal hernias. Axial hiatus hernias can sometimes cause extrinsic compression at the crural diaphragm, potentially leading to dysphagia [26].

The association between esophageal body motor abnormalities and dysphagia is not consistent in GERD. Motor abnormalities in the esophageal body and LES can be seen to a higher degree in GERD, especially in the presence of reflux esophagitis or BE [27, 28]. Esophageal body hypomotility can impair clearance of esophageal refluxate, and thus result in more profound gastroesophageal reflux [29, 30], although it is unclear if esophageal body hypomotility causes more severe GERD, or if severe GERD results in more profound hypomotility. While esophageal hypomotility may improve with the healing of esophagitis in animal models [31], a similar improvement has not been demonstrated in patients with reflux esophagitis treated with acid suppressive medications [32, 33]. Therefore, it remains unclear whether chronic esophageal acid exposure may contribute to esophageal motor injury, or a primary esophageal motor abnormality may precede GERD [34]. In either instance, the relationship to dysphagia is not definitive or consistent. Despite this, the absence of esophageal contraction reserve following multiple rapid swallow (MRS) during pre-operative esophageal high-resolution manometry (HRM) predicts post-fundoplication dysphagia [35, 36]. Therefore, this MRS maneuver may help with surgical planning by guiding the tailoring of fundoplication (i.e., partial vs complete 360-degree wrap) to minimize the risk of post-operative dysphagia [Level 3 Recommendation]. Further, patients with intact contraction reserve prior to antireflux surgery are more likely to resolve ineffective esophageal motility after surgery, compared to those without contraction reserve on MRS [37], though the relationship between these manometric findings and post-operative dysphagia is less clear.

Rather than weak contraction amplitude, breaks in esophageal peristaltic integrity have been reported more often in patients with non-obstructive dysphagia. When patients with non-obstructive dysphagia were compared to asymptomatic controls, small (2–5 cm) and large (>5 cm) breaks in esophageal body peristaltic integrity on HRM were seen more frequently in patients with dysphagia, though rates of failed peristalsis were similar between these groups [38]. Similarly, dysphagia was found more frequently among patients with more profound ineffective esophageal motility (IEM) on esophageal HRM (at least 50% ineffective liquid swallows) versus those with less profound IEM (30–50% ineffective liquid swallows; 25% vs 12%, $p = 0.08$) [39].

Dysphagia can develop after surgical therapy for GERD. Dysphagia is encountered more often following laparoscopic fundoplication compared to pharmacologic GERD therapy (short-term, 13% vs 4%, RR 3.6; medium-term 10% vs 2%, RR 5.4) [40]. Persistent post-fundoplication dysphagia can arise from morphologic esophagogastric junction (EGJ) abnormalities or esophageal body dysmotility. Dysphagia can also be seen following magnetic lower esophageal sphincter augmentation; dysphagia was initially noted in over two-thirds of patients post-operatively, but decreased to 11% at 1 year, and 4% at 3 years [41, 42].

The likelihood of post-fundoplication dysphagia may be related to a lack of effective esophageal peristaltic performance and type of fundoplication. Among patients with post-myotomy fundoplication, rates of dysphagia at 6-year follow-up were higher for Nissen compared to partial fundoplication (39% vs 10%, $p = 0.03$) [43]. Among patients with esophageal dysmotility and GERD, rates of dysphagia 2 years after fundoplication were higher for Nissen fundoplication compared to partial Toupet fundoplication [44]. Although data are limited, severe esophageal body hypomotility should prompt a partial fundoplication over a complete fundoplication to minimize post-operative dysphagia [Level 4 Recommendation], although the definition of "severe" hypomotility continues to be debated.

Endoscopic ablative approaches for dysplastic BE, particularly radiofrequency ablation (RFA), inflict esophageal mucosal injury, potentially leading to stricture formation with associated dysphagia. Studies of dysplastic BE treated with RFA have quantified this risk: 6% of patients had esophageal strictures by 12 months in an American cohort [45], and 12% had esophageal strictures by 3 years in a European cohort [46]. Meta-analysis of RFA in dysplastic BE suggested that the pooled rate of stricture development among 37 included studies (representing 9200 patients) was 5.6% [47].

Dysphagia from Disorders Mimicking GERD

Medications can induce esophageal mucosal injury, typically from direct contact with the esophageal mucosa resulting in caustic or hyperosmolar toxicity; this condition is termed pill esophagitis. Pill esophagitis can manifest as esophageal ulceration and exudate, and can mimic GERD in endoscopic findings (ulceration, exudates) or symptoms (dysphagia, odynophagia). Offending medications can include antibiotics (especially doxycycline), non-steroidal anti-inflammatory drugs (NSAIDs), acetaminophen, amlodipine, Ramipril, bisphosphonates, and glimepiride, among others [48]. Additionally, in the setting of esophageal strictures and/or esophageal hypomotility, pills may be retained in the esophagus in the presence of strictures and/or esophageal hypomotility, prolonging mucosal contact times and contributing to esophageal manifestations and symptoms [49].

Eosinophilic esophagitis (EoE), an increasingly common allergen/immune-mediated illness, is caused by eosinophilic infiltration into the esophageal mucosa. Typical symptoms can consist of dysphagia, food bolus impaction, heartburn, or chest pain [50]. Although there is wide geographic variation, meta-analyses suggest an overall EoE incidence of 7/100,000 persons/year and pooled prevalence of 43.4/100,000 among adults [51]. Diagnosis of EoE among patients undergoing endoscopy for dysphagia is higher, in the order of at least 10–15%, and increasing in recent years [52–54]. Symptoms of EoE can overlap with GERD. Additionally, GERD can also result in esophageal eosinophilia on biopsies as well as esophageal strictures. Similar to GERD, initial treatment for esophageal eosinophilia includes PPI therapy [50, 55, 56]. Recent work has suggested that esophageal eosinophilia responsive to PPI therapy is clinically and endoscopically indistinguishable from esophageal eosinophilia not responsive to PPI [57], indicating that PPI therapy should be the primary treatment option for when esophageal eosinophilia is encountered [50]. In patients with suspected reflux symptoms refractory to PPI, especially dysphagia, EoE should be ruled out with esophageal mucosal biopsies from the distal and proximal esophagus during endoscopy.

Symptoms of GERD, such as heartburn, regurgitation, and chest pain, can resemble symptoms of achalasia spectrum disorders, where relaxation of the LES is impaired. Patients who have achalasia can be mislabeled as GERD; therefore, esophageal HRM represents a valuable diagnostic modality in patients with suspected GERD symptoms who do not report symptomatic improvement with PPI therapy [58]. For example, achalasia spectrum disorders were found in 2.5% of a cohort of >1000 patients undergoing HRM studies prior to antireflux surgery [59]. Similarly, in a cohort of >100 patients with presumed reflux symptoms not responsive to PPI, >30% had alternate diagnoses besides GERD, which included 2% with achalasia [60].

Infectious esophagitis typically presents with dysphagia or odynophagia but can also manifest as retrosternal burning or discomfort, and overlap with symptoms of GERD. Although infectious esophagitis is more common in immunocompromised states, certain infectious processes, especially herpes esophagitis and esophageal candidiasis, can also be encountered in immunocompetent individuals. The most common causes of infectious esophagitis include candida species, herpes simplex virus, and cytomegalovirus [61].

Other less commonly encountered disorders can also mimic GERD. Lichen planus, a T-cell mediated immunologic phenomenon that typically involves the skin or nails, can rarely involve the esophagus. Presenting symptoms can include dysphagia, and esophageal manifestations on endoscopy can be misdiagnosed as reflux esophagitis [62]. The diagnosis can be confirmed by biopsy and histopathologic examination. Acute esophageal necrosis, or the so-called black esophagus, represents a rare phenomenon where ischemia leads to diffuse circumferential black-appearing mucosa with abrupt demarcation at the gastroesophageal junction. Patients with black esophagus are typically older and have multiple co-morbidities. Presentation can consist of upper gastrointestinal hemorrhage, but the condition can be sometimes encountered on the endoscopic evaluation of esophageal symptoms including dysphagia. Stricture formation can also occur upon healing of the necrosis [63, 64]. Ingestion of caustic substances, particularly strong alkalis (such as concentrated sodium hydroxide) but also acids, can damage the esophageal mucosa via liquefaction necrosis, with subsequent stricture formation after 2–3 weeks as the primary complication [65, 66]. Accidental ingestions are typically seen in children; caustic ingestions as part of a suicide attempt have been reported in adults.

If all testing is negative, functional dysphagia can be diagnosed. According to Rome IV criteria, functional dysphagia requires exclusion of esophageal mucosal processes including eosinophilic esophagitis, gastroesophageal reflux disease, and major motor disorders [9]. In one large series assessing diagnostic evaluation of dysphagia at a tertiary care center, 2.4% of patients with esophageal dysphagia were eventually diagnosed with functional dysphagia after testing was negative in the setting of persistent symptoms [67]. Widespread use of endo-FLIP has potential to identify structural or motor mechanisms of dysphagia even when alternate testing is negative, further reducing the proportion of patients with functional dysphagia [68].

Diagnosis of GERD in Dysphagia Presentations

Esophageal evaluation in dysphagia presentations is modulated by the patient's history, and typically starts with an upper endoscopy (Fig. 4.2). Esophageal function testing is often performed for the documentation of abnormal reflux burden, especially in the evaluation of atypical GERD symptoms including dysphagia [69, 70]. Persisting esophageal symptoms despite empiric PPI therapy also requires esophageal physiologic testing, including HRM and ambulatory reflux monitoring [8]. HRM evaluates for and excludes achalasia spectrum disorders in the setting of persisting GERD symptoms, and assesses esophageal peristaltic performance [71].

Metrics extracted from ambulatory reflux monitoring, including distal esophageal acid exposure times (AET) and symptoms association with impedance-detected reflux events predict symptomatic response to antireflux therapy [72]. These two metrics may be used to phenotype GERD (Fig. 4.3); elevated AET with or without reflux-symptom association is seen with pathologic GERD. Reflux-symptom association alone with physiologic acid exposure suggests reflux hypersensitivity, while physiologic AET with negative reflux-symptom association points away from

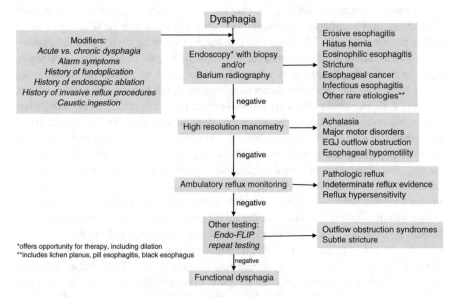

Fig. 4.2 Algorithm for evaluation of dysphagia. A careful history helps direct evaluation, which typically starts with an endoscopy and/or barium radiography. Ambulatory reflux monitoring and esophageal manometry are performed concurrently, as manometry is used to direct placement of pH and pH-impedance probes. Endoscopic functional lumen imaging probe (endo-FLIP) evaluation may add value to esophageal testing in dysphagia presentations. Tests such as barium radiography and high resolution manometry may need to be repeated if symptoms persist with otherwise negative evaluation, the former incorporating solid bolus or a timed upright protocol, and the latter incorporating provocative testing including solid swallows, rapid drink challenge, and a test meal. If all testing is negative, functional dysphagia is considered

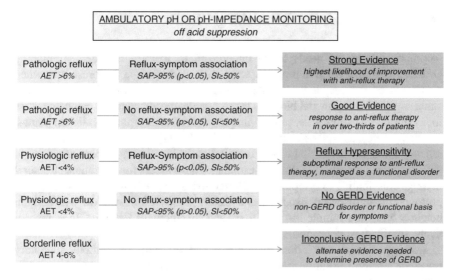

Fig. 4.3 GERD phenotypes using acid exposure time (AET) and reflux-symptom association. Elevated AET > 6% signifies pathologic reflux, with or without reflux-symptom association (strong or good evidence for GERD, respectively). AET < 4% constitutes physiologic reflux. If reflux-symptom association is identified with physiologic reflux, reflux hypersensitivity is diagnosed. Physiologic reflux with negative reflux-symptom association indicates lack of GERD evidence and fulfils criteria for functional heartburn in the absence of eosinophilic esophagitis on esophageal biopsies, and major motor disorders on esophageal high-resolution manometry. AET values between 4% and 6% are inconclusive for pathologic reflux, and findings from alternate testing are needed to sway clinical opinion toward or away from pathologic reflux

GERD-related mechanisms for symptoms [72–74]. While these metrics have been extensively studied in typical GERD presentations, data in atypical presentations are not as robust, particularly in the setting of dysphagia without endoscopic or motor pathology.

Novel reflux metrics have been introduced to augment the value of pH-impedance monitoring. Baseline distal esophageal impedance values have been documented to be low in the setting of mucosal damage from reflux [75]. Baseline impedance values can be extracted from ambulatory pH-impedance studies during three 10-minute periods during night-time sleep, when there are no artifacts, reflux episodes, or swallows [76]. The averaged value, termed mean nocturnal baseline impedance (MNBI), has been demonstrated to segregate pathologic reflux from functional esophageal syndromes, and to predict symptom response from antireflux therapy [77–79]. Postreflux swallow-induced peristaltic wave (PSPW) is a reflux-induced primary peristaltic wave associated with salivation, which functions to clear esophageal refluxate and resolve esophageal mucosal acidification [76]. When quantified as the ratio of the number of reflux episodes followed within 30 seconds by a PSPW to the total number of reflux episodes on 24-hour impedance tracings, this index may segregate erosive GERD, non-erosive GERD, and patients without GERD [76].

Diagnosis of Disorders Mimicking GERD

Appropriate work-up needs to be undertaken to identify disorders mimicking GERD, especially when alarm symptoms such as dysphagia are present or when symptoms do not respond adequately to antisecretory therapy [6, 8, 80]. Upper endoscopy with esophageal biopsies is the first diagnostic step and can help assess for eosinophilic esophagitis, pill esophagitis, infectious esophagitis, lichen planus, and malignancy, as well as complications of GERD [7]. Upper endoscopy does not reliably evaluate esophageal motor function, only identifying at best one-third of patients with achalasia [81]. Barium esophagograms assess for prominent structural findings contributing to symptoms (profound strictures, malignancies) and diagnose profound motor disorders like achalasia [82]. A timed barium swallow with column height > 5 cm at 1 minute has sensitivity and specificity of 94% and 76%, respectively, for diagnosing achalasia [83].

Esophageal high-resolution manometry (HRM) with or without stationary impedance (high resolution impedance manometry, HRIM) is the next step when symptoms persist, and endoscopy and/or barium radiography are normal [70, 82]. Integrated relaxation pressure (IRP), the HRM metric nadir residual pressure during lower esophageal sphincter relaxation, has a sensitivity of 93–98% and specificity of 96–98% for a diagnosis of achalasia [84, 85]. Provocative maneuvers performed at HRM may increase the diagnostic yield of HRM. The rapid drink challenge test (which consists of free drinking of 100–200 mL of liquid through a straw in the sitting position) may improve the detection of latent EGJ outflow obstruction [86–88]. Single solid swallows and standardized test meals may also demonstrate esophageal motility disorders not diagnosed with single wet swallows alone, though the clinical utility of these findings warrant further study [89].

Endo-FLIP simultaneously measures pressure and diameter within hollow viscus using a distensible balloon with pairs of impedance sensors and can provide distensibility measurements at the esophagogastric junction. A newer version also evaluates esophageal body contractility in addition to EGJ distensibility [68], providing valuable information in achalasia spectrum disorders [90]. However, endo-FLIP is not utilized in routine assessment of GERD, as EGJ distensibility does not consistently correlate with esophageal reflux parameters; it is a useful tool in further evaluation of unexplained dysphagia [68, 91, 92].

Management of Dysphagia in GERD Presentations

Acid Suppression

Typical GERD presentations prompt empiric PPI therapy in the absence alarm symptoms. In this setting, PPIs represent the mainstay of pharmacologic GERD management [93]. Best-practice advice from the American Gastroenterological Association recommends that patients with proven GERD (with evidence of mucosal disease or complications on endoscopy and/or positive ambulatory reflux monitoring) should be treated with PPIs for short-term healing and for long-term symptom control [94] (Level 1A Recommendation). On meta-analyses, short-term (12 weeks or less) PPI treatment heals erosive esophagitis in more than 80% of patients [93, 95] (Level 1A Recommendation). In a cohort of 12,000 patients with reflux esophagitis, dysphagia resolved in 83% after once-daily proton pump inhibitor (PPI) therapy, and resolution of dysphagia was strongly associated with healing of erosive esophagitis (odds of healing 3.37 higher for those with resolution of dysphagia compared to those with persistent dysphagia) [11]. Therefore, long-term PPI therapy is recommended in dysphagia-predominant presentations within the GERD context, both for the healing of esophagitis and for dysphagia relief.

Dilation of Peptic Strictures

The cornerstone of management of symptomatic peptic strictures is endoscopic dilation. Dilation may be performed with catheter-mounted through-the-scope balloons, or with graded bougie dilators that can be wire-guided (Savary) or blind (Maloney or Hurst) [96]. The commonly cited "rule of three" described by H. Worth Boyce in 1977 refers to limiting dilation at any one session to a maximum of three increments in dilator diameter after encountering resistance, to minimize the feared complication of perforation [97]. However, his recommendations preceded the development of balloon dilators (from which there is limited appreciation of resistance), and a retrospective study found no increased risk of perforation with dilations performed to a higher diameter than the "rule of three" [98].

When strictures are refractory to endoscopic dilation, especially if they re-develop at short intervals following dilation, injection of corticosteroids into rents created by dilation can prolong dysphagia relief. In randomized studies evaluating peptic strictures resistant to standard endoscopic dilation despite maintenance PPI therapy, injection of triamcinolone decreased the need for repeat dilation and time to repeat dilation compared to sham injections [99, 100] (Level 1D Recommendation). Therefore, the option of intralesional steroid injections can be considered in patients with refractory peptic strictures presenting with troublesome dysphagia. Further, endoscopic incisional therapy, such as with needle-knife, may provide advantages over bougie dilation in refractory esophageal strictures but has not been well studied. Esophageal stenting, while primarily utilized for palliation in the setting of malignant strictures, may have a role in refractory peptic strictures, when temporary esophageal stents can be sutured in place. Meta-analysis suggests response rates of about 40% with a single session of stenting but with higher risks of complications (such as stent migration in 29% and other adverse events in 21%) [101]. Other options include self-bougienage or surgery as salvage therapy [102].

Although the management of esophageal strictures centers on endoscopic dilation, randomized trials have shown that maintenance PPI therapy improves dysphagia symptoms and lowers the need for repeated endoscopic dilations, compared to H2 antagonists [103, 104] (Level 1A Recommendation). This augments the cost-effectiveness of PPI therapy in dysphagia predominant presentations.

Antireflux Surgery

Surgical antireflux options are often considered for GERD in the setting of persistent symptoms or mucosal damage despite optimal pharmacologic therapy, especially with significant hiatus hernia, and/or a preference for surgery. In well-defined GERD, antireflux surgery is comparable to PPI therapy in providing symptom relief [105, 106] (Level 1A Recommendation). Antireflux surgery carries a higher risk of post-operative dysphagia compared to medical therapy. If dysphagia develops following antireflux surgery, early dysphagia (<6 weeks after surgery) can be managed conservatively, with only 3.5% requiring endoscopic intervention in one study [107]. In contrast, in patients with late post-operative dysphagia in the same study (>6 weeks after surgery), >90% of the patients had symptomatic benefit with endoscopic dilation [107].

Management of Specific Conditions

Management of EoE is covered in greater detail in Chap. 6. Briefly, management centers on pharmacologic therapy with PPI or topical corticosteroids, dietary therapy with elimination diets, and/or endoscopic therapy with dilation [56, 108].

Pill esophagitis typically responds to discontinuation of the offending medication. Acid suppression with PPI, topical therapy with sucralfate, and dilation of peptic stricture when present are additional management avenues [48].

Treatment of infectious esophagitis is specific to the causative organism, taking into account the immune status of the patient and severity of infection. Especially in immunocompromised individuals, esophageal candidiasis is treated with oral systemic antifungal therapy (i.e., fluconazole) in immunocompromised individuals, while mild infections in immunocompetent individuals can be treated with swallowed nystatin [109]. In viral esophagitis, targeted antiviral therapy is effective (acyclovir for herpes simplex virus, ganciclovir or foscarnet for cytomegalovirus) [110], although immunocompromised patients may require extensions or re-treatment for herpes simplex virus esophagitis and treatment of concomitant candida esophagitis when present [111]. However, in immunocompetent hosts, herpes simplex virus esophagitis appears to be self-limiting; the benefits of antiviral therapy in this setting are unknown, though it may shorten the duration of symptoms [112].

Although lacking definitive recommendations given its rarity, lichen planus responds to systemic and topical steroids; associated esophageal strictures require endoscopic dilation [113–115].

Treatment of acute esophageal necrosis (black esophagus) centers on restoration of hemodynamic stability, correction of coexisting medical conditions, and intravenous antisecretory therapy, but mortality remains high [63, 64].

Conclusions

Dysphagia can be encountered in the context of GERD, and evaluation targets GERD complications, GERD-related mechanisms, and disorders mimicking GERD. A careful history can elucidate etiologic factors that can modulate investigation. Evaluation starts with an upper endoscopy and can include esophageal function tests, barium radiography, and endo-FLIP. Provocative maneuvers during manometry can be of complementary value. Management generally starts with acid suppression and is targeted toward etiologic mechanisms. If investigation is negative in the setting of persisting dysphagia, functional dysphagia can be diagnosed.

Conflict of Interest Disclosures   AP discloses no conflicts. CPG discloses consulting and speakers' bureau relationships with Medtronic and Diversatek, and consulting relationships with Ironwood, Torax, and Quintiles.

References

1. El-Serag HB, Sweet S, Winchester CC, et al. Update on the epidemiology of gastro-oesophageal reflux disease: a systematic review. Gut. 2014;63:871–80.
2. Peery AF, Crockett SD, Murphy CC, et al. Burden and cost of gastrointestinal, liver, and pancreatic diseases in the United States: update 2018. Gastroenterology. 2019;156:254–72, e11.
3. Peery AF, Crockett SD, Barritt AS, et al. Burden of gastrointestinal, liver, and pancreatic diseases in the United States. Gastroenterology. 2015;149:1731–41. e3
4. Shaheen NJ, Hansen RA, Morgan DR, et al. The burden of gastrointestinal and liver diseases, 2006. Am J Gastroenterol. 2006;101:2128–38.
5. Vakil N, van Zanten SV, Kahrilas P, et al. The Montreal definition and classification of gastroesophageal reflux disease: a global evidence-based consensus. Am J Gastroenterol. 2006;101:1900–20; quiz 1943.
6. Katz PO, Gerson LB, Vela MF. Guidelines for the diagnosis and management of gastroesophageal reflux disease. Am J Gastroenterol. 2013;108:308–28; quiz 329.
7. Shaheen NJ, Weinberg DS, Denberg TD, et al. Upper endoscopy for gastroesophageal reflux disease: best practice advice from the clinical guidelines committee of the American College of Physicians. Ann Intern Med. 2012;157:808–16.
8. Savarino E, Bredenoord AJ, Fox M, et al. Expert consensus document: advances in the physiological assessment and diagnosis of GERD. Nat Rev Gastroenterol Hepatol. 2017;14:665–76.
9. Aziz Q, Fass R, Gyawali CP, et al. Functional esophageal disorders. Gastroenterology. 2016;150:1368–79.
10. Richter JE, Rubenstein JH. Presentation and epidemiology of gastroesophageal reflux disease. Gastroenterology. 2018;154:267–76.

11. Vakil NB, Traxler B, Levine D. Dysphagia in patients with erosive esophagitis: prevalence, severity, and response to proton pump inhibitor treatment. Clin Gastroenterol Hepatol. 2004;2:665–8.
12. Armstrong D, Bennett JR, Blum AL, et al. The endoscopic assessment of esophagitis: a progress report on observer agreement. Gastroenterology. 1996;111:85–92.
13. Lundell LR, Dent J, Bennett JR, et al. Endoscopic assessment of oesophagitis: clinical and functional correlates and further validation of the Los Angeles classification. Gut. 1999;45:172–80.
14. Triadafilopoulos G. Nonobstructive dysphagia in reflux esophagitis. Am J Gastroenterol. 1989;84:614–8.
15. Singh S, Stein HJ, DeMeester TR, et al. Nonobstructive dysphagia in gastroesophageal reflux disease: a study with combined ambulatory pH and motility monitoring. Am J Gastroenterol. 1992;87:562–7.
16. Ruigomez A, Garcia Rodriguez LA, Wallander MA, et al. Esophageal stricture: incidence, treatment patterns, and recurrence rate. Am J Gastroenterol. 2006;101:2685–92.
17. Said A, Brust DJ, Gaumnitz EA, et al. Predictors of early recurrence of benign esophageal strictures. Am J Gastroenterol. 2003;98:1252–6.
18. Wang A, Mattek NC, Holub JL, et al. Prevalence of complicated gastroesophageal reflux disease and Barrett's esophagus among racial groups in a multi-center consortium. Dig Dis Sci. 2009;54:964–71.
19. Rex DK, Cummings OW, Shaw M, et al. Screening for Barrett's esophagus in colonoscopy patients with and without heartburn. Gastroenterology. 2003;125:1670–7.
20. Sharma P. Review article: prevalence of Barrett's oesophagus and metaplasia at the gastro-oesophageal junction. Aliment Pharmacol Ther. 2004;20(Suppl 5):48–54; discussion 61-2.
21. Johansson J, Hakansson HO, Mellblom L, et al. Prevalence of precancerous and other metaplasia in the distal oesophagus and gastro-oesophageal junction. Scand J Gastroenterol. 2005;40:893–902.
22. Pohl H, Welch HG. The role of overdiagnosis and reclassification in the marked increase of esophageal adenocarcinoma incidence. J Natl Cancer Inst. 2005;97:142–6.
23. Lagergren J, Bergstrom R, Lindgren A, et al. Symptomatic gastroesophageal reflux as a risk factor for esophageal adenocarcinoma. N Engl J Med. 1999;340:825–31.
24. Spechler SJ, Sharma P, Souza RF, et al. American Gastroenterological Association technical review on the management of Barrett's esophagus. Gastroenterology. 2011;140:e18–52; quiz e13.
25. Shaheen NJ, Falk GW, Iyer PG, et al. ACG clinical guideline: diagnosis and management of Barrett's Esophagus. Am J Gastroenterol. 2016;111:30–50; quiz 51.
26. Philpott H, Sweis R. Hiatus hernia as a cause of dysphagia. Curr Gastroenterol Rep. 2017;19:40.
27. Savarino E, Gemignani L, Pohl D, et al. Oesophageal motility and bolus transit abnormalities increase in parallel with the severity of gastro-oesophageal reflux disease. Aliment Pharmacol Ther. 2011;34:476–86.
28. Meneghetti AT, Tedesco P, Damani T, et al. Esophageal mucosal damage may promote dysmotility and worsen esophageal acid exposure. J Gastrointest Surg. 2005;9:1313–7.
29. Ribolsi M, Balestrieri P, Emerenziani S, et al. Weak peristalsis with large breaks is associated with higher acid exposure and delayed reflux clearance in the supine position in GERD patients. Am J Gastroenterol. 2014;109:46–51.
30. Lin S, Ke M, Xu J, et al. Impaired esophageal emptying in reflux disease. Am J Gastroenterol. 1994;89:1003–6.
31. Zhang X, Geboes K, Depoortere I, et al. Effect of repeated cycles of acute esophagitis and healing on esophageal peristalsis, tone, and length. Am J Physiol Gastrointest Liver Physiol. 2005;288:G1339–46.
32. Xu JY, Xie XP, Song GQ, et al. Healing of severe reflux esophagitis with PPI does not improve esophageal dysmotility. Dis Esophagus. 2007;20:346–52.
33. Timmer R, Breumelhof R, Nadorp JH, et al. Oesophageal motility and gastro-oesophageal reflux before and after healing of reflux oesophagitis. A study using 24 hour ambulatory pH and pressure monitoring. Gut. 1994;35:1519–22.

34. Gyawali CP, Roman S, Bredenoord AJ, et al. Classification of esophageal motor findings in gastro-esophageal reflux disease: conclusions from an international consensus group. Neurogastroenterol Motil. 2017;29

35. Shaker A, Stoikes N, Drapekin J, et al. Multiple rapid swallow responses during esophageal high-resolution manometry reflect esophageal body peristaltic reserve. Am J Gastroenterol. 2013;108:1706–12.

36. Stoikes N, Drapekin J, Kushnir V, et al. The value of multiple rapid swallows during preoperative esophageal manometry before laparoscopic antireflux surgery. Surg Endosc. 2012;26: 3401–7.

37. Mello MD, Shriver AR, Li Y, et al. Ineffective esophageal motility phenotypes following fundoplication in gastroesophageal reflux disease. Neurogastroenterol Motil. 2016;28:292–8.

38. Roman S, Lin Z, Kwiatek MA, et al. Weak peristalsis in esophageal pressure topography: classification and association with Dysphagia. Am J Gastroenterol. 2011;106:349–56.

39. Blonski W, Vela M, Safder A, et al. Revised criterion for diagnosis of ineffective esophageal motility is associated with more frequent dysphagia and greater bolus transit abnormalities. Am J Gastroenterol. 2008;103:699–704.

40. Garg SK, Gurusamy KS. Laparoscopic fundoplication surgery versus medical management for gastro-oesophageal reflux disease (GORD) in adults. Cochrane Database Syst Rev. 2015:CD003243.

41. Ganz RA, Edmundowicz SA, Taiganides PA, et al. Long-term outcomes of patients receiving a magnetic sphincter augmentation device for gastroesophageal reflux. Clin Gastroenterol Hepatol. 2016;14:671–7.

42. Ganz RA, Peters JH, Horgan S, et al. Esophageal sphincter device for gastroesophageal reflux disease. N Engl J Med. 2013;368:719–27.

43. Zhu ZJ, Chen LQ, Duranceau A. Long-term result of total versus partial fundoplication after esophagomyotomy for primary esophageal motor disorders. World J Surg. 2008;32:401–7.

44. Strate U, Emmermann A, Fibbe C, et al. Laparoscopic fundoplication: Nissen versus Toupet two-year outcome of a prospective randomized study of 200 patients regarding preoperative esophageal motility. Surg Endosc. 2008;22:21–30.

45. Shaheen NJ, Sharma P, Overholt BF, et al. Radiofrequency ablation in Barrett's esophagus with dysplasia. N Engl J Med. 2009;360:2277–88.

46. Phoa KN, van Vilsteren FG, Weusten BL, et al. Radiofrequency ablation vs endoscopic surveillance for patients with Barrett esophagus and low-grade dysplasia: a randomized clinical trial. JAMA. 2014;311:1209–17.

47. Qumseya BJ, Wani S, Desai M, et al. Adverse events after radiofrequency ablation in patients with Barrett's esophagus: a systematic review and meta-analysis. Clin Gastroenterol Hepatol. 2016;14:1086–95. e6

48. Kim SH, Jeong JB, Kim JW, et al. Clinical and endoscopic characteristics of drug-induced esophagitis. World J Gastroenterol. 2014;20:10994–9.

49. Seminerio J, McGrath K, Arnold CA, et al. Medication-associated lesions of the GI tract. Gastrointest Endosc. 2014;79:140–50.

50. Dellon ES, Hirano I. Epidemiology and natural history of eosinophilic esophagitis. Gastroenterology. 2018;154:319–32. e3

51. Arias A, Perez-Martinez I, Tenias JM, et al. Systematic review with meta-analysis: the incidence and prevalence of eosinophilic oesophagitis in children and adults in population-based studies. Aliment Pharmacol Ther. 2016;43:3–15.

52. Prasad GA, Talley NJ, Romero Y, et al. Prevalence and predictive factors of eosinophilic esophagitis in patients presenting with dysphagia: a prospective study. Am J Gastroenterol. 2007;102:2627–32.

53. Mackenzie SH, Go M, Chadwick B, et al. Eosinophilic oesophagitis in patients presenting with dysphagia--a prospective analysis. Aliment Pharmacol Ther. 2008;28:1140–6.

54. Murray IA, Joyce S, Palmer J, et al. Incidence and features of eosinophilic esophagitis in dysphagia: a prospective observational study. Scand J Gastroenterol. 2016;51:257–62.

55. Dellon ES, Gonsalves N, Hirano I, et al. ACG clinical guideline: evidenced based approach to the diagnosis and management of esophageal eosinophilia and eosinophilic esophagitis (EoE). Am J Gastroenterol. 2013;108:679–92; quiz 693.
56. Dellon ES, Liacouras CA, Molina-Infante J, et al. Updated international consensus diagnostic criteria for eosinophilic esophagitis: proceedings of the AGREE Conference. Gastroenterology. 2018;155:1022–33. e10.
57. Dellon ES, Speck O, Woodward K, et al. Clinical and endoscopic characteristics do not reliably differentiate PPI-responsive esophageal eosinophilia and eosinophilic esophagitis in patients undergoing upper endoscopy: a prospective cohort study. Am J Gastroenterol. 2013;108:1854–60.
58. Patel A, Posner S, Gyawali CP. Esophageal high-resolution manometry in gastroesophageal reflux disease. JAMA. 2018;320:1279–80.
59. Chan WW, Haroian LR, Gyawali CP. Value of preoperative esophageal function studies before laparoscopic antireflux surgery. Surg Endosc. 2011;25:2943–9.
60. Herregods TV, Troelstra M, Weijenborg PW, et al. Patients with refractory reflux symptoms often do not have GERD. Neurogastroenterol Motil. 2015;27:1267–73.
61. Ahuja NK, Clarke JO. Evaluation and management of infectious esophagitis in immunocompromised and immunocompetent individuals. Curr Treat Options Gastroenterol. 2016;14:28–38.
62. Katzka DA, Smyrk TC, Bruce AJ, et al. Variations in presentations of esophageal involvement in lichen planus. Clin Gastroenterol Hepatol. 2010;8:777–82.
63. Gurvits GE. Black esophagus: acute esophageal necrosis syndrome. World J Gastroenterol. 2010;16:3219–25.
64. Gurvits GE, Cherian K, Shami MN, et al. Black esophagus: new insights and multicenter international experience in 2014. Dig Dis Sci. 2015;60:444–53.
65. Mas E, Breton A, Lachaux A. Management of caustic esophagitis in children. Arch Pediatr. 2012;19:1362–8.
66. Uygun I. Caustic oesophagitis in children: prevalence, the corrosive agents involved, and management from primary care through to surgery. Curr Opin Otolaryngol Head Neck Surg. 2015;23:423–32.
67. Bill J, Rajagopal S, Kushnir V, et al. Diagnostic yield in the evaluation of dysphagia: experience at a single tertiary care center. Dis Esophagus. 2018;31
68. Carlson DA, Kahrilas PJ, Lin Z, et al. Evaluation of esophageal motility utilizing the functional lumen imaging probe. Am J Gastroenterol. 2016;111:1726–35.
69. Roman S, Gyawali CP, Savarino E, et al. Ambulatory reflux monitoring for diagnosis of gastroesophageal reflux disease: update of the Porto consensus and recommendations from an international consensus group. Neurogastroenterol Motil. 2017;29
70. Gyawali CP, Bredenoord AJ, Conklin JL, et al. Evaluation of esophageal motor function in clinical practice. Neurogastroenterol Motil. 2013;25:99–133.
71. Kahrilas PJ, Bredenoord AJ, Fox M, et al. Expert consensus document: Advances in the management of oesophageal motility disorders in the era of high-resolution manometry: a focus on achalasia syndromes. Nat Rev Gastroenterol Hepatol. 2017;14:677–88.
72. Patel A, Sayuk GS, Gyawali CP. Parameters on esophageal pH-impedance monitoring that predict outcomes of patients with gastroesophageal reflux disease. Clin Gastroenterol Hepatol. 2015;13:884–91.
73. Patel A, Sayuk GS, Gyawali CP. Prevalence, characteristics, and treatment outcomes of reflux hypersensitivity detected on pH-impedance monitoring. Neurogastroenterol Motil. 2016;28:1382–90.
74. Patel A, Sayuk GS, Kushnir VM, et al. GERD phenotypes from pH-impedance monitoring predict symptomatic outcomes on prospective evaluation. Neurogastroenterol Motil. 2016;28:513–21.
75. Kandulski A, Weigt J, Caro C, et al. Esophageal intraluminal baseline impedance differentiates gastroesophageal reflux disease from functional heartburn. Clin Gastroenterol Hepatol. 2014.

76. Frazzoni M, Savarino E, de Bortoli N, et al. Analyses of the post-reflux swallow-induced peristaltic wave index and nocturnal baseline impedance parameters increase the diagnostic yield of impedance-pH monitoring of patients with reflux disease. Clin Gastroenterol Hepatol. 2016;14:40–6.
77. de Bortoli N, Martinucci I, Savarino E, et al. Association between baseline impedance values and response proton pump inhibitors in patients with heartburn. Clin Gastroenterol Hepatol. 2015;13:1082–8. e1
78. Frazzoni L, Frazzoni M, de Bortoli N, et al. Postreflux swallow-induced peristaltic wave index and nocturnal baseline impedance can link PPI-responsive heartburn to reflux better than acid exposure time. Neurogastroenterol Motil. 2017;29
79. Patel A, Wang D, Sainani N, et al. Distal mean nocturnal baseline impedance on pH-impedance monitoring predicts reflux burden and symptomatic outcome in gastro-oesophageal reflux disease. Aliment Pharmacol Ther. 2016;44:890–8.
80. Savarino E, de Bortoli N, Bellini M, et al. Practice guidelines on the use of esophageal manometry - A GISMAD-SIGE-AIGO medical position statement. Dig Liver Dis. 2016;48:1124–35.
81. Vaezi MF, Pandolfino JE, Vela MF. ACG clinical guideline: diagnosis and management of achalasia. Am J Gastroenterol. 2013;108:1238–49; quiz 1250.
82. Gyawali CP, de Bortoli N, Clarke J, et al. Indications and interpretation of esophageal function testing. Ann N Y Acad Sci. 2018;1434:239–53.
83. Blonski W, Kumar A, Feldman J, et al. Timed barium swallow: diagnostic role and predictive value in untreated achalasia, esophagogastric junction outflow obstruction, and non-achalasia dysphagia. Am J Gastroenterol. 2018;113:196–203.
84. Ghosh SK, Pandolfino JE, Rice J, et al. Impaired deglutitive EGJ relaxation in clinical esophageal manometry: a quantitative analysis of 400 patients and 75 controls. Am J Physiol Gastrointest Liver Physiol. 2007;293:G878–85.
85. Roman S, Huot L, Zerbib F, et al. High-resolution manometry improves the diagnosis of esophageal motility disorders in patients with dysphagia: a randomized multicenter study. Am J Gastroenterol. 2016;111:372–80.
86. Carlson DA, Roman S. Esophageal provocation tests: are they useful to improve diagnostic yield of high resolution manometry? Neurogastroenterol Motil. 2018;30:e13321.
87. Ang D, Hollenstein M, Misselwitz B, et al. Rapid drink challenge in high-resolution manometry: an adjunctive test for detection of esophageal motility disorders. Neurogastroenterol Motil. 2016;
88. Marin I, Serra J. Patterns of esophageal pressure responses to a rapid drink challenge test in patients with esophageal motility disorders. Neurogastroenterol Motil. 2016;28:543–53.
89. Ang D, Misselwitz B, Hollenstein M, et al. Diagnostic yield of high-resolution manometry with a solid test meal for clinically relevant, symptomatic oesophageal motility disorders: serial diagnostic study. Lancet Gastroenterol Hepatol. 2017;2:654–61.
90. Hirano I, Pandolfino JE, Boeckxstaens GE. Functional lumen imaging probe for the management of esophageal disorders: expert review from the Clinical Practice Updates Committee of the AGA Institute. Clin Gastroenterol Hepatol. 2017;15:325–34.
91. Carlson DA, Lin Z, Hirano I, et al. Evaluation of esophageal distensibility in eosinophilic esophagitis: an update and comparison of functional lumen imaging probe analytic methods. Neurogastroenterol Motil. 2016;28:1844–53.
92. Carlson DA, Lin Z, Kahrilas PJ, et al. The functional lumen imaging probe detects esophageal contractility not observed with manometry in patients with achalasia. Gastroenterology. 2015;149(7):1742–51.
93. Gyawali CP, Fass R. Management of gastroesophageal reflux disease. Gastroenterology. 2018;154(2):302–18.
94. Freedberg DE, Kim LS, Yang YX. The risks and benefits of long-term use of proton pump inhibitors: expert review and best practice advice from the American Gastroenterological Association. Gastroenterology. 2017;152:706–15.

95. Chiba N, De Gara CJ, Wilkinson JM, et al. Speed of healing and symptom relief in grade II to IV gastroesophageal reflux disease: a meta-analysis. Gastroenterology. 1997;112:1798–810.
96. Ravich WJ. Endoscopic management of benign esophageal strictures. Curr Gastroenterol Rep. 2017;19:50.
97. Boyce HW Jr. Precepts of safe esophageal dilation. Gastrointest Endosc. 1977;23:215.
98. Grooteman KV, Wong Kee Song LM, Vleggaar FP, et al. Non-adherence to the rule of 3 does not increase the risk of adverse events in esophageal dilation. Gastrointest Endosc. 2017;85:332–7, e1.
99. Ramage JI Jr, Rumalla A, Baron TH, et al. A prospective, randomized, double-blind, placebo-controlled trial of endoscopic steroid injection therapy for recalcitrant esophageal peptic strictures. Am J Gastroenterol. 2005;100:2419–25.
100. Altintas E, Kacar S, Tunc B, et al. Intralesional steroid injection in benign esophageal strictures resistant to bougie dilation. J Gastroenterol Hepatol. 2004;19:1388–91.
101. Fuccio L, Hassan C, Frazzoni L, et al. Clinical outcomes following stent placement in refractory benign esophageal stricture: a systematic review and meta-analysis. Endoscopy. 2016;48:141–8.
102. de Wijkerslooth LR, Vleggaar FP, Siersema PD. Endoscopic management of difficult or recurrent esophageal strictures. Am J Gastroenterol. 2011;106:2080–91; quiz 2092.
103. Smith PM, Kerr GD, Cockel R, et al. A comparison of omeprazole and ranitidine in the prevention of recurrence of benign esophageal stricture. Restore Investigator Group. Gastroenterology. 1994;107:1312–8.
104. Marks RD, Richter JE, Rizzo J, et al. Omeprazole versus H2-receptor antagonists in treating patients with peptic stricture and esophagitis. Gastroenterology. 1994;106:907–15.
105. Galmiche JP, Hatlebakk J, Attwood S, et al. Laparoscopic antireflux surgery vs esomeprazole treatment for chronic GERD: the LOTUS randomized clinical trial. JAMA. 2011;305:1969–77.
106. Mehta S, Bennett J, Mahon D, et al. Prospective trial of laparoscopic nissen fundoplication versus proton pump inhibitor therapy for gastroesophageal reflux disease: seven-year follow-up. J Gastrointest Surg. 2006;10:1312–6; discussion 1316-7.
107. Hasak S, Brunt LM, Wang D, et al. Clinical characteristics and outcomes of patients with postfundoplication dysphagia. Clin Gastroenterol Hepatol. 2019;17(10):1982–90.
108. Dellon ES, Jensen ET, Martin CF, et al. Prevalence of eosinophilic esophagitis in the United States. Clin Gastroenterol Hepatol. 2014;12(4):589–96.e1.
109. Mathieson R, Dutta SK. Candida esophagitis. Dig Dis Sci. 1983;28:365–70.
110. Wilcox CM, Karowe MW. Esophageal infections: etiology, diagnosis, and management. Gastroenterologist. 1994;2:188–206.
111. Hoversten P, Kamboj AK, Wu TT, et al. Variations in the clinical course of patients with herpes simplex virus esophagitis based on immunocompetence and presence of underlying esophageal disease. Dig Dis Sci. 2019;64(7):1893–900.
112. Ramanathan J, Rammouni M, Baran J Jr, et al. Herpes simplex virus esophagitis in the immunocompetent host: an overview. Am J Gastroenterol. 2000;95:2171–6.
113. Ynson ML, Forouhar F, Vaziri H. Case report and review of esophageal lichen planus treated with fluticasone. World J Gastroenterol. 2013;19:1652–6.
114. Chryssostalis A, Gaudric M, Terris B, et al. Esophageal lichen planus: a series of eight cases including a patient with esophageal verrucous carcinoma. A case series. Endoscopy. 2008;40:764–8.
115. Donnellan F, Swan MP, May GR, et al. Fluticasone propionate for treatment of esophageal lichen planus. A case series. Dis Esophagus. 2011;24:211–4.

Chapter 5
Non-Reflux-Mediated Esophageal Strictures

Sajiv Sethi and Joel E. Richter

Introduction

Strictures are a common disease of the esophagus. They may develop from a variety of underlying disease processes such as developmental, inflammatory, neuromuscular, or iatrogenic causes [1]. The development of esophageal inflammation and ulceration results in the deposition of collagen fibers which contracts over time and causes narrowing of the esophageal lumen [2]. Typically, patients with strictures present with the primary symptom of solid food dysphagia. Weight loss is often a characteristic feature of malignant esophageal strictures, while patients with benign strictures usually have a good appetite and do not lose weight unless the esophagus is markedly compromised [3]. Esophageal dilation is indicated for the management of esophageal narrowing. The goal of endoscopic therapy is to allow the patient to eat a solid diet and tolerate liquids. Typically, once a stricture is successfully dilated to 15–18 mm, patients are able to tolerate a solid diet [4]. While patients with a narrowed esophageal lumen are undergoing therapy, it is important to monitor their nutritional status. If unable to tolerate the intake of solid foods, nutrition can be maintained via liquids or percutaneous gastrostomy tube (PEG) feedings. The goal of therapy is to relieve symptoms while avoiding complications and to prevent recurrence.

Esophageal strictures can broadly be classified into benign or malignant types (Fig. 5.1). It is important to note that malignant strictures have an increased rate of perforations regardless of the device or method of dilation used. Benign strictures may

S. Sethi
University of South Florida Division of Digestive Diseases and Nutrition, Tampa, FL, USA

J. E. Richter (✉)
Division of Digestive Diseases and Nutrition, Joy Mccann Culverhouse Center for Swallowing Disorders, Joy Culverhouse Center for Swallowing Disorders, Division of Digestive Diseases and Nutrition, Tampa, FL, USA
e-mail: jrichte1@health.usf.edu

© Springer Nature Switzerland AG 2020
D. A. Patel et al. (eds.), *Evaluation and Management of Dysphagia*,
https://doi.org/10.1007/978-3-030-26554-0_5

Fig. 5.1 Esophageal Stricture Types

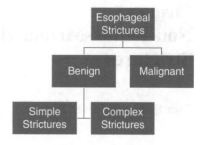

Table 5.1 Common Etiologies of Strictures

Simple Strictures	Complex Strictures
Schatzki Rings	Anastomotic
Esophageal Webs	ESR/EMR
Peptic Strictures	Ischemic
Cricopharyngeal Bar	Zollinger–Ellison Syndrome
Lichen Planus	Nasogastric tube
Eosinophilic Esophagitis	

further be categorized into simple or complex strictures (Table 5.1). Simple strictures are typically short (1–2 cm long), focal, straight strictures that often allow the passage of a normal diameter (9–10 mm) adult endoscope [4]. They result from mucosal and submucosal fibrosis and typically are able to tolerate an increased degree of dilation in a single session [5]. Examples of simple strictures include Schatzki rings, esophageal webs, and peptic strictures [3]. This type of stricture responds well to endoscopic dilation and most patients require 1–3 dilation sessions. A study of simple strictures noted that 95% of patients responded to five dilations or less [5]. Conversely, complex strictures demonstrate a longer (>2 cm) length and are more angulated or irregular with a narrowed diameter (typically <10 mm). They are long standing in duration, have minimal endoscopic inflammation, and demonstrate deep transmural fibrosis. These strictures present a greater therapeutic challenge making them more difficult to treat and more likely to recur. Complex strictures include circular, anastomotic strictures, post-endoscopy strictures, ischemic strictures, and strictures aggravated by nasogastric tube intubation or Zollinger–Ellison syndrome [6].

Device Choice

In general, dilation may be performed with a balloon or bougie dilator. The name bougie derives from French, meaning candle. Bougie dilators are further subdivided into wire-guided and non-wire-guided dilators. Several varieties of wire-guided bougie dilators are available such as Savary-Gilliard (Cook Medical, Winston-Salem, North Carolina, USA) dilators which are made with a radio-opaque band at the widest point of the dilator to provide fluoroscopic guidance, while American Dilatation

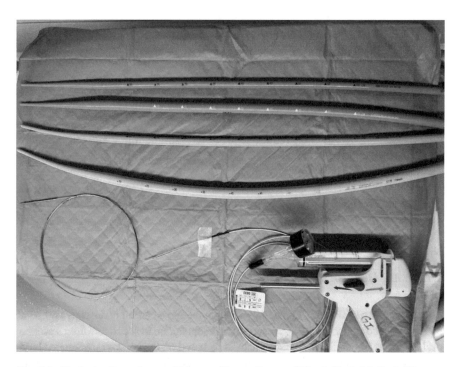

Fig. 5.2 Clockwise from the top: Maloney dilators, Savary–Gilliard (Cook Medical, Winston-Salem, North Carolina, USA) dilators, balloon inflation device with TTS balloon dilator and a guidewire

System (ConMed, Utica, New York, USA) and SafeGuide dilators (Medovations, Milwaukee, USA) are similar but radiopaque (Fig. 5.2). Such push dilators consist of a central channel to accommodate a guidewire and a tapered tip. Using a guidewire with or without fluoroscopic guidance, these bougies are best used for tight and complex strictures. These dilators cost approximately $4000–$5000 per set and come with a 5-year warranty. Across dilators, external markings are present on the dilators however their measurements have an important difference. External markings can be from the tip such as in the American system, or from the point of maximal diameter in the Savary-Gilliard or both (SafeGuide). The Maloney dilators are the most commonly used example of a non-wire-guided bougie. These dilators are weighted with tungsten and are passed blindly. They are best used for larger (>12 mm) simple strictures. Bougie dilation has the distinct advantage of being able to provide a fixed diameter dilation across the entire length of the esophagus which in turn provides a better tactile assessment of lumen narrowing.

An older system of dilators, the Eder-Puestow, a series of graduated metal olives, is now rarely used.

Through-the-scope (TTS) balloon dilators are designed to pass through the endoscope with or without wire guidance which allows real-time visualization of stricture dilation. They are the most commonly used dilators in community practice.

While push dilators generate radial and longitudinal shearing forces, balloon dilators were developed to generate only radial forces within a stricture, as it was believed that this may decrease complications. However, this has not been shown in clinical practice and no difference in outcomes has been seen between wire-guided bougie and balloon dilators [7, 8]. A disadvantage of balloon dilation is that they under-dilate transmural fibrotic strictures. Balloons are adequate for simple strictures; however, they consistently under-dilate transmural fibrotic strictures and are cumbersome and time-consuming because they require repositioning several times with long stricture. One must also consider that balloons are expensive, often costing $125–$175 each in the American marketplace, and not reusable.

Either balloon or wire-guided bougie dilators may be used to perform esophageal dilatation (GRADE of evidence: high; strength of recommendation: strong. Level 1C.

Choosing the Correct Initial Dilator Size

Prior to esophageal dilation, all patients should undergo a careful endoscopy and some patients with complex strictures need a barium esophagram to accurately assess esophageal anatomy. Initial dilator diameter should be based on the known or estimated baseline stricture diameter, length, and the underlying pathology. It is important to consider limiting the initial dilation diameter to 10–12 mm (30–36 Fr) in cases of very narrow strictures not traversed by the adult endoscope [2]. Some authorities and guidelines have recommended a rule of three to guide the number of dilations or size increments per session. This guideline recommends using no more than 3 successively larger diameter dilators in a single session. We shall discuss this further in the next section.

Limit the initial dilation diameter to 10–12 mm for very narrow strictures. GRADE of evidence: very low; strength of recommendation: weak. Level 5

The Rule of Three

The exact origin of the rule of three appears to be unclear. Early reference to this rule was made by one of the pioneers of esophageal dilation Dr. Worth Boyce in 1977 [9, 10]. This guideline recommends the passage of no more than three dilators per session if moderate to severe resistance is encountered. This rule was first proposed in the period of bougie dilator use. Thus, one limitation to this rule is that it requires tactile sensation and as a result may not be applicable in the use of hydrostatic balloon dilators [4]. Over time, this rule has gone from a practical rule to one that is incorporated in recent esophageal guidelines [11].

Recent literature has challenged the "rule of three." A 2017 study of 297 patients undergoing 2216 esophageal bougie or balloon dilations found that nonadherence to the rule of three did not increase the risk of adverse events including esophageal perforation [12]. These results were also confirmed by a separate study of 164 patients with esophageal strictures of various etiologies which found that dilation without adherence to the rule of three was not associated with increased risk of complications [13]. The study found that gender, complex strictures, location of the stricture, type of dilator, and additional interventions were not associated with adverse events. However, malignant strictures were associated with an increased rate of perforation regardless of the device or methods used. Other alternatives such as the "rule of six" have been proposed as well, however, the best approach is a personalized strategy that accounts for each stricture's unique characteristics.

In general, safe dilation takes precedence over fast dilation. Safety is of utmost importance because a perforation in the setting of a complex stricture can result in cicatricial scarring necessitating lifelong dilation or even death. In practical experience, for very tight or very long strictures it may be prudent to limit initial dilation to 1 or 2 size increments only, especially if the endoscopist faces significant resistance. Conversely, in our practice, larger dilation increments can safely be used for less tight strictures.

No more than three dilators should be passed per session. GRADE of evidence: low; strength of recommendation: low. Level 5

Timing of Dilation

The interval between dilations is a subjective approach that must be personalized to each individual patient. The degree of active inflammation versus mature collagen is key to the success of dilation. Inflammatory strictures require frequent dilation until the inflammation resolves, while mature strictures respond well as the collagen is stretched and disrupted. While some simple strictures can be successfully dilated in a single session, other complex strictures may require multiple sessions to ensure a patent esophageal lumen. Depending on the degree of lumen narrowing, some complex strictures may require dilation every few days, but most can be gradually dilated every 2–3 weeks to a planned diameter and patient satisfaction. Repeated dilations can occur on a set schedule or when symptoms recur.

Strictures may be dilated at intervals of days to months depending on their etiology and individual characteristics. GRADE of evidence: low; strength of recommendation: moderate. Level 5

Simple Strictures

Cricopharyngeal Bar

Upper esophageal sphincter (UES) dysfunction can cause oropharyngeal dysphagia. The cricopharyngeus or cricopharyngeal (CP) muscle is the major component of the UES. Approximately 5–10% of patients undergoing dynamic pharyngeal radiography demonstrate a CP bar. They are more common in old patients as muscle tissue is replaced by collagen. This presents as a prominent, persistent, posterior indentation at the level of the lower third of the cricoid cartilage, best visualized in a lateral radiograph [14]. Traditionally, these have been managed with myotomy, however, endoscopic dilation is now the preferred management [15]. A single dilation session with either balloon or bougie dilation can produce long-term symptom relief for some patients, especially those without other causes of oropharyngeal dysphagia [15].

Esophageal dilation is an effective treatment option for cricopharyngeal bar. GRADE of evidence: low; strength of recommendation: moderate. Level 4

Lichen Planus

Lichen planus is a disease affecting the mucus membranes of middle-aged patients, especially women. The most common site of involvement is the mouth, however, other organs such as the skin, vulva, penis, and esophagus can be affected [16, 17]. Etiology of this disease may be related to drug reaction or an autoimmune process [18]. Esophageal involvement presents with symptoms of dysphagia or odynophagia and some patients may have food impactions as well. The esophagus can either be the presenting site or a delayed manifestation of the disease [16]. Strictures can occur across the entire length of the esophagus; however, the proximal esophagus is most often affected. Although data on therapy is sparse, esophageal dilation is an effective treatment option. Other modalities such as systemic and injectional steroids, tacrolimus, and cyclosporin have been tried in limited case reports as well [19]. A hallmark feature consistent across literature is the delayed identification of this disease after onset of symptoms [17].

Esophageal dilation is an effective treatment option for lichen planus. GRADE of evidence: low; strength of recommendation: low. Level 4

Schatzki's Ring

A Schatzki's ring is an annular constriction at the gastro-esophageal mucosal junction, consisting of squamous epithelium on the proximal side and gastric mucosa on the distal aspect [20]. It was described in 1953 by Richard Schatzki on barium swallow and has been found to occur in 6–14% of barium swallow examinations, often in asymptomatic patients [21, 22]. It is a common cause of intermittent dysphagia to solids and may cause food bolus impaction in up to two thirds of patients [23]. Ring diameters of ≤13 mm usually cause dysphagia while diameters greater than 20 mm rarely cause symptoms. In patients with ring diameters between 13 mm and 20 mm, symptoms are less consistently observed. Radiographic examination is superior to endoscopic visualization because the latter is dependent on proper distension of the esophagogastric region beyond the caliber of the ring, which is often difficult to accomplish.

Schatzki's rings often exist with other esophageal disorders, such as hiatal hernias, reflux esophagitis, and esophageal webs [23]. The association between Schatzki's rings and gastroesophageal reflux may explain why patients on long-term acid suppressive therapy have lower rates of ring recurrence after esophageal dilation [24]. A prospective randomized study of 44 patients from Greece with symptomatic Schatzki's rings noted that acid suppression after Schatzki ring dilation prevented relapse of the ring (Fig. 5.3) [24]. While a small study, it demonstrated an absolute risk reduction (ARR) of 40% with acid suppression and a number needed to treat of 3.

While esophageal dilation is the preferred therapy for patients, especially those with symptoms, a small retrospective case series of 9 patients demonstrated improvement in ring lumen diameter and passage of a 13 mm barium tablet in patients treated with oral proton pump inhibitor therapy alone [25]. Dilation therapy for Schatzki's rings is safe and effective. Dilation is directed toward achieving rupture of the ring. In many cases, a single dilation with passage of a large bougie (16–20 mm) with ring rupture is adequate to alleviate symptoms [26].

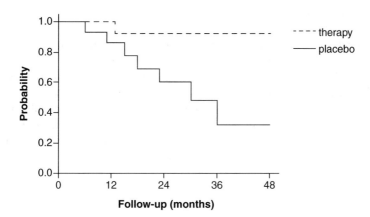

Patients at risk	0	12	24	36	48
Therapy	15	14	11	9	4
Placebo	15	11	7	3	1

Fig. 5.3 Actuarial probability of remaining free from relapse of a Schatzki's ring following successful endoscopic treatment, in terms of prophylactic antisecretory therapy versus placebo. The difference between the two groups was significant (log-rank: 7.07, $p = 0.008$). (Adapted from: Sgouros et al. [24])

An alternative therapeutic option is four quadrant electrosurgical incision of the ring which has similar efficacy as a single large diameter dilation in randomized trials [27]. In this technique, three to four incisions are made radially to the esophageal wall using a standard needle-knife papillotome with a 5 mm cutting wire [28]. Incisions using standard endoscopic submucosal dissection (ESD) needle knife, IT knife, or argon plasma coagulation have also been described [2]. One advantage of electrosurgical incision is that patients have a longer period of symptom-free remission as compared to bougie dilation [28]. Thus, this may be the therapeutic option of choice in patients with recurrent rings [29]. An alternative treatment technique using jumbo biopsy forceps to cause obliteration of Schatzki rings has been shown to be safe and effective in a pilot study of 10 patients. Patients demonstrated improvement in dysphagia without serious complications with a mean follow-up time of 379 days [30].

Do not offer dilatation for incidentally discovered asymptomatic Schatzki's rings (GRADE of evidence: low; strength of recommendation: strong). Level 5

PPI therapy after dilatation is recommended, as this reduces the risk of relapse of Schatzki's ring (GRADE of evidence: moderate; strength of recommendation: strong). Level 1C

Electrosurgical incision is an effective alternative treatment to esophageal dilatation for treatment of Schatzki's rings (GRADE of evidence: high; strength of recommendation: strong). Level 1D

Esophageal Webs

Esophageal webs are thin membranous structures that obstruct the esophageal lumen. These have been classically associated with Plummer–Vinson syndrome (PVS) in which a cervical esophageal web occurs in patients with iron deficiency anemia [31]. However, PVS is rarely seen the western world and most webs are not associated with anemia. Patients with webs typically present with solid food dysphagia. Esophageal dilation with either bougie or balloon dilation can produce favorable results [1]. Esophageal webs typically do not recur after disruption.

Esophageal dilation is an effective treatment of esophageal webs (GRADE of evidence: low; strength of recommendation: low). Level 4

Complex Strictures

Post-Endoscopic Therapy Strictures

Strictures causing esophageal stenosis can occur after endoscopic mucosal ablation, endoscopic mucosal resection (EMR), or endoscopic submucosal dissection (ESD). Esophageal stenosis is known to occur once the mucosal or submucosal resection comprises more than 75% of the esophageal circumference [32–34]. Additionally, longer mucosal defects, especially those longer than 30 mm are associated with greater severity of stenosis requiring increased number of dilations [32]. These strictures respond well to esophageal treatment with either bougie or balloon dilation [35]. Dilation is both safe and effective with a reported success rate of 90% and low perforation rate [36, 37]. Other rare complications of post esophageal resection strictures are bleeding and bacteremia [34]. Rarely, some strictures may not respond to repeated dilation. In these cases, there are reports of successful treatment with esophageal stents or steroid injection [34, 35]. These therapies are discussed in detail under the management of refractory strictures.

All patients undergoing endoscopic resection should be placed on PPI therapy to reduce the risk of stricture formation. A randomized, controlled, open label study from Japan found that prophylactic injection of steroids following extensive ESD did not decrease the frequency of stricture formation but did lead to significantly fewer dilation sessions as compared to the control group [38]. Other studies have also noted that use of oral prednisolone in patients after large EMR or ESD decreases the need for repeat dilations [39, 40].

There exists a high chance of developing symptomatic stricture requiring endoscopic dilatation following EMR or ESD after resection of more than 75% of the esophageal circumference; and a longitudinal resection length of > 30 mm (GRADE of evidence: moderate; strength of recommendation: strong). Level 2

Dilation should be considered for the management of symptomatic post-mucosal resection strictures (GRADE of evidence: moderate; strength of recommendation: strong). Level 2

Post-Ablative Strictures

Photodynamic therapy (PDT) was the first-line therapy for patients with Barrett's esophagus in the 1980s and 1990s before being supplanted by radiofrequency ablation (RFA) as the "gold standard" approach [41]. One of the main drawbacks of PDT was the high rate of stricture formation, approaching 36%. These strictures were typically managed with repeated dilations [42].

RFA is an accepted treatment for patients with dysplastic Barrett's esophagus. It may be used alone or in combination with endoscopic resection [41]. RFA treatment causes the formation of esophageal ulceration which may lead to stricture formation. A distinct advantage of RFA is the ability to ablate to a depth of 500 μm, which is not possible with other ablation techniques. Randomized and database registry data have reported a post-treatment stricture rate of approximately 6–9% [43, 44]. These strictures respond remarkably well to dilation and most patients require between 1 and 2.6 total sessions [44]. Patients who undergo EMR before RFA are more likely to develop strictures then those who did not. The rates of stricture development are higher, as high as 20% in patients who undergo RFA for early squamous cell neoplasia [45]. PPI treatment is known to reduce the risk of stricture formation and thus is recommended for patients undergoing RFA.

There exists a high risk of stricture formation particularly after photodynamic therapy (PDT), EMR before ablation and after RFA for early squamous cell neoplasia (GRADE of evidence: moderate; strength of recommendation: strong). Level 2

PPI therapy should be offered to patients after ablation to reduce stricture occurrence *(GRADE of evidence: low; strength of recommendation: strong). Level 5*

Eosinophilic Esophagitis

Eosinophilic Esophagitis (EoE) was initially thought to be an inflammatory disease of the esophagus associated with mucosal eosinophilia; however, it is now known to cause esophageal strictures, especially in adult patients [46]. Studies have shown that esophageal strictures are present in 30–80% of adults with EoE with their presence and severity directly proportional to the longer duration of disease [46]. We now recognize EoE to have both an inflammatory and fibrostenotic component [47]. The inflammatory portion of the disease may be controlled with PPIs, steroids, and food elimination diet; however, symptoms persist until the fibrostenosis is disrupted by esophageal dilation. Although initially considered dangerous in EoE treatment, esophageal dilation has slowly been recognized as an extremely effective and safe treatment for those with fibrostenotic disease [47]. Patients typically respond very well to esophageal dilation and require a mean number of 2 dilations. Adverse events such as perforation (0.03–0.3%), hemorrhage (0.03–0.05%), and hospitalization for pain (0.6%) are rare complications [48, 49]. The rate of perforation has been found to be similar regardless of TTS balloon or bougie dilator use [49].

All patients should undergo endoscopy to assess the location of obvious strictures and estimate esophageal diameter. Endoscopy has poor sensitivity (14.7%) and only modest specificity (79.2%) for identifying esophageal strictures. Thus, we believe all patients with EoE should undergo some degree of dilation [50]. Endoscopy has a sensitivity of only 25% in detecting an esophagus narrowed to ≤15 mm in diameter [50]. It is recommended to start low with small diameter dilators and gradually dilate to a goal of 16–18 mm at which point patients should be able to tolerate a regular diet [51]. Patients may require multiple sessions which may be separated by 3–4 weeks. Moderate resistance to bougie passage, blood on the dilator, or significant tears are indications to stop the dilation session. Once the patient has been dilated to a goal of 16–18 mm, they may need further dilations if symptoms of dysphagia reoccur. Symptom-free interval may last from 1 to 3 years [51, 52]. Chest pain after dilation is common in EoE patients, with a broad range (0.6–100%) reported irrespective of the technique used [48]. Some patients may require narcotic analgesia; however, most patients easily respond to reassurance and nonsteroidal anti-inflammatory drugs (NSAIDs). It is important to dilate the entire length of the esophagus because multiple strictures may not be obvious to the endoscopist's eye. Both TTS and bougie dilators are acceptable therapeutic options

[53]. If a TTS balloon is used, it must be followed by a pull-through technique to ensure dilation of the entire length of the esophagus [53].

Esophageal dilation should be offered to all patients with EoE, especially those with dysphagia (GRADE of evidence: high; strength of recommendation: strong). Level 1A

Dilatation of EoE is no more dangerous than dilatation for other esophageal diseases, with similar rates of perforation (GRADE of evidence: high; strength of recommendation: strong). Level 2

Esophageal dilation may be repeated as needed. (GRADE of evidence: high; strength of recommendation: strong). Level 2

Dilation of the entire esophagus with a bougie dilator or TTS balloon dilation with pull through is recommended. (GRADE of evidence: high; strength of recommendation: strong). Level 3

Postoperative Strictures

Surgery, especially those with resection and creation of an esophageal anastomosis, has the potential for fibrotic stricture formation. Esophagectomy with esophago-gastrostomy for esophageal or gastric cardiac malignancy can lead to stricturing disease in 4–66% of cases [54, 55]. These strictures typically are short and straight but may occasionally be complicated. Ensuring maximum vascularization of the anastomosis during surgery is important to prevent esophageal anastomotic strictures [2, 56–58]. Anastomotic leaks are frequently complicated by periesophageal inflammation, fibrosis, and difficult to manage strictures. If patients report dysphagia after surgery, investigation with barium swallow and endoscopy is recommended. Dysphagia after fundoplication is typically due to a tight wrap, slipped wrap, or paraesophageal hernia and less likely due to strictures [59, 60].

Postoperative strictures may be successfully treated with either bougie or balloon dilation [61]. Dilation may be performed with or without fluoroscopy since there exists no data to suggest an optimal technique [55, 62]. Patients typically respond well to dilation, with symptom improvement after the first session and require a median of four sessions. Treatment success can be seen between 62% and 100% of patients [54, 61]. Delayed gastric emptying may be a risk factor for stricture formation. Pyloroplasty or pyloromyotomy can help reduce the frequency of dilations required to treat anastomotic strictures [63]. The results of steroid injections in these papers are controversial. In a Dutch study of 60 patients, steroid injection before bougie dilation did not show a statistically significant decrease in the frequency of dilations or number of dilations. Additionally, injection of steroids led to an increase in the number of complications, especially esophageal candidiasis [64]. More recently, a Japanese study examined intralesional triamcinolone injection compared to placebo for the balloon dilation of anastomotic strictures after esophagectomy. The authors randomized 65 patients and noted patients in

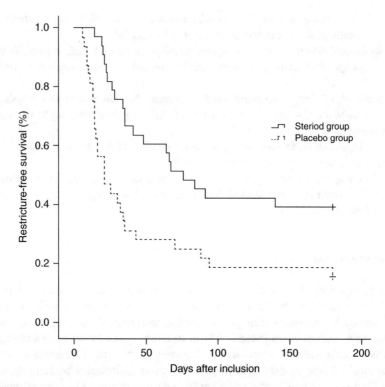

Fig. 5.4 Comparison of restricture-free survival in the steroid group and placebo group. During the 6-month follow-up, the restricture-free survival rate in the steroid group was significantly better than that in the placebo group (39.4 vs. 15.6%, respectively; $p = 0.002$). (Adapted from: Hanaoka et al. [65])

the steroid group required fewer dilations and had a longer recurrence-free interval (Fig. 5.4) [65]. Needle knife incision has been studied as primary therapy; however, it was not shown to have any advantage over bougie dilation in the overall success rate or mean number of dilations required. Complication rates for the treatment of postoperative strictures have been reported around 30%, however, frank perforation during dilation appears to be no more common than other types of strictures [62].

In patients with dysphagia after surgery, consider performing upper GI endoscopy and barium swallow first. (GRADE of evidence: moderate; strength of recommendation: strong). Level 3

Consider treatment of concurrent delayed gastric emptying in order to reduce the need for redilatations. (GRADE of evidence: low; strength of recommendation: weak). Level 4

Steroids as an adjunct therapy may decrease the number of dilations required and improve disease-free interval. (GRADE of evidence: moderate; strength of recommendation: strong). Level 1D

Radiation-Induced Strictures

Radiation therapy is an increasingly used therapeutic modality for the treatment of various malignancies. It is well known to cause stricturing of the esophagus. Radiation leads to tissue ischemia, fibrosis, and subsequent development of stenosis. The fibrosis seen in this disease leads to the development of a non-compliant mediastinum, resulting in the formation of refractory and progressive strictures [2]. The risk of stricture formation is dependent on the tumor invasion, T score, and degree of circumferential tumor involvement [66]. The risk of stricture formation is increased with a higher dose of radiation or concurrent chemoradiation administration [67–70]. Occasionally, patients can develop complete or nearly complete esophageal obstruction [71, 72]. Stricture formation can occur early in treatment course due to inflammation and true fibrous scarring evolved over many years.

Esophageal dilation is a successful and safe therapeutic option for these patients [68]. Successful dilation is achieved in up to 95% of patients [73]. The complication rate for dilation of radiation strictures has been reported around 9% for all events and 4% for frank perforation [73]. Successful dilation and luminal restoration can be achieved via an anterograde or retrograde approach [72, 74]. Placement of a gastrostomy tube should be considered in all patients to aid nutrition. Gastrostomy tubes offer an alternative channel for retrograde dilation in patients where anterograde guidewire placement is unsuccessful [72]. A combined anterograde retrograde dilation (CARD) approach has been shown to be successful as well. Although this technique may decrease the need for invasive surgery, it does carry a risk of esophageal perforation [75]. An anterograde endoscope is inserted and advanced to the proximal portion of the stricture. A second endoscope is then inserted through the gastrostomy site and transillumination of the stricture is performed in order to identify the obstructed lumen. A guidewire may be passed from the distal esophagus proximally under fluoroscopic guidance. The wire may puncture through the obstructed lumen and is retrieved per oral [75, 76]. A needle knife, straight catheter, or an EUS fine aspiration needle may be used to traverse this stricture as well [77]. Upon successful guidewire passage, bougie or balloon can be used to dilate the stricture. Repeat dilations through this method can be performed as well. In some patients, placement off a metal stent may help to maintain esophageal lumen patency [78].

A combined anterograde and retrograde dilatation (CARD) may be used as an alternative to surgery. (*GRADE of evidence: moderate; strength of recommendation: weak*). Level 3

A guidewire may be used to navigate the esophageal lumen for severe strictures. (*GRADE of evidence: low; strength of recommendation: strong*). Level 4

After gaining luminal patency using the CARD procedure, perform subsequent dilatation using either balloon or bougie dilation (*GRADE of evidence: moderate; strength of recommendation: strong*). Level 4

Caustic Strictures

Ingestion of a caustic substance can lead to stricture formation. In Western countries, alkaline materials account for most caustic ingestions, whereas in developing countries, acid ingestion is more common [79]. Acid ingestion causes coagulation necrosis with eschar formation which may limit substance penetration and injury depth. Alkaline materials combine with tissue proteins causing liquefactive necrosis and saponification. They penetrate deeper into tissues and are helped by their higher viscosity and longer duration of esophageal wall contact. Alkali agents may be absorbed into blood vessels leading to thrombosis and decreased blood supply to already damaged tissue [79, 80]. Thus, alkaline ingestion is typically associated with more serious injury; however, ingestion of strong acids can also lead to rapid full thickness esophageal injury. Strong acid indigestion is more frequently associated with systemic complications such as renal failure, liver dysfunction, disseminated intravascular coagulation, and hemolysis [80].

Evaluation with a CT scan can offer information about the depth of esophageal wall involvement, extent of necrosis, and stomach perforation [81]. After radiographic assessment is complete, an upper endoscopy with gentle air insufflation or preferably with CO_2 should be considered within the first 96 hours of caustic ingestion. Endoscopy is performed to determine the degree of injury, prognosis, management, stricture formation, and need for dilation [82]. Contraindications to endoscopy include radiographic concern for perforation and burns to the supraglottic and epiglottic areas [83]. Caution is recommended in patients with frank necrosis of the esophagus or complete obliteration of the esophageal lumen due to massive edema [82]. A CT grading system for caustic lesions has been proposed; however, limited clinical data has restricted its widespread use [81]. Increased maximum esophageal wall thickness, as seen on CT scan, has been associated with a higher number of sessions required for adequate dilation [84]. Caustic ingestion leads to impairment of the lower esophageal sphincter pressure producing increased gastroesophageal reflux which may further incite stricture formation [85]. Oral steroids, antibiotics, mitomycin C, and stent placement have been studied to prevent stricture formation; however, data on their efficacy remains limited [86–88].

Dilation may be performed with balloon or bougie dilators. In the acute early setting, esophageal rupture has been reported in as high as 31% of balloon dilation cases. Balloon inflation has the potential to cause mechanical compression of the trachea or obstruction at the endotracheal tube tip [89, 90]. The choice of therapy is mostly dependent on physician preference [91–93]. Overall complication rate for dilation of caustic strictures is higher than other types of benign strictures being reported between 0.47% and 32% [92]. The timing of dilation is important as late management has been associated with esophageal wall fibrosis and collagen deposition [94]. Between 1 and 3 weeks after injury, dilation is most hazardous, and some avoid this time interval. After week 3, scar retraction and stricture formation begin. The initial interval between dilation sections should be short, less than 2–3 weeks. Patients typically require 3–4 sessions, however some may require a significantly higher number of dilations [79, 95]. Delayed presentation and treatment may affect outcomes and the success of dilation. Those admitted with significant delay after injury have been found to have most severe recurrent strictures [95, 96]. If esophageal dilation fails, surgical therapy must be considered [96].

Perform upper gastrointestinal tract endoscopy within the first 96 hours after caustic ingestion. *(GRADE of evidence: moderate; strength of recommendation: strong)*. Level 4

Consider avoiding dilatation within 3 weeks of initial caustic ingestion *(GRADE of evidence: low; strength of recommendation: weak)*. Level 4

Consider a time interval between dilatations of <2 weeks *(GRADE of evidence: very low; strength of recommendation: weak)*. Level 5

Nasogastric Tube Strictures

The long-term placement of nasogastric tubes (NGT) has been implicated as an iatrogenic cause of esophageal strictures [97]. Such patients typically have NGTs placed for weeks to months. This is followed by the development of dysphagia due to an underlying stricture. The development of a stricture in such patients is typically multifactorial secondary to mucosal trauma from longstanding NGT use, induced gastroesophageal reflux, impaired esophageal clearance, high gastric acid output, and use of steroids [98]. These strictures may be treated with balloon or bougie dilation [99]. Depending on the degree of esophageal lumen narrowing, patients may require multiple dilations to achieve sustained esophageal lumen patency [99].

Strictures secondary to NG tube placement may be treated with balloon or bougie dilation (GRADE of evidence: very low; strength of recommendation: weak). Level 4

Refractory Strictures

The Kochman criteria defines refractory or recurrent strictures as those with an anatomic restriction due to a cicatricial luminal compromise or fibrosis resulting in clinical symptoms of dysphagia in the absence of endoscopic evidence of inflammation [6]. Refractory strictures are those without resolution of an anatomic problem to a diameter of at least 14 mm over 5 sessions at 2-week intervals. Recurrent strictures are the result of an inability to maintain a satisfactory luminal diameter for 4 weeks once the target diameter of 14 mm has been achieved. This definition does not apply to inflammatory strictures which require treatment of the underlying inflammation and those patients having dysphagia due to neuromuscular dysfunction [6, 100]. Complex strictures, those >2 centimeters, angulated, irregular, severely narrowed diameter, are difficult to treat and are more likely to be refractory despite therapy [3]. Bougie or balloon dilators with or without fluoroscopy may be used for dilation of refractory strictures. Many adjunctive therapies have been studied for the management of refractory strictures.

Steroid injection combined with balloon dilation has been studied to prevent stricture recurrence. It was initially described in 1966 showing promise in the treatment of peptic strictures [101]. This technique involves injection of 0.5 mL aliquots of 40 mg/mL triamcinolone to all four quadrants of the stricture. There is debate regarding the injection of steroids before or after dilation. Most experts recommend pre-dilation before steroid injection for maximal tissue penetration and efficacy; however, there exist no studies comparing both techniques against each other. In our practice, we prefer to inject steroids after dilation. In studies of peptic strictures, injection of a steroid into the stricture combined with acid suppression was found to decrease the need for repeat dilation and increase the interval between dilations [102]. In a smaller study of corrosive strictures, patients were allocated to steroid injection versus placebo groups. There was no difference in the dilation frequency or recurrent dysphagia between the groups [103]. In a cohort of patients with anastomotic strictures after esophagectomy, patients who underwent steroid injection in addition to dilation did not have a decrease in the frequency or interval of dilations compared to dilation therapy alone [64]. In this study, patients were also noted to have an increased number of complications, primarily candida esophagitis, in the steroid injection group. A newer Japanese randomized controlled trial, however, reported different results. A total of 65 patients undergoing endoscopic balloon dilation were randomized into steroid or placebo group. Patients in the steroid injection had a longer stricture recurrence-free interval [65].

Incisional therapy using a needle or IT knife was first reported in the treatment of Schatzki rings [104]. In this procedure, performed under direct visualization with or without a transparent cap, radial incisions of refractory strictures parallel to the longitudinal axis of the esophagus are made [105]. Incisional therapy has been found to be most efficacious for short strictures. In head-to-head studies, no significant difference was found between incisional and dilation therapy [106]. Since no complications were observed with incisional therapy either, it may be considered as an alternative treatment option.

Temporary stent placement has been increasingly used for refractory esophageal strictures. At the time of this writing, self-expandable plastic stents are FDA approved for this indication [107]. Fully covered self-expandable metal stents, although not FDA approved, are used to treat benign strictures as well [108]. Unlike metal and plastic stents, biodegradable stents have the distinct advantage of not requiring removal [109]. In a meta-analysis of 18 studies of patients who underwent stent placement, 40% of patients reported complete relief of dysphagia [110]. Stent migration rate was reported at 29%. The majority of patients respond to stent placement for 4–8 weeks, although in some patients stents were placed for as long as 3 months [110]. Long-term stent placement can lead to tissue growth around the stent causing it to become embedded in the esophageal wall. Up to 70% of patients develop stricture recurrence after stent removal, particularly in patients with strictures >7 cm [111].

In comparison to plastic stents, metal stents have lower migration rates and decreased need for re-intervention [112]. Complications of stent placement include tissue ingrowth and new stricture formation, pain, stent migration, pain, fistula formation, and gastroesophageal reflux [113]. Partially covered or uncovered metal stents have a risk of embedding into the esophageal wall and, thus, should be avoided.

Placement of a single biodegradable metal stent offers only temporary relief of symptoms [109, 114]. However, sequential placement of a first, second, and then third biodegradable stent resulted in a mean dysphagia-free period of 90, 55, and 106 days, respectively [114]. Dysphagia recurred in all patients suggesting that biodegradable stents are not an effective long-term solution.

Overall, the management of refractory benign esophageal strictures (RBES) can be a challenge. A multicenter study of 70 patients with RBES over a 15-year period noted that patients underwent a median of 15.5 dilation sessions per patient. Authors noted RBES resolution in only 31.4% of patients with a mean dysphagia-free period of 3.3 months for patients treated with dilation and 2.4 months for patients treated with stent placement [115] (Fig. 5.5).

In patients with short, proximal strictures, self-dilation is a safe an effective therapeutic option [116]. This may be performed in the presence of a physician or, in the case of a well-trained patient, at home. This technique, in which patients learn to pass a polyvinyl dilator orally on a routine basis, has been used since at least the 1970s [117]. In patients requiring frequent dilations this may reduce the burden of hospitalization and surgery [118]. A retrospective review of 52 patients from the Mayo clinic who were treated with self-dilation reported decreased need for endoscopic procedures, increased intervention-free interval, and improvement of dysphagia scores after self-dilation. Furthermore, 85% of their patients who received enteral nutrition prior to self-dilation had their feeding tubes removed [117]. The median number of endoscopic interventions was reduced from 9.5 to 0 within 12 months before and after self-dilation, respectively. Patients undergoing self-dilation increased interval time between endoscopic interventions to approximately 417 days. These results are supported by a Dutch study of patients with refractory post-surgical and caustic strictures

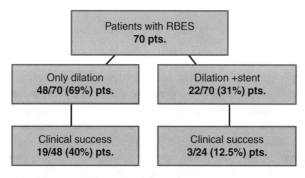

Fig. 5.5 Clinical outcome of patients with refractory benign esophageal strictures according to endoscopic therapy. RBES, refractory benign esophageal stricture; OR odds ratio, CI confidence interval. (Adapted from: Repici et al. [115])

undergoing self-dilation which noted a decrease in the number of endoscopic dilation procedures in a 9 month period from 17 to 1.5. They were able to teach 16 of 17 total patients self-dilation and all 16 patients were able to tolerate solid food at the end of the study [119].

Mitomycin C is a chemotherapeutic agent which has antifibrotic properties for the treatment of refractory strictures. A study of 74 patients with anastomotic or post-endoscopic mucosal dissection (ESD) strictures divided patients into three groups (intralesional mitomycin C with dilation, intralesional dexamethasone with dilation, or normal saline plus dilation alone). The study found that intramuscular injection of mitomycin C or dexamethasone increased the duration of symptom relief compared with dilation alone [120]. Another prospective study compared mitomycin C to intralesional triamcinolone injection and found that mitomycin C reduced the number of dilations required [121]. Patients who do not respond to all measures should be considered for surgery [122].

Intralesional steroid injection combined with dilatation should be considered for refractory strictures with evidence of inflammation (GRADE of evidence: high; strength of recommendation: strong). Level 1A

Consider incisional therapy in patients with refractory Schatzki's rings and anastomotic strictures (GRADE of evidence: very low; strength of recommendation: weak). Level 4

Temporary placement of fully covered self-expanding removable stents should be considered in patients who have failed other methods of therapy (GRADE of evidence: high; strength of recommendation: weak). Level 1C

The optimum duration of stent placement is usually between 4 and 8 weeks but individual factors such as stricture anatomy and type of stent must be accounted (GRADE of evidence: very low; strength of recommendation: weak). Level 4

A select group of patients who are self-directed and have short strictures can be candidates for self-dilation. (GRADE of evidence: very low; strength of recommendation: weak). Level 4

Conclusion

In conclusion, esophageal strictures are a common clinical entity. Strictures can occur due to various etiologies giving rise to either complex or simple strictures. While a variety of endoscopic therapies exist, esophageal dilation is the mainstay of treatment in these patients. Currently, the majority of data is limited to retrospective studies. There exists a paucity of prospective and randomized studies comparing different techniques and outcomes. Several options for dilation exist and careful selection of the type of dilator and technique is important. The choice of therapy must be individualized for each patient and based on underlying etiology and anatomy of the stricture. Overall, esophageal dilation is a safe and effective therapeutic modality. Future research should focus on complex and refractory strictures with randomized studies comparing different modalities.

References

1. Ravich WJ. Endoscopic management of benign esophageal strictures. Curr Gastroenterol Rep. 2017;19(10):50.
2. Sami SS, Haboubi HN, Ang Y, et al. UK guidelines on oesophageal dilatation in clinical practice. Gut. 2018;67(6):1000–23.
3. van Boeckel PG, Siersema PD. Refractory esophageal strictures: what to do when dilation fails. Curr Treat Options Gastroenterol. 2015;13(1):47–58.
4. Richter JE. Rule of three for esophageal dilation: like the tortoise versus the rabbit, low and slow is our friend and our patients' win. Gastrointest Endosc. 2017;85(2):338–9.
5. Pereira-Lima JC, Ramires RP, Zamin I Jr, Cassal AP, Marroni CA, Mattos AA. Endoscopic dilation of benign esophageal strictures: report on 1043 procedures. Am J Gastroenterol. 1999;94(6):1497–501.
6. Kochman ML, McClave SA, Boyce HW. The refractory and the recurrent esophageal stricture: a definition. Gastrointest Endosc. 2005;62(3):474–5.
7. Saeed ZA, Winchester CB, Ferro PS, Michaletz PA, Schwartz JT, Graham DY. Prospective randomized comparison of polyvinyl bougies and through-the-scope balloons for dilation of peptic strictures of the esophagus. Gastrointest Endosc. 1995;41(3):189–95.
8. Scolapio JS, Pasha TM, Gostout CJ, et al. A randomized prospective study comparing rigid to balloon dilators for benign esophageal strictures and rings. Gastrointest Endosc. 1999;50(1):13–7.
9. Boyce HW Jr. Precepts of safe esophageal dilation. Gastrointest Endosc. 1977;23(4):215.
10. Tulman AB, Boyce HW Jr. Complications of esophageal dilation and guidelines for their prevention. Gastrointest Endosc. 1981;27(4):229–34.
11. Standards of Practice C, Egan JV, Baron TH, et al. Esophageal dilation. Gastrointest Endosc. 2006;63(6):755–60.
12. Grooteman KV, Wong Kee Song LM, Vleggaar FP, Siersema PD, Baron TH. Non-adherence to the rule of 3 does not increase the risk of adverse events in esophageal dilation. Gastrointest Endosc. 2017;85(2):332–7. e331.
13. Benites Goni HE, Arcana Lopez R, Bustamante Robles KY, et al. Factors associated with complications during endoscopic esophageal dilation. Rev Esp Enferm Dig. 2018;110(7):440–5.
14. Williams RB, Grehan MJ, Hersch M, Andre J, Cook IJ. Biomechanics, diagnosis, and treatment outcome in inflammatory myopathy presenting as oropharyngeal dysphagia. Gut. 2003;52(4):471–8.
15. Wang AY, Kadkade R, Kahrilas PJ, Hirano I. Effectiveness of esophageal dilation for symptomatic cricopharyngeal bar. Gastrointest Endosc. 2005;61(1):148–52.
16. Katzka DA, Smyrk TC, Bruce AJ, Romero Y, Alexander JA, Murray JA. Variations in presentations of esophageal involvement in lichen planus. Clin Gastroenterol Hepatol. 2010;8(9):777–82.
17. Fox LP, Lightdale CJ, Grossman ME. Lichen planus of the esophagus: what dermatologists need to know. J Am Acad Dermatol. 2011;65(1):175–83.
18. Eisen D. The clinical features, malignant potential, and systemic associations of oral lichen planus: a study of 723 patients. J Am Acad Dermatol. 2002;46(2):207–14.
19. Rao B, Gulati A, Jobe B, Thakkar S. Esophageal lichen planus: understanding a potentially severe stricturing disease. Case Rep Gastrointest Med. 2017;2017:5480562.
20. Goyal RK, Bauer JL, Spiro HM. The nature and location of lower esophageal ring. N Engl J Med. 1971;284(21):1175–80.
21. Kramer P. Frequency of the asymptomatic lower esophageal contractile ring. N Engl J Med. 1956;254(15):692–4.
22. Patel B, Han E, Swan K. Richard Schatzki: a familiar ring. AJR Am J Roentgenol. 2013;201(5):W678–82.
23. Muller M, Gockel I, Hedwig P, et al. Is the Schatzki ring a unique esophageal entity? World J Gastroenterol. 2011;17(23):2838–43.

24. Sgouros SN, Vlachogiannakos J, Karamanolis G, et al. Long-term acid suppressive therapy may prevent the relapse of lower esophageal (Schatzki's) rings: a prospective, randomized, placebo-controlled study. Am J Gastroenterol. 2005;100(9):1929–34.
25. Novak SH, Shortsleeve MJ, Kantrowitz PA. Effective treatment of symptomatic lower esophageal (Schatzki) rings with acid suppression therapy: confirmed on barium esophagography. AJR Am J Roentgenol. 2015;205(6):1182–7.
26. Eckardt VF, Kanzler G, Willems D. Single dilation of symptomatic Schatzki rings. A prospective evaluation of its effectiveness. Dig Dis Sci. 1992;37(4):577–82.
27. Ibrahim A, Cole RA, Qureshi WA, et al. Schatzki's ring: to cut or break an unresolved problem. Dig Dis Sci. 2004;49(3):379–83.
28. Wills JC, Hilden K, Disario JA, Fang JC. A randomized, prospective trial of electrosurgical incision followed by rabeprazole versus bougie dilation followed by rabeprazole of symptomatic esophageal (Schatzki's) rings. Gastrointest Endosc. 2008;67(6):808–13.
29. DiSario JA, Pedersen PJ, Bichis-Canoutas C, Alder SC, Fang JC. Incision of recurrent distal esophageal (Schatzki) ring after dilation. Gastrointest Endosc. 2002;56(2):244–8.
30. Gonzalez A, Sullivan MF, Bonder A, Allison HV, Bonis PA, Guelrud M. Obliteration of symptomatic Schatzki rings with jumbo biopsy forceps (with video). Dis Esophagus. 2014;27(7):607–10.
31. Hirose T, Funasaka K, Furukawa K, et al. A case of Plummer-Vinson syndrome with esophageal web formation in which detailed endoscopic images were obtained. Intern Med. 2019; 58:785–9.
32. Katada C, Muto M, Manabe T, Boku N, Ohtsu A, Yoshida S. Esophageal stenosis after endoscopic mucosal resection of superficial esophageal lesions. Gastrointest Endosc. 2003;57(2):165–9.
33. Mizuta H, Nishimori I, Kuratani Y, Higashidani Y, Kohsaki T, Onishi S. Predictive factors for esophageal stenosis after endoscopic submucosal dissection for superficial esophageal cancer. Dis Esophagus. 2009;22(7):626–31.
34. Isomoto H, Yamaguchi N, Minami H, Nakao K. Management of complications associated with endoscopic submucosal dissection/endoscopic mucosal resection for esophageal cancer. Dig Endosc. 2013;25(Suppl 1):29–38.
35. Pouw RE, Seewald S, Gondrie JJ, et al. Stepwise radical endoscopic resection for eradication of Barrett's oesophagus with early neoplasia in a cohort of 169 patients. Gut. 2010;59(9):1169–77.
36. Takahashi H, Arimura Y, Okahara S, et al. Risk of perforation during dilation for esophageal strictures after endoscopic resection in patients with early squamous cell carcinoma. Endoscopy. 2011;43(3):184–9.
37. Yoda Y, Yano T, Kaneko K, et al. Endoscopic balloon dilatation for benign fibrotic strictures after curative nonsurgical treatment for esophageal cancer. Surg Endosc. 2012;26(10):2877–83.
38. Takahashi H, Arimura Y, Okahara S, et al. A randomized controlled trial of endoscopic steroid injection for prophylaxis of esophageal stenoses after extensive endoscopic submucosal dissection. BMC Gastroenterol. 2015;15:1.
39. Sato H, Inoue H, Kobayashi Y, et al. Control of severe strictures after circumferential endoscopic submucosal dissection for esophageal carcinoma: oral steroid therapy with balloon dilation or balloon dilation alone. Gastrointest Endosc. 2013;78(2):250–7.
40. Yamaguchi N, Isomoto H, Shikuwa S, et al. Effect of oral prednisolone on esophageal stricture after complete circular endoscopic submucosal dissection for superficial esophageal squamous cell carcinoma: a case report. Digestion. 2011;83(4):291–5.
41. Shaheen NJ, Falk GW, Iyer PG, Gerson LB, American College of G. ACG clinical guideline: diagnosis and management of Barrett's esophagus. Am J Gastroenterol. 2016;111(1):30–50; quiz 51.
42. Overholt BF, Lightdale CJ, Wang KK, et al. Photodynamic therapy with porfimer sodium for ablation of high-grade dysplasia in Barrett's esophagus: international, partially blinded, randomized phase III trial. Gastrointest Endosc. 2005;62(4):488–98.
43. Shaheen NJ, Sharma P, Overholt BF, et al. Radiofrequency ablation in Barrett's esophagus with dysplasia. N Engl J Med. 2009;360(22):2277–88.

44. Haidry RJ, Dunn JM, Butt MA, et al. Radiofrequency ablation and endoscopic mucosal resection for dysplastic barrett's esophagus and early esophageal adenocarcinoma: outcomes of the UK National Halo RFA registry. Gastroenterology. 2013;145(1):87–95.
45. Haidry RJ, Butt MA, Dunn J, et al. Radiofrequency ablation for early oesophageal squamous neoplasia: outcomes form United Kingdom registry. World J Gastroenterol. 2013;19(36):6011–9.
46. Richter JE. Esophageal dilation in eosinophilic esophagitis. Best Pract Res Clin Gastroenterol. 2015;29(5):815–28.
47. Richter JE. Endoscopic treatment of eosinophilic esophagitis. Gastrointest Endosc Clin N Am. 2018;28(1):97–110.
48. Moawad FJ, Molina-Infante J, Lucendo AJ, Cantrell SE, Tmanova L, Douglas KM. Systematic review with meta-analysis: endoscopic dilation is highly effective and safe in children and adults with eosinophilic oesophagitis. Aliment Pharmacol Ther. 2017;46(2):96–105.
49. Dougherty M, Runge TM, Eluri S, Dellon ES. Esophageal dilation with either bougie or balloon technique as a treatment for eosinophilic esophagitis: a systematic review and meta-analysis. Gastrointest Endosc. 2017;86(4):581–91. e583.
50. Gentile N, Katzka D, Ravi K, et al. Oesophageal narrowing is common and frequently underappreciated at endoscopy in patients with oesophageal eosinophilia. Aliment Pharmacol Ther. 2014;40(11–12):1333–40.
51. Richter JE. Esophageal dilation for eosinophilic esophagitis: it's safe! Why aren't we doing more dilations? Gastrointest Endosc. 2017;86(4):592–4.
52. Lee GS, Craig PI, Freiman JS, de Carle D, Cook IJ. Intermittent dysphagia for solids associated with a multiringed esophagus: clinical features and response to dilatation. Dysphagia. 2007;22(1):55–62.
53. Madanick RD, Shaheen NJ, Dellon ES. A novel balloon pull-through technique for esophageal dilation in eosinophilic esophagitis (with video). Gastrointest Endosc. 2011;73(1):138–42.
54. Fukagawa T, Gotoda T, Oda I, et al. Stenosis of esophago-jejuno anastomosis after gastric surgery. World J Surg. 2010;34(8):1859–63.
55. Williams VA, Watson TJ, Zhovtis S, et al. Endoscopic and symptomatic assessment of anastomotic strictures following esophagectomy and cervical esophagogastrostomy. Surg Endosc. 2008;22(6):1470–6.
56. Honkoop P, Siersema PD, Tilanus HW, Stassen LP, Hop WC, van Blankenstein M. Benign anastomotic strictures after transhiatal esophagectomy and cervical esophagogastrostomy: risk factors and management. J Thorac Cardiovasc Surg. 1996;111(6):1141–6; discussion 1147-1148.
57. Pierie JP, de Graaf PW, Poen H, van der Tweel I, Obertop H. Incidence and management of benign anastomotic stricture after cervical oesophagogastrostomy. Br J Surg. 1993;80(4): 471–4.
58. Briel JW, Tamhankar AP, Hagen JA, et al. Prevalence and risk factors for ischemia, leak, and stricture of esophageal anastomosis: gastric pull-up versus colon interposition. J Am Coll Surg. 2004;198(4):536–41; discussion 541-532.
59. Hui JM, Hunt DR, de Carle DJ, Williams R, Cook IJ. Esophageal pneumatic dilation for postfundoplication dysphagia: safety, efficacy, and predictors of outcome. Am J Gastroenterol. 2002;97(12):2986–91.
60. Pessaux P, Arnaud JP, Delattre JF, Meyer C, Baulieux J, Mosnier H. Laparoscopic antireflux surgery: five-year results and beyond in 1340 patients. Arch Surg. 2005;140(10):946–51.
61. Marjanovic G, Schrag HJ, Fischer E, Hopt UT, Fischer A. Endoscopic bougienage of benign anastomotic strictures in patients after esophageal resection: the effect of the extent of stricture on bougienage results. Dis Esophagus. 2008;21(6):551–7.
62. Lee J, Song HY, Ko HK, et al. Fluoroscopically guided balloon dilation or temporary stent placement for patients with gastric conduit strictures after esophagectomy with esophagogastrostomy. AJR Am J Roentgenol. 2013;201(1):202–7.

63. Sutcliffe RP, Forshaw MJ, Tandon R, et al. Anastomotic strictures and delayed gastric emptying after esophagectomy: incidence, risk factors and management. Dis Esophagus. 2008;21(8):712–7.
64. Hirdes MM, van Hooft JE, Koornstra JJ, et al. Endoscopic corticosteroid injections do not reduce dysphagia after endoscopic dilation therapy in patients with benign esophagogastric anastomotic strictures. Clin Gastroenterol Hepatol. 2013;11(7):795–801. e791.
65. Hanaoka N, Ishihara R, Motoori M, et al. Endoscopic balloon dilation followed by intralesional steroid injection for anastomotic strictures after esophagectomy: a randomized controlled trial. Am J Gastroenterol. 2018;113(10):1468–74.
66. Atsumi K, Shioyama Y, Nakamura K, et al. Predictive factors of esophageal stenosis associated with tumor regression in radiation therapy for locally advanced esophageal cancer. J Radiat Res. 2010;51(1):9–14.
67. Alevronta E, Ahlberg A, Mavroidis P, et al. Dose-response relations for stricture in the proximal oesophagus from head and neck radiotherapy. Radiother Oncol. 2010;97(1):54–9.
68. Caudell JJ, Schaner PE, Desmond RA, Meredith RF, Spencer SA, Bonner JA. Dosimetric factors associated with long-term dysphagia after definitive radiotherapy for squamous cell carcinoma of the head and neck. Int J Radiat Oncol Biol Phys. 2010;76(2):403–9.
69. Tuna Y, Kocak E, Dincer D, Koklu S. Factors affecting the success of endoscopic bougia dilatation of radiation-induced esophageal stricture. Dig Dis Sci. 2012;57(2):424–8.
70. Caudell JJ, Schaner PE, Meredith RF, et al. Factors associated with long-term dysphagia after definitive radiotherapy for locally advanced head-and-neck cancer. Int J Radiat Oncol Biol Phys. 2009;73(2):410–5.
71. Francis DO, Hall E, Dang JH, Vlacich GR, Netterville JL, Vaezi MF. Outcomes of serial dilation for high-grade radiation-related esophageal strictures in head and neck cancer patients. Laryngoscope. 2015;125(4):856–62.
72. Boyce HW, Estores DS, Gaziano J, Padhya T, Runk J. Endoscopic lumen restoration for obstructive aphagia: outcomes of a 25-year experience. Gastrointest Endosc. 2012;76(1):25–31.
73. Chapuy CI, Annino DJ, Tishler RB, Haddad RI, Snavely A, Goguen LA. Success of endoscopic pharyngoesophageal dilation after head and neck cancer treatment. Laryngoscope. 2013;123(12):3066–73.
74. Garcia A, Flores RM, Schattner M, et al. Endoscopic retrograde dilation of completely occlusive esophageal strictures. Ann Thorac Surg. 2006;82(4):1240–3.
75. Dellon ES, Cullen NR, Madanick RD, et al. Outcomes of a combined antegrade and retrograde approach for dilatation of radiation-induced esophageal strictures (with video). Gastrointest Endosc. 2010;71(7):1122–9.
76. Langerman A, Stenson KM, Ferguson MK. Retrograde endoscopic-assisted esophageal dilation. J Gastrointest Surg. 2010;14(7):1186–9.
77. Moyer MT, Stack BC Jr, Mathew A. Successful recovery of esophageal patency in 2 patients with complete obstruction by using combined antegrade retrograde dilation procedure, needle knife, and EUS needle. Gastrointest Endosc. 2006;64(5):789–92.
78. Gonzalez JM, Vanbiervliet G, Gasmi M, Grimaud JC, Barthet M. Efficacy of the endoscopic rendez-vous technique for the reconstruction of complete esophageal disruptions. Endoscopy. 2016;48(2):179–83.
79. Contini S, Scarpignato C. Caustic injury of the upper gastrointestinal tract: a comprehensive review. World J Gastroenterol. 2013;19(25):3918–30.
80. Mamede RC, de Mello Filho FV. Ingestion of caustic substances and its complications. Sao Paulo Med J. 2001;119(1):10–5.
81. Ryu HH, Jeung KW, Lee BK, et al. Caustic injury: can CT grading system enable prediction of esophageal stricture? Clin Toxicol (Phila). 2010;48(2):137–42.
82. Zargar SA, Kochhar R, Mehta S, Mehta SK. The role of fiberoptic endoscopy in the management of corrosive ingestion and modified endoscopic classification of burns. Gastrointest Endosc. 1991;37(2):165–9.

83. Isbister GK, Page CB. Early endoscopy or CT in caustic injuries: a re-evaluation of clinical practice. Clin Toxicol (Phila). 2011;49(7):641–2.
84. Lahoti D, Broor SL, Basu PP, Gupta A, Sharma R, Pant CS. Corrosive esophageal strictures: predictors of response to endoscopic dilation. Gastrointest Endosc. 1995;41(3):196–200.
85. Mutaf O, Genc A, Herek O, Demircan M, Ozcan C, Arikan A. Gastroesophageal reflux: a determinant in the outcome of caustic esophageal burns. J Pediatr Surg. 1996;31(11):1494–5.
86. Wang RW, Zhou JH, Jiang YG, et al. Prevention of stricture with intraluminal stenting through laparotomy after corrosive esophageal burns. Eur J Cardiothorac Surg. 2006;30(2):207–11.
87. Pelclova D, Navratil T. Do corticosteroids prevent oesophageal stricture after corrosive ingestion? Toxicol Rev. 2005;24(2):125–9.
88. Berger M, Ure B, Lacher M. Mitomycin C in the therapy of recurrent esophageal strictures: hype or hope? Eur J Pediatr Surg. 2012;22(2):109–16.
89. Gercek A, Ay B, Dogan V, Kiyan G, Dagli T, Gogus Y. Esophageal balloon dilation in children: prospective analysis of hemodynamic changes and complications during general anesthesia. J Clin Anesth. 2007;19(4):286–9.
90. Doo EY, Shin JH, Kim JH, Song HY. Oesophageal strictures caused by the ingestion of corrosive agents: effectiveness of balloon dilatation in children. Clin Radiol. 2009;64(3):265–71.
91. Ilkin Naharci M, Tuzun A, Erdil A, et al. Effectiveness of bougie dilation for the management of corrosive esophageal strictures. Acta Gastroenterol Belg. 2006;69(4):372–6.
92. Singhal S, Kar P. Management of acid- and alkali-induced esophageal strictures in 79 adults by endoscopic dilation: 8-years' experience in New Delhi. Dysphagia. 2007;22(2):130–4.
93. Kim JH, Song HY, Kim HC, et al. Corrosive esophageal strictures: long-term effectiveness of balloon dilation in 117 patients. J Vasc Interv Radiol. 2008;19(5):736–41.
94. Gumaste VV, Dave PB. Ingestion of corrosive substances by adults. Am J Gastroenterol. 1992;87(1):1–5.
95. Contini S, Scarpignato C, Rossi A, Strada G. Features and management of esophageal corrosive lesions in children in Sierra Leone: lessons learned from 175 consecutive patients. J Pediatr Surg. 2011;46(9):1739–45.
96. Panieri E, Rode H, Millar AJ, Cywes S. Oesophageal replacement in the management of corrosive strictures: when is surgery indicated? Pediatr Surg Int. 1998;13(5–6):336–40.
97. Graham J, Barnes N, Rubenstein AS. The nasogastric tube as a cause of esophagitis and stricture. Am J Surg. 1959;98(1):116–9.
98. Zaninotto G, Bonavina L, Pianalto S, Fassina A, Ancona E. Esophageal strictures following nasogastric intubation. Int Surg. 1986;71(2):100–3.
99. Yoon YS, Kim JY, Lee KJ, Yu KP, Lee MS. Balloon dilatation for an esophageal stricture by long-term use of a nasogastric tube: a case report. Ann Rehabil Med. 2014;38(4):581–4.
100. Siersema PD, de Wijkerslooth LR. Dilation of refractory benign esophageal strictures. Gastrointest Endosc. 2009;70(5):1000–12.
101. Ashcraft KW, Holder TM. The expeimental treatment of esophageal strictures by intralesional steroid injections. J Thorac Cardiovasc Surg. 1969;58(5):685–91. passim.
102. Ramage JI Jr, Rumalla A, Baron TH, et al. A prospective, randomized, double-blind, placebo-controlled trial of endoscopic steroid injection therapy for recalcitrant esophageal peptic strictures. Am J Gastroenterol. 2005;100(11):2419–25.
103. Camargo MA, Lopes LR, Grangeia Tdc A, Andreollo NA, Brandalise NA. Use of corticosteroids after esophageal dilations on patients with corrosive stenosis: prospective, randomized and double-blind study. Rev Assoc Med Bras (1992). 2003;49(3):286–92.
104. Burdick JS, Venu RP, Hogan WJ. Cutting the defiant lower esophageal ring. Gastrointest Endosc. 1993;39(5):616–9.
105. Hordijk ML, Siersema PD, Tilanus HW, Kuipers EJ. Electrocautery therapy for refractory anastomotic strictures of the esophagus. Gastrointest Endosc. 2006;63(1):157–63.
106. Hordijk ML, van Hooft JE, Hansen BE, Fockens P, Kuipers EJ. A randomized comparison of electrocautery incision with Savary bougienage for relief of anastomotic gastroesophageal strictures. Gastrointest Endosc. 2009;70(5):849–55.

107. Pungpapong S, Raimondo M, Wallace MB, Woodward TA. Problematic esophageal stricture: an emerging indication for self-expandable silicone stents. Gastrointest Endosc. 2004;60(5):842–5.
108. Wadhwa RP, Kozarek RA, France RE, et al. Use of self-expandable metallic stents in benign GI diseases. Gastrointest Endosc. 2003;58(2):207–12.
109. Repici A, Vleggaar FP, Hassan C, et al. Efficacy and safety of biodegradable stents for refractory benign esophageal strictures: the BEST (biodegradable esophageal stent) study. Gastrointest Endosc. 2010;72(5):927–34.
110. Fuccio L, Hassan C, Frazzoni L, Miglio R, Repici A. Clinical outcomes following stent placement in refractory benign esophageal stricture: a systematic review and meta-analysis. Endoscopy. 2016;48(2):141–8.
111. Kim JH, Song HY, Choi EK, Kim KR, Shin JH, Lim JO. Temporary metallic stent placement in the treatment of refractory benign esophageal strictures: results and factors associated with outcome in 55 patients. Eur Radiol. 2009;19(2):384–90.
112. Canena JM, Liberato MJ, Rio-Tinto RA, et al. A comparison of the temporary placement of 3 different self-expanding stents for the treatment of refractory benign esophageal strictures: a prospective multicentre study. BMC Gastroenterol. 2012;12:70.
113. Hirdes MM, Vleggaar FP, Siersema PD. Stent placement for esophageal strictures: an update. Expert Rev Med Devices. 2011;8(6):733–55.
114. Hirdes MM, Siersema PD, van Boeckel PG, Vleggaar FP. Single and sequential biodegradable stent placement for refractory benign esophageal strictures: a prospective follow-up study. Endoscopy. 2012;44(7):649–54.
115. Repici A, Small AJ, Mendelson A, et al. Natural history and management of refractory benign esophageal strictures. Gastrointest Endosc. 2016;84(2):222–8.
116. Wong KK, Hendel D. Self-dilation for refractory oesophageal strictures: an Auckland City Hospital study. N Z Med J. 2010;123(1321):49–53.
117. Qin Y, Sunjaya DB, Myburgh S, et al. Outcomes of oesophageal self-dilation for patients with refractory benign oesophageal strictures. Aliment Pharmacol Ther. 2018;48(1):87–94.
118. Zehetner J, DeMeester SR, Ayazi S, Demeester TR. Home self-dilatation for esophageal strictures. Dis Esophagus. 2014;27(1):1–4.
119. van Halsema EE, t Hoen CA, de Koning PS, Rosmolen WD, van Hooft JE, Bergman JJ. Self-dilation for therapy-resistant benign esophageal strictures: towards a systematic approach. Surg Endosc. 2018;32(7):3200–7.
120. Zhang Y, Wang X, Liu L, Chen JP, Fan ZN. Intramuscular injection of mitomycin C combined with endoscopic dilation for benign esophageal strictures. J Dig Dis. 2015;16(7):370–6.
121. Mendez-Nieto CM, Zarate-Mondragon F, Ramirez-Mayans J, Flores-Flores M. Topical mitomycin C versus intralesional triamcinolone in the management of esophageal stricture due to caustic ingestion. Rev Gastroenterol Mex. 2015;80(4):248–54.
122. Javed A, Pal S, Dash NR, Sahni P, Chattopadhyay TK. Outcome following surgical management of corrosive strictures of the esophagus. Ann Surg. 2011;254(1):62–6.

Chapter 6
Eosinophilic Esophagitis

Betty H. Li, Nina Gupta, and Robert T. Kavitt

Introduction

Eosinophilic esophagitis (EoE) is a chronic immune-mediated condition of the esophagus with increasing incidence and prevalence worldwide. It is now identified as a cause of food impaction, dysphagia, and upper gastrointestinal symptoms in both the pediatric and the adult population. While EoE has not been associated with increased mortality or cancer risk, it is a progressive disease that causes significant morbidity. Since its recognition as a distinct clinical entity in the 1990s, research has expanded our understanding of its pathogenesis. Diagnostic criteria and treatment modalities have thus evolved considerably in the last two decades. This chapter will review the epidemiology, pathophysiology, diagnosis, and management of EoE.

B. H. Li
Department of Medicine, University of Chicago, Chicago, IL, USA

N. Gupta
Section of Gastroenterology, Hepatology, and Nutrition, University of Chicago, Chicago, IL, USA
e-mail: nina.gupta@uchospitals.edu

R. T. Kavitt (✉)
Center for Esophageal Diseases, Section of Gastroenterology, Hepatology, and Nutrition, University of Chicago, Chicago, IL, USA
e-mail: rkavitt@bsd.uchicago.edu

© Springer Nature Switzerland AG 2020
D. A. Patel et al. (eds.), *Evaluation and Management of Dysphagia*,
https://doi.org/10.1007/978-3-030-26554-0_6

Epidemiology

Incidence and Prevalence

Population-based studies investigating the incidence of EoE have mostly been conducted in North America and Europe. The incidence of EoE ranges from 2.1 to 12.8 new cases per 100,000 persons per year [1]. A systematic review with meta-analysis of population-based studies observed a significant rise in the pooled incidence rates of EoE from 2.8/100,000 to 7.2/100,000 inhabitants/year [2]. While some studies attribute the rise to increased disease recognition, other studies have shown that the incidence of EoE outpaces that of endoscopic biopsies by several fold [1, 3–5]. Recent data suggests that the incidence is truly rising and not an artifact of increase detection. Overall, disease distribution and presentation vary according to several individual and community determinants.

The reported prevalence of EoE is affected by study methodology, population examined, and clinical practice patterns. The majority of information gathered as population-based estimates arise from data in North America and Europe, with some data from Australia and Asia. Currently, the estimated prevalence of EoE worldwide ranges between 13 and 49 cases per 100,000, although there is significant regional heterogeneity, and has been reported to be as high as 90.7 per 100,000 [1, 6]. As EoE is a non-fatal condition, studies universally report an increasing prevalence of EoE. It should be noted that the majority of studies prior to 2017 excluded patients whose disease responded to proton-pump inhibitor (PPI) therapy. Recent consensus guidelines on the diagnosis of EoE do not include this distinction, therefore studies likely underestimate the burden of disease.

Age

EoE can affect persons of all ages including infants, adolescents, and adults. The majority of EoE cases are seen in adults age 18–65 years [7]. A large number of EoE patients are under the age of 50, with a particularly high incidence near the third decade of life [5, 8, 9]. Pediatric cases account for about 25% of all EoE cases and usually occur between 5 and 10 years of age, though cases in very young children are also reported [10]. A large study of 30 million US patients estimated the prevalence of EoE in the adult population at 30.0/100,000, with prevalence in pediatric patients (age < 18) at 25.1/100,000 persons [7]. EoE is less common in the elderly (age > 65) with an incidence of approximately 12–18 cases per 100,000 in the USA [7, 9, 11].

Gender

Men are more frequently diagnosed with EoE than women, with a male to female ratio of 3:1 [9, 12–14]. A meta-analysis of five population-based studies found the pooled prevalence of EoE in male patients to be 53.8 per 100,000 compared with

20.1 per 100,000 in female patients [2]. Additionally, males more commonly report symptoms of dysphagia and food impaction [15]. A greater proportion of males are also diagnosed in childhood than compared with females [13, 16]. A large multicenter study found similar gender differences, with men noted to have a longer duration of symptoms and more esophageal strictures than women [17]. While this gender bias has been consistently observed in the literature, the reason for this discrepancy is incompletely understood as no significant differences are observed in endoscopic or histologic features [13].

Race

In the USA, EoE is particularly seen in Caucasians, who represent the majority of cases and account for approximately 80–96% of cases worldwide [14]. In a 2012 study conducted by Sperry et al., very few differences between Caucasian patients and African-American patients were observed. However, the authors did find that African Americans tended to present at a younger age with failure to thrive, while Caucasians often presented at an older age with symptoms of dysphagia [13]. A large retrospective study of 793 patients and several other smaller population studies reported similar findings [17]. Data regarding EoE in other racial groups are more limited, but the available data confirms lower rates of disease in these groups than in Caucasians. A large population study conducted at Kaiser Permanente of Southern California found EoE was 8 times more prevalent in Caucasians compared to Hispanics (11.6/10,000 vs 1.4/10,000) [18]. Another study conducted at two different institutions with a primarily Hispanic patient population found that EoE was 2–7 times more common among Caucasian patients than Hispanic patients [19].

Geography and Climate

The incidence and prevalence of EoE vary by geographic region, with the highest burden of disease in North America, Western Europe, and Australia [20]. A population-based analysis reported the incidence of EoE to be 5.4 per 100,000 inhabitants per year in North America and 1.7 in Europe [2]. The same study also found the pooled prevalence of EoE to be 1.9 times greater in North America than in Europe. Comparatively, the prevalence of EoE in Western Australia was found to be about half of that of Europe in a 2004 study [21]. Regardless of geographic location, a steady rise in EoE incidence and prevalence rates were observed upon comparison of studies conducted before and after 2008 [2].

Information on the epidemiology of EoE in other regions of the world including Central and South America, Asia, and Africa are scarce. In a large systematic review of EoE in Asian countries, a total of 217 patients were identified. More than half of the studies were performed in Japan, followed by Korea, Turkey, Saudi Arabia, China, and Taiwan [22]. One study of 1021 asymptomatic adult patients undergoing endoscopic evaluation conducted in Shanghai, China, only had 4 cases of

EoE [23]. In Japan, the prevalence of EoE is of similar magnitude, estimated to be about 0.01% [22]. Interestingly, even with lower rates of incidence and prevalence in Asian countries, the age and gender ratios of the reported cases were similar to those reported in Western countries [24]. Regional variations are not clearly understood and may be partly due to the result of access to endoscopic resources, physician awareness, or environmental exposures.

In addition to global variations, the prevalence of EoE also seems to vary by locality. For example, in the USA, population density is reported to have a strong inverse association with esophageal eosinophilia [25]. Additionally, patients diagnosed with EoE were almost twice as likely to live in cold climate zones than tropical climate zones in the USA [26]. There is also some evidence that seasonal variations affect symptoms attributed to EoE. Fogg and colleagues reported worsening symptoms attributed to EoE and increased eosinophilic infiltration on esophageal biopsies during the pollen season, with subsequent improvement during the winter months [27]. These results suggest that environmental flora and aeroallergens may play a role in pathogenesis and the disease course of EoE.

Pathogenesis

The understanding of EoE has significantly evolved over the last two decades and the pathogenesis is still being extensively studied. A hallmark feature of EoE is abnormal infiltration of eosinophils in the esophagus causing acute inflammation and chronic changes. Diagnostic criteria include several clinical and histological features that will be discussed further in later sections. This section aims to summarize current understanding of the interaction between genetic, environmental, and cellular factors in the pathogenesis of the disease. These pathways are the basis of targeted treatment in EoE.

Genetic Etiology

Prior familial studies have observed significantly increased risk of EoE among young, male first-degree relatives [28]. However, the mode of inheritance of EoE is complex and is not consistent with a traditional Mendelian pattern [29]. Multiple genes have been identified as likely contributors to the development of EoE and may have synergistic effects. Gene variants involved in general atopic disease, such as thymic stromal lymphopoietin (TSLP) that regulates Th2 cell development and activates eosinophils, are implicated in EoE. Genes specific to the pathogenesis of EoE have also been identified, such as CCL26 which encodes a potent eosinophil chemoattractant eotaxin-3 and CAPN14 which has a role in esophageal epithelial barrier function [30–32]. Although genetic factors may contribute to the development of EoE, the rapid rise in EoE incidence indicates a larger role for environmental factors in disease risk. A familial study conducted by Alexander et al. demonstrated that "heritability" estimates changed greatly by twin analysis when accounting for common environment, where environmental factors contributed 81.0% of total phenotypic variance [29]. These results suggest that research on EoE designed to study nuclear families are likely overestimating the heritability of EoE and interpretation of these results are limited as common environmental exposures confound heritability analysis. By including common environment in the full model, heritability is estimated at 14.5% [29]. It is proposed that both genetic and environmental factors play an important role in the development of EoE and may be linked via epigenetic regulation [33]. Such regulation has been demonstrated for the strongly associated EoE genes CCL26 and CAPN14 [34]. Lifetime exposures likely potentiate a genetically susceptible individual for the development of EoE.

Role of Allergens

Strong evidence suggests that an allergic etiology is an underlying mechanism of EoE. The pathogenesis of EoE has similarities to that of other atopic disorders, such as asthma or atopic dermatitis [35]. Food and environmental allergens trigger a diverse esophageal inflammatory response, leading to a pathologic cycle of tissue damage and repair in EoE. However, the pathways by which the disease evolves over time remains a topic of investigation. Experimental models have shown that EoE can be induced in mice by means of allergen exposure to common culprits such as peanuts, inhaled aspergillus, or dust mite antigen [36]. Approximately 70% of diagnosed patients exhibited concomitant atopic diseases and sensitization to one or more foods and aeroallergens [37–39]. Furthermore, a wealth of literature has documented the benefit of allergen elimination through strict exclusion diets, particularly in children with EoE. In a sensitized individual, allergens react with IgE bound to mast cells and lead to localized mast cell degranulation. Mast cells release histamine and chemotactic factors that recruit eosinophils to the esophagus and induce eosinophilic degranulation. Eosinophilic granules release a variety of chemokines, cytokines, and cytotoxic proteins, which ultimately cause inflammation and tissue damage [35]. Even in patients who do not have manifestations of atopy or show positivity to allergy skin testing, studies have shown that they still exhibit classic cellular markers of allergy in the esophagus including immunoglobulin (Ig)-E bearing mast cells [40]. Due to the high rate of sensitization and the clinical response to elimination diets, food-specific IgE were initially suggested as a possible driver of EoE. However, the determination of specific IgE and/or skin prick tests have been inadequate in identifying causative allergens in EoE [41]. Diets geared toward eliminating specific type I allergens do not result in significant histologic or symptomatic improvements in all patients. Additionally, small trials using a specific anti-IgE antibody (omalizumab) only induced remission in a limited number of patients, did not significantly reduce eosinophil counts, and had variable endoscopic response despite reduction in IgE levels [42, 43]. In line with these findings, studies using animal models have demonstrated that EoE can be induced with B-cell-deficient mice but not in mice that are T lymphocyte deficient [44, 45]. Therefore, mounting data suggests that while EoE is often associated with IgE sensitization, the disease is not a purely IgE-mediated allergy.

Impaired Epithelial Barrier and Th2

There is increasing evidence that the development of EoE is associated with epithelial barrier dysfunction and subsequent T helper type 2 (Th2) predominant inflammation. Epithelial barrier impairment can develop due to a number of reasons including genetic predisposition, reflux disease, microbial imbalance, or food intake. Increased barrier permeability can allow microbes and allergens to attach and invade, resulting in activation of the immune system, cytokine release, and inflammation. Once the inflammation is established, impaired mucosal integrity may promote further allergen exposure thus perpetuating the cycle of cytokine release and a leaky epithelial barrier.

Desmoglein (DSG)-1, an intercellular adhesion molecule responsible for epithelial integrity, is one of the most strongly downregulated genes in EoE [46]. Other barrier function genes including Filaggrin, SPRR3, and keratins are also downregulated in esophageal tissue cells of active EoE [47]. Furthermore, both TSLP and CAPN14 have been shown to be overexpressed by the esophageal epithelia in patients with EoE [48]. TSLP regulates Th2 responses, especially those involving interleukin (IL)-13 production and have been implicated in atopic diseases [31]. In vitro, increased CAPN14 expression results in architectural changes indicative of barrier impairment [34, 49]. In active EoE, in addition to IgE-bound mast cells and eosinophils in the esophagus, tissue and serum have increased levels of type 2 allergic inflammatory mediators such as IL-5 and IL-13 [50]. IL-5 promotes eosinophil development, activation, survival, and recruitment to sites of inflammation. IL-13 is a key regulator of DSG and epithelial barrier genes. When overexpressed in mouse models, it has been shown to result in an EoE-like inflammation [51]. These various mediators are all part of the Th2 cascade which is central to mucosal eosinophilia and tissue remodeling in EoE.

EoE is a disease in which a dysregulated esophageal mucosal environment leads to Th2-predominant inflammation and disease development in response to food allergens and aeroallergens. A number of genetic and epigenetic factors can predispose to the development of EoE. Studies have started to uncover the role of activated eosinophils, mast cells, and the cytokines IL-5 and IL-13 as mediators of disease.

Diagnosis

Clinical Manifestations

The predominant symptoms of EoE can vary between adults and children. Infants and toddlers often present with non-specific symptoms of feeding intolerance, nausea, vomiting, and failure to thrive [38]. In contrast, as patients get older, dysphagia and food impaction tend to be the most common presenting symptoms. Approximately 33–54% of adult patients with EoE present for endoscopic management due to food impaction [52]. Other commonly reported symptoms include heartburn (30–60% of patients) and non-cardiac chest pain (8–44%) [53]. The progression of symptoms from childhood to adulthood are thought to be associated with progressive esophageal tissue remodeling that occurs with chronic inflammation. A retrospective study of 379 cases of EoE found that for every ten-year increase in age, the odds of having fibrostenotic changes on endoscopy more than doubled [54]. As symptoms persist, many adults develop food aversions and adaptive feeding mechanisms such that elucidating dysphagia can be difficult. Patients can develop subconscious behaviors including eating slowly, prolonged periods of mastication, increased fluid intake with food, crushing pills, or taking small bites to cope with their narrowed esophageal caliber. Clinicians should therefore obtain a careful history paying particular attention to eating and swallowing habits with any patient who presents with symptoms suggestive of EoE. Importantly, symptom frequency and severity do not always correlate with the degree of eosinophilia or histologic disease activity, therefore diagnosis and monitoring require endoscopic evaluation [55].

When diagnosed with EoE at a young age, a significant percentage of patients can achieve symptomatic resolution. However, over time a large subset of these patients also experience relapse of symptoms. One study of 89 pediatric EoE patients found that 66% had resolution of symptoms with time but 79% later relapsed after a mean follow-up of 3 ± 1.4 years [38]. Two retrospective survey-based studies also suggested that symptoms associated with EoE diagnosed in childhood commonly persist into adulthood with approximately 40% of patients requiring ongoing medical therapy and ongoing care by a gastroenterologist [56, 57].

Symptom Scoring Systems

Several scoring systems have been proposed to standardize the evaluation of EoE symptoms and assess response to treatment. However, EoE clinical guidelines do not endorse the use of any specific scoring system, and thus many studies do not use a scoring system or use their own non-validated indices. While a uniformly adopted scoring system could reduce variability in symptoms assessment, many scoring systems previously used, including the Mayo Dysphagia Questionnaire-30 Day (MDQ-30) and the Straumann Dysphagia Index, are criticized for their cumbersome nature, lack of validation, and poor clinical applicability [58]. To address this, simplified scoring systems have been developed such as the Dysphagia Symptom Questionnaire (DSQ). This 3-question patient-reported outcome form is administered daily for 30 consecutive days [59]. When tested with both pediatric and adult patients, compliance and acceptance was excellent. However, the DSQ is limited by its focus on dysphagia.

The Eosinophilic Esophagitis Activity Index (EEsAI) PRO instrument is another scoring system that has been validated and can be used in adult patients. Symptoms from 183 adult EoE patients in Switzerland and the USA were studied and used to develop the 7-item questionnaire. The scoring system requires patients to recount dysphagia symptoms over a 7-day recall period taking into account behavioral adaptations [60]. However, a recent prospective multicenter study showed that endoscopic or histologic remission was only predicted with 60–65% accuracy using an EEsAI score of 20 as an arbitrary cutoff [55].

Comorbid Conditions

Patients diagnosed with EoE have also been found to have higher rates of concomitant allergic diseases such as atopic dermatitis, atopic rhinitis/sinusitis, asthma, and food allergies [38]. A meta-analysis and systematic review of 21 studies that included 53,542 EoE patients and controls found that allergic rhinitis was significantly more common among patients with EoE compared with control subjects (odds ratio [OR] 5.09), as was bronchial asthma (OR 3.01) and eczema (OR 2.85) [61]. Up to 50–80% of children with EoE have been reported to have atopy, with a somewhat lower rate in adults [62]. In patients with dysphagia, the presence of concomitant allergic symptoms should raise the index of suspicion for EoE.

Aside from atopic disorders, reports have suggested the association of EoE with multiple autoimmune conditions, most notably connective tissue disease. Individuals with connective tissue disease have been found to have an 8-fold risk of having EoE in retrospective analysis [63]. Larger prospective studies have not been conducted to confirm this association. EoE has also been reported with celiac disease and inflammatory bowel disease (IBD), although more recent research indicates that EoE is likely independent of these diseases. A large retrospective, cross-sectional study conducted with data from a US national pathology database demonstrated only a weak association between EoE and celiac disease, with an adjusted odds ratio of 1.26 (95% confidence interval: 0.98–1.60) [64]. Additionally, an association between EoE and IBD has only been made in case reports. Researchers examining the phenotype of eosinophils in patients with IBD and EoE found distinct features in the expression of surface markers that provide evidence for the independence of these two diseases [65].

Diagnostic Criteria

The diagnosis of EoE includes both clinical and histologic criteria. The first consensus guidelines for the diagnosis of EoE were published in 2007. In the subsequent decade, substantial changes have been made to the diagnostic algorithm

Table 6.1 Diagnostic criteria for eosinophilic esophagitis (EoE)

1. Symptoms of esophageal dysfunction (e.g., dysphagia, food impaction, heartburn, chest discomfort, regurgitation)
2. ≥15 eosinophils (eos) per high-power microscopy field (hpf) on esophageal biopsy (~60 eos/mm²). Eosinophilic infiltration should be isolated to the esophagus.
3. Assessment for non-EoE disorders that could cause or potentially contribute to esophageal eosinophilia (see Table 6.2)

Table 6.2 Other causes of esophageal eosinophilia

Hypereosinophilic syndrome
Eosinophilic gastroenteritis
Infection
Vasculitis
Celiac Disease
Crohn's Disease
Connective tissue disease

based on evolving clinical experience and research studies. The most recent 2018 expert consensus statement set forth three specific criteria to diagnose EoE (see Table 6.1) [66].

Of note, increased eosinophilia on biopsy cannot in isolation be equated to a diagnosis of EoE. There is significant phenotypic variability in the presentation of EoE and clinicians must take this into account with the diagnosis.

The principal update in the 2018 consensus statement was the removal of the requisite that mucosal eosinophilia be refractory to a trial of high-dose proton pump inhibitors (PPI). Historically, both clinicians and researchers struggled with the diagnostic challenge of differentiating EoE from gastroesophageal reflux disease (GERD). Like EoE, GERD can also be associated with esophageal eosinophilia and can present with similar clinical symptoms of esophageal dysfunction. It was assumed that GERD and EoE were independent conditions, but the lack of a standard criterion for the diagnosis of GERD made its exclusion extremely difficult. Previously, a response to PPI therapy was used as criteria favoring reflux disease rather than EoE. However, a large body of research has suggested that EoE and GERD have a complex intersecting relationship rather than a mutually exclusive one. For example, acid reflux can induce mucosal injury thereby promoting cytokine release and eosinophilic infiltration while EoE may alter esophageal motility and structure thereby increasing the risk of GERD. The acid-reflux injury to the mucosal barrier then increases exposure to antigens thought to contribute to the pathogenesis of EoE [67]. According to the 2018 Updated International Consensus Diagnostic Criteria for Eosinophilic Esophagitis, concurrent diagnoses of GERD and EoE can be made [66].

A new condition termed PPI-responsive esophageal eosinophilia (PPI-REE) has also been the subject of debate. The term PPI-REE was derived when clinicians observed that about one-third to one-half of patients who had clinical and histologic findings of esophageal eosinophilia responded to PPI treatment but did not have typical symptoms of GERD. For several years, it was unclear whether PPI-REE was a subtype of EoE or a distinct clinical entity. Experts proposed that patients with PPI-REE be distinguished from those with EoE based on their initial response to eight weeks of acid suppression treatment [68]. However, a number of ensuing studies examining the differences between EoE and PPI-REE concluded that baseline features (before PPI therapy) were essentially indistinguishable. Clinical presentation, endoscopic findings, histologic features, inflammatory markers, and even RNA expression profiles were largely similar between the two conditions [69–71]. Cases also emerged where patients diagnosed with PPI-REE, after stopping PPI treatment, exhibited recurrence of esophageal eosinophilia and responded to classic EoE therapy of elimination diet and topical steroids [72]. These data suggest that PPI-REE and EoE have the same immunological mechanisms. Thus, 2017 guidelines on eosinophilic esophagitis no longer consider PPI-REE as a separate clinical entity [6]. It remains uncertain why some experience complete remission on PPI therapy while others do not.

Endoscopic Findings

Endoscopic esophageal assessment with biopsy is necessary for the diagnosis of EoE. Distinct endoscopic findings in EoE are usually only seen when the underlying histologic inflammatory cascade has been present for long enough to cause tissue remodeling. These findings, summarized in Table 6.3, Fig. 6.1, include fixed esophageal rings (trachealization), transient esophageal rings (felinization), white exudates, longitudinal furrows, edema, esophageal stenosis, stricture, and friable mucosa (crêpe-paper esophagus) [52]. In a meta-analysis conducted by Kim et al. of over 4600 patients with EoE, the overall pooled prevalence was as follows: esophageal rings, 44%; strictures, 21%; stenosis/stricture, 9%; linear furrows, 48%; white plaques, 27%; and pallor/decreased vasculature, 41%. In prospective studies, at least one abnormality was detected by endoscopy in 93% of patients [73]. Additionally, endoscopic findings vary between children and adults. Children more commonly have either a normal-appearing esophagus or inflammatory findings such as edematous mucosa with loss of vascular markings, pallor, or white plaques [73, 74]. Adults typically have endoscopic findings related to fibrostenotic changes including fixed rings, stenosis, and strictures [54]. Approximately 7–10% of adult EoE patients and 32% of pediatric patients will present with a normal appearing esophagus [73, 75].

Endoscopic assessment of disease activity is emerging as a therapeutically relevant outcome measure. However, there is a paucity of validated clinical tools to evaluate endoscopic features of EoE. The use of a uniform nomenclature to facilitate comparison of studies and communication between clinicians is recognized as

Table 6.3 Common Findings in EoE

Endoscopic	Exudates/white spots
	Pale, edematous mucosa, decreased vascularity
	Longitudinal furrows/ridges
	Rings or "trachealization"
	Stenosis/stricture or narrow caliber esophagus
	Friable mucosa with lacerations upon passing of the endoscope or "crêpe-paper esophagus"
Histologic	Eosinophil infiltration/abscess formation
	Dilated intercellular spaces (spongiosis)
	Epithelial desquamation/dyskeratosis
	Basal zone hyperplasia
	Rete peg elongation
	Lamina propria fibrosis

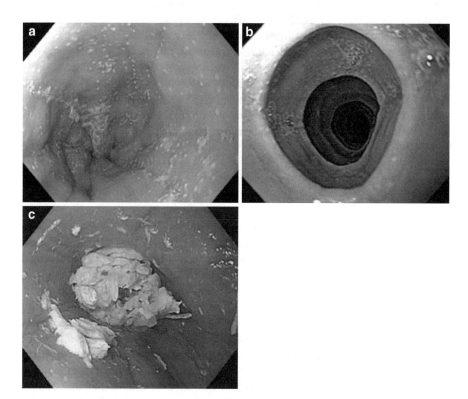

Fig. 6.1 Endoscopic images of patients with eosinophilic esophagitis. (**a**) White specks of esophageal mucosa consistent with eosinophilic microabscesses. (**b**) Ringed appearance of the esophagus. (**c**) Esophageal food impaction in setting of eosinophilic esophagitis

an area in need of advancement. Recently, a novel classification system was proposed called the EoE endoscopic reference score (EREFS). The acronym reflects the major components of the score: exudates, rings, edema, furrows, and strictures. It showed fair to good interobserver agreement among practicing and academic gastroenterologists [76].

In both the pediatric and adult population, improvement in endoscopic finding has been shown to correlate with histological remission after EoE treatment [77]. A tool such as EREFS therefore has the potential to standardize recognition and reporting of disease activity in EoE. However, data regarding the EREFS score is equivocal. In a prospective endoscopic study of adults with EoE, those who had a robust histologic response to treatment were found to have a significant decrease in EREFS scores [78]. The study also found that inflammatory components had the most prominent improvement after treatment. However, a prospective multicenter study of 145 EoE patients found that correlation of EREFS score with histological activity and clinical symptoms via the Dysphagia Symptom Score was poor. Based on the study, only exudates correlated with peak eosinophil count and histological outcome, whereas furrows and edema persisted in 50–70% of patients despite histological proven remission after treatment. Likewise, the study noted that none of the endoscopic findings were able to adequately predict dysphagia severity [79]. Another study exhibited similar results, suggestive of modest accuracy of the EREFS score in clinical practice [80]. These mixed results may be due to variability in endoscopist experience and practice. In order to optimize the predictive value of EREFS, the component features may need to be modified.

Histologic Features

While clinical presentation and endoscopic findings can raise suspicion for EoE, histologic confirmation of eosinophilia is necessary for the diagnosis. When obtaining biopsies, a minimum of 2–4 esophageal biopsies should be obtained from the distal esophagus and 2–4 from the proximal esophagus with a minimum of six biopsies in areas that appear grossly inflamed [6, 81]. This maximizes the likelihood of detecting eosinophilia since EoE can affect the esophagus in a patchy manner [66, 74, 82]. While the distal esophagus has been shown to have a denser eosinophilic infiltrate than the mid-esophagus in pediatric patients, this difference has been inconsistently demonstrated in adults [83–85]. When present, the likelihood of diagnosing EoE increases when multiple biopsies are taken from multiple esophageal regions. The current eosinophil density threshold to diagnose EoE is 15 eosinophils per high power field (hpf) in esophageal mucosa (peak concentration in the specimens examined). The level of 15 eosinophils/hpf is somewhat arbitrary and different cut-off values were used in earlier studies. Using 15 eos/hpf as a threshold, one study identified diagnostic sensitivities of 84%, 97%, and

100% when obtaining 2, 3, and 6 biopsy specimens, respectively [86]. While the threshold of 15 eos/hpf is highly sensitive, lower levels of eosinophilia have been reported in patients with EoE [82]. It is also important to consider several other potential etiologies of abnormal esophageal eosinophilia including gastroesophageal reflux, eosinophilic gastrointestinal diseases, Crohn's disease, celiac disease, and infection, among others. During upper endoscopy, biopsy specimens should be obtained from the gastric antrum and duodenum to rule out eosinophilic gastroenteritis in children, as well as in adults with potential gastric or intestinal symptoms [12, 74].

Histologic eosinophilia is a key feature of EoE with eosinophils typically layered in the epithelium or aggregated in microabscesses [87]. Disruption of epithelial tight junctions can cause dilation of the interepithelial space, termed spongiosis, that may progress to the formation of small "lakes" in the epithelium. These observed changes can lead to epithelial acanthosis with basal zone hyperplasia. Additionally, eosinophilic infiltration can extend to the lamina propria or deeper tissue layers causing collagen deposition and ultimately macroscopic tissue remodeling [88, 89]. In adults, eosinophilic microabscesses and lamina propria fibrosis were found to be most specific for eosinophilic esophagitis (98% and 97%, respectively), however they are not sensitive (56% and 27%, respectively) and are quite rare findings [82].

Imaging

Barium esophagography can be used in adolescents and adults to identify anatomic and mucosal abnormalities that have developed from tissue remodeling in EoE. This modality is most helpful in certain cases, such as when esophageal stenosis or stricture is suspected, and endoscopic dilation may be needed. The study can help characterize the length and diameter of complicated esophageal strictures. The indication for an esophagram should be discussed with the radiologist in advance to ensure the entire esophagus, including the caliber and distensibility of the esophageal lumen, is fully assessed. There is currently no role for CT or MRI in the diagnosis or disease monitoring of EoE.

Novel Diagnostic Modalities

Although EoE is best diagnosed by endoscopy and esophageal biopsy, the cost and risk of repeated endoscopy to monitor histologic response to treatment is burdensome. Therefore, there has been significant interest in identifying novel methods that are less expensive, more reliable, and/or less invasive.

Mucosal Impedance

One proposed mechanism in the pathogenesis of EoE is a loss of mucosal integrity leading to sensitization to food antigens. Dilation of intercellular spaces results in increased epithelial permeability which is thought to facilitate antigen exposure. This process can also allow free trans-epithelial transport of small molecules and electrolytes. As a result, electrical conductance across the epithelium increases and mucosal impedance decreases [90]. Using stationary transnasal intraluminal pH/impedance probe, van Rhijin et al. found a decreased baseline impedance value throughout the esophagus in EoE patients but not in healthy controls [91]. A follow-up prospective study by the same group using electrical tissue impedance spectroscopy also showed that electrical tissue impedance and transepithelial electrical resistance were reduced in EoE patients [92]. Recently, a through-the-scope probe that can measure mucosal impedance was developed, allowing for more precise and efficient assessment. It has been hypothesized that this mucosal impedance device could be used to measure the activity of EoE. In a study of 20 patients, point impedance measurements showed excellent inverse correlation to the number of eosinophils per high-power field taken from corresponding biopsy specimens. Using an impedance cut-off value of 2300 Ω, sensitivity and specificity were found to be 90% and 91%, respectively. It was also noted that once eosinophil count was greater than the threshold of 15 eos/hpf, there was a marked decrease in esophageal impedance reflecting active disease [93]. Larger prospective controlled trials are needed to investigate whether impedance measurement could replace esophageal biopsies in the future.

Esophageal Distensibility (Impedance Planimetry)

Symptoms in EoE are often related to tissue remodeling and fibrosis rather than active eosinophilic inflammation. The extent of fibrosis is difficult to quantify by standard esophageal biopsies due to its patchy distribution and lack of depth to include the lamina propria. Endoscopy often underestimates stricture presence and extent compared with barium esophagography.

The introduction of high-resolution impedance planimetry has enabled direct evaluation of esophageal mechanical properties and distensibility. The functional luminal imaging probe (FLIP) is an orally passed catheter with an infinitely compliant inflatable balloon and multiple electrodes that measure luminal cross-sectional area and intra-luminal pressure to render a three-dimensional approximation of esophageal anatomy [94]. Pressure volume characteristics are determined from step-wise distension of the balloon, which allows for objective measurements of esophageal narrowing. The balloon catheter is easily passed during endoscopy and no perforations have thus far been reported. The use of FLIP has been evaluated in a number of esophageal disorders including achalasia, GERD, and EoE

[94]. One study of thirty-three EoE patients has shown that esophageal distensibility, defined by the change in the narrowest measurable cross-sectional area over the change in intraluminal pressure, was significantly reduced in EoE patients compared with controls [95]. Another study reported an association of reduced distensibility with clinical outcomes including future food impaction and requirement for esophageal dilation [96]. Despite these findings and the commercial availability of FLIP, current recommendations for clinical use are limited by the low level of evidence and lack of standardized protocols. Currently, diagnostic and treatment decisions are not recommended to be based on Endo-FLIP findings [97]. However, whether the addition of FLIP would enhance the current care of EoE warrants further investigation.

Esophageal String

In addition to mucosal eosinophils, the presence of other molecules such as eosinophil-derived granule proteins (EDP) and related Th2 cytokines can be markers of disease activity [98, 99]. Thus, there has been interest in measuring the level of these biomarkers in esophageal secretions to estimate mucosal inflammation. Furuta and colleagues developed a mechanism by which to obtain and measure these proteins using the Esophageal String Test (EST) [100]. The device consists of a capsule filled with approximately 90 cm of string. The proximal end of the string is taped to the cheek and then the capsule is swallowed to deploy the string into the duodenum. After overnight incubation, the string is withdrawn so luminal secretions from the proximal portion can be scraped and analyzed for eosinophil-derived proteins. When tested in 41 children, the levels of luminal eosinophil-derived proteins in string samples significantly differentiated children with active EoE from those with EoE in remission, GERD, and normal esophagus. Furthermore, levels of proteins correlated with peak and mean esophageal eosinophils/HPF on biopsy. The benefits of this bedside test include its minimally invasive nature and ability to provide detailed biochemical information that may be able to differentiate disease phenotypes in the future. However, the data needs to be validated with larger studies.

Cytosponge

The ideal technique to monitor EoE would obviate the need for endoscopy yet adequately sample the esophageal mucosa for analysis. Researchers have examined the role of the Cytosponge (University of Cambridge) as a minimally invasive method for collecting esophageal tissue. The Cytosponge was originally invented for detecting Barrett's esophagus [101]. It consists of an ingestible gelatin capsule that is swallowed to dissolve and release a 3-cm diameter spherical mesh. The mesh is withdrawn through the mouth by traction of an attached string, and tissue specimens are collected from the sponge for analysis. In a prospective two-center cross-sectional study of 57 adults with active EoE and 44 adults with inactive EoE, the sensitivity and specificity of the Cytosponge was 75% and 86%, respectively, when using a cutoff of 15 eos/HPF [102]. The tissue samples had very good correlation with mucosal eosinophil density on subsequent esophageal biopsies. The procedure successfully obtained adequate tissue samples in 95% of EoE patients and was well tolerated with no adverse events or sponge detachments. While these results suggest Cytosponge may be a promising device in the assessment of EoE, further research is required to understand its efficacy prior to incorporating it into routine practice.

Allergy Testing

Previous expert consensus statements recommended that patients diagnosed with EoE be evaluated by allergist or immunologist to assess the presence of concomitant disorders such as asthma, rhinitis, eczema, or food allergies [74]. This recommendation was made due to high rates (about 50–60%) of concurrent allergic diatheses found in patients with EoE [74]. However, the evidence for the benefit of allergy testing in the diagnosis and management of EoE remains unclear. Clinical decisions based on the interpretation of allergy testing have shown modest results at best. There are 3 types of allergy testing currently available: skin prick testing (SPT), atopy patch testing (APT), and serum food-specific IgE (sIgE) testing. SPT is a standardized and validated technique to study immediate allergic reactions medicated by mast cell-bound IgE [103]. In contrast, APT is used to assess the presence of non-IgE, cell-mediated reactions, but performance is not standardized and interpretation is subject to significant interobserver variation [104].

A systematic meta-analysis by González-Cervera and colleagues concluded that the predisposition of atopy to EoE is unproven, despite the extensively described association [61]. Allergy testing therefore has no role in the diagnosis of EoE. However, there is continued interest in establishing whether SPT and APT would be beneficial in assessing treatment response and in disease monitoring.

Esophageal Prick Testing

Skin tests and serum IgE levels do not accurately identify foods for elimination diets in patients with EoE. This may be because inflammation in EoE is localized to the esophagus. To further investigate this, Warners and colleagues evaluated direct esophageal response to food allergens. In a small prospective pilot study of 8 patients, the researchers injected allergen extracts into local esophageal mucosa and assessed for immediate and delayed response with repeat endoscopy. The study found that compared with SPT and serum IgE testing, the sensitization patterns identified through esophageal prick testing (EPT) correlated more accurately with culprit foods in EoE patients [105]. This study was the first to demonstrate the feasibility and safety of EPT. Given the results, the authors advocate for further exploration of EPT and its potential to guide elimination diets.

Plasma Markers

Biomarkers from peripheral blood, breath sampling, oropharyngeal swabs, stool, and urine have also been assessed as a means of non-invasive EoE monitoring [106]. Currently, only 3 randomized controlled studies (RCT) have been completed, and no meta-analysis has been published. A limitation of using biomarker testing is the lack of reliability and reproducibility. Several biomarkers have been studied in patients with EoE, but none have been incorporated into treatment guidelines or clinical practice. The most common biomarker assessed were peripheral blood absolute eosinophil count (AEC) and IgE [106]. Both serum IgE levels and peripheral eosinophilia are frequently elevated in EoE patients, but neither has adequate sensitivity and specificity to utilize in clinical practice.

Approximately 70% of patients with EoE have elevated total IgE values on endoscopy [107]. However, despite evidence of increased IgE production in the esophageal epithelium, it seems to be insufficient to cause a significant increase at peripheral levels. Studies have shown poor correlation between serum total IgE levels and the number of eosinophils found in esophageal biopsies [108, 109]. Additionally, IgE-targeted therapies have yielded less promising results than expected [41, 110, 111]. Total serum IgE testing therefore has a limited role in the diagnosis and management of EoE.

The AEC is a simple and inexpensive serum test. Peripheral blood eosinophilia has been described in EoE patients (defined as >300/mm^3) [112, 113] and a number of studies have found that the percentage of peripheral blood eosinophils has high positive correlation with esophageal eosinophil density in pediatric and adult patients [112–114]. However, the use of AEC in the diagnosis and monitoring of EoE is thought to be imperfect due to possible confounders such as atopy, infection, and other inflammatory conditions. Only 5 small studies compared peripheral AEC between EoE patients and atopic patients with no significant difference noted [65, 112–114]. Min et al. conducted a prospective cohort analysis of 42 pediatric and adult patients and found the level of AEC was associated with a diagnosis of EoE, even after controlling for age, sex, allergic rhinitis, asthma, eczema, and seasonal allergies. Additionally, in the longitudinal analyses AEC alone predicted tissue eosinophilia post treatment [115]. Overall, evidence suggests that AEC may have value in the assessment of EoE. However, a majority of studies are small and have not demonstrated sufficient accuracy for clinical use.

Given the shortcomings of using absolute eosinophil count as an EoE disease activity marker, an approach using eosinophil surface makers, eosinophil-derived proteins, and pro-eosinophil cytokine levels has also been evaluated. It has been hypothesized that circulating eosinophils display distinct phenotypes in various disorders. The markers of greatest interest in this area of research include eosinophilic cationic protein (ECP), eosinophil-derived neurotoxin (EDN), eotaxin-3, chemokine protein levels, chemokine receptor-3 on eosinophils (CCR3), and interleukin (IL)-5. ECP and EDN have shown promise in a number of studies while the other mediators have shown variable results in the literature, particularly in prospective studies [116, 117]. Some investigators have proposed increasing sensitivity and specificity of biomarkers by using them in combination (e.g., plasma AEC with EDN, or AEC and ECP, etc.) [112, 115]. However, larger and more longitudinal studies are needed to clarify the role of these biomarkers in the diagnosis and management of EoE. At present, there is inadequate data to support the use of serologic markers as a surrogate disease indicator in patients with EoE and it is not recommended to base therapeutic decisions on these markers.

Treatment Options

Currently, there are a number of treatment modalities for patients diagnosed with EoE (summarized in Table 6.4). These include proton pump inhibitors, corticosteroids, and elimination diets (elemental or empiric). These treatments can be used alone or in combination. None of the medical therapies discussed for EoE are approved by the US Food and Drug Administration, and thus they are used off label. For patients who develop advanced symptoms such as esophageal narrowing, endoscopic dilation can be used to alleviate symptoms. Treatment should be individualized according to each patient's concerns and lifestyles, prior therapy, and the severity of presentation. The efficacy of any therapy should be checked by a follow-up endoscopy after a 6- to 12-week initial course [6]. The goal is to improve symptoms and minimize the risk of complications from chronic inflammation. Although the impact of successful therapy on the natural history of EoE has not been elucidated, effective treatment has been shown to reverse long-term complications including subepithelial fibrosis [118]. Therefore, timely treatment is of utmost importance [54].

One endpoint of therapy is a reduction of esophageal eosinophilia to fewer than 15 eosinophils/HPF in biopsies, although a discrete cut-off has not been clearly recommended in clinical guidelines. Controversy remains regarding treatment endpoints and long-term management. Data suggests that patients may experience recurrence and even progression of symptoms when treatments are discontinued [83, 119]. This causes uncertainty regarding when to stop acute therapy. Current expert consensus recommends maintenance therapy for patients with evidence of chronic esophageal remodeling, a history of food impactions, severe symptoms, or rapid recurrence of symptoms while not undergoing therapy.

Table 6.4 Treatment options for eosinophilic esophagitis (EoE)[a]

Treatment Type	Therapy	Description/Drug dosing	Estimated effectiveness as induction therapy	Grade of Evidence
Pharmacologic	Proton Pump Inhibitors	Omeprazole or Esomeprazole: 20–40 mg twice a day (initial dose)	30–60%	Level 1A
	Swallowed topical corticosteroids	Fluticasone via metered dose inhaler: 880–1760 mcg/day typically in divided doses	55–80%	Level 1A
		Budesonide viscous suspension: 2 mg/day typically in divided doses		Level 1A
	Oral corticosteroids [b]	Prednisone 1–2 mg/kg/day		Level 1D
Diet	Elemental	Amino acid–based, allergen-free formula followed by slow reintroduction of foods	70–95%	Level 1B
	Empiric elimination diet	Six most commonly allergenic food groups (milk, wheat, egg, soy, peanut/tree nuts, shellfish/fish) are removed from the diet and individually reintroduced after a symptomatic and histologic response	55–75%	Level 1C
Conservative Dilation [c]	Through-the-scope balloon or bougie dilator	Minimum target diameter between 15 and 20 mm over multiple sessions	80–95% (symptomatic relief only)	Level 1C

[a]No therapies for eosinophilic esophagitis have been approved by the US Food and Drug Administration to date. The dosing listed in the table is largely based on the 2013 American College of Gastroenterology guidelines
[b]Reserved for refractory or severe cases
[c] Reserved for patients who relapse on dietary or pharmacologic therapy. First-line therapy if high-grade strictures are present

Pharmacologic Therapies

Proton Pump Inhibitors In prior years, a response to PPI trial was used to exclude PPI-REE or GERD in patients with esophageal eosinophilia. However, given recent data, experts agree that PPI-responsive esophageal eosinophilia should be regarded as a clinical sub-phenotype of EoE and not as a distinct entity [6, 66]. EoE and GERD are now thought to be different entities that likely coexist, either in an unrelated fashion or in a complex bidirectional relationship. A PPI trial is no longer required for EoE diagnosis but rather PPI therapy is recommended as a first-line treatment for EoE (grade of evidence 1A). Since the early 2000s, retrospective studies observed a clinical and histological response to PPI therapy in patients diagnosed with esophageal eosinophilia. Evidence now supports that PPIs likely improve EoE by conferring both acid-suppressive benefits as well as anti-inflammatory effects via cytokine release [120, 121]. A recent systematic review with meta-analysis found that PPI therapy induced histological remission in about 50% of the patients (defined as peak eosinophil counts <15 eosinophils/hpf) and clinical remission in approximately 60% [122]. Importantly, PPI improved symptoms and histologic measures even in patients without acid-reflux symptoms and negative pH testing [122]. Four different PPIs were included in the meta-analysis: lansoprazole, rabeprazole, omeprazole, and esomeprazole. However, some studies have not specified the type and doses of PPI used, which limits the ability to directly compare acid-suppressing agents. There was a trend toward increased efficacy when PPI was administered twice daily compared to once daily; however, this evidence is derived mainly from retrospective studies and case reports. The current recommendation for initiation of PPI therapy in adults with EoE is omeprazole 20 or 40 mg twice daily or equivalent for 8–12 weeks followed by both symptom assessment and endoscopy with biopsies to assess response [74].

While PPIs are efficacious in inducing remission in many EoE patients, their role in the long-term treatment remains unclear. They have been shown to maintain remission in patients who initially respond to the PPI therapy, however the optimal duration of PPI treatment is unclear since limited long-term data exists. The first study evaluating long-term PPI therapy was published in 2015 and included 75 adult patients [123]. The majority of patients (73%) maintained histological remission at least 1 year on a minimum effective clinical dose. A significant portion of patients (27%) had a loss of response on maintenance therapy but a majority regained histological remission after dose escalation. There were 16 patients who temporarily discontinued PPI therapy, and all had symptom and/or histological relapse, suggesting that a subgroup of patients may require maintenance high-dose PPI. It may be reasonable to adopt a treatment strategy of progressively tapering PPI dose to maintain disease remission [6].

Topical Corticosteroids Current guidelines recommend topical corticosteroids as first-line pharmacologic treatment of EoE (grade of evidence 1A). Several systematic reviews have found that both fluticasone propionate and budesonide induce histologic remission in pediatric and adult patients when compared to placebo [124–127]. Murali et al. found that topical steroids are effective in inducing complete histologic remission in 57.8% (OR 20.8) and partial histologic remission in 82.1% (OR 32.2) of patients when compared to 4.1% and 14.4% with placebo [124]. Another analysis by Chuang et al. also found significant reduction in esophageal eosinophil counts after topical steroid treatment when compared to controls. In subgroup analysis, histologic response was only significant in trials that excluded PPI responders [125]. Topical corticosteroids thus appear to be most effective in patients without a diagnosis of GERD and in patients with a normal pH status. While RCTs showed excellent histologic response to topical steroid therapy, clinical improvement did not reach statistical significance [124]. This may be in part due to a lack of a standard symptom-scoring tool among RCTs assessing clinical response. It also may also be explained by a lag time between histologic and clinical response, since topical therapy is more likely to be effective against the acute inflammatory changes of EoE rather than the advanced fibrostenotic disease which often causes symptoms.

A meta-analysis performed by Lipka et al. found no statistically significant difference between PPI, budesonide, and fluticasone for the treatment of EoE [127]. However, due to heterogeneity in the studies regarding inclusion criteria, daily dose (fluticasone either 440 µg or 880 µg twice daily, budesonide 1–4 mg daily depending on age), duration of treatment (2 weeks to 3 months), and delivery system (swallowed aerosolized formulation, oral suspension, viscous slurry, effervescent tablets), it is difficult to make direct comparisons. Two prospective randomized controlled trials have been completed to compare PPI versus topical corticosteroids in adult patients with an EoE. The first by Peterson et al. in 2010 compared an 8-week esomeprazole (40 mg daily) treatment to aerosolized, swallowed fluticasone (440 mcg twice a day) found no differences between dysphagia symptoms or magnitude of eosinophil infiltration between the two treatment arms [128]. The second was a similar but larger study of 42 patients by Moawad et al. in 2013, which also found that patients treated with esomeprazole 40 mg once daily had similar histologic and clinical response to patients treated with fluticasone 440 mcg twice daily [129]. Poor histologic response was noted in patients with GERD who were randomized to the topical steroid arm. Due to low cost, good safety profile, convenience, and possibility of concomitant GERD, some experts recommend the consideration of PPI therapy early or as initial treatment [74, 130].

Topical steroids are swallowed and can be administered in an aerosolized or slurry form. Acceptable regimens include fluticasone given by mouth with a metered-dose inhaler (without a spacer) and swallowed budesonide administered as either an oral viscous preparation or nebulized [68]. A single prospective, open-label RCT compared budesonide 1 mg twice daily for 8 weeks given in nebulized and viscous preparations. Complete histologic remission was higher (64% vs. 27%) in the oral viscous budesonide group [131]. It was suspected that drug to mucosal contact time could be an important factor in treatment outcomes. A recent 12-week RCT using a novel muco-adherent topical oral formulation of budesonide reported that 31% of patients in the treatment group achieved <1 eos/hpf vs none in the placebo group [132].

The duration of maintenance treatment and optimal dose of topical corticosteroid necessary to keep patients in remission are yet to be clearly defined. An RCT following 28 patients for 50 weeks showed that low dose swallowed budesonide (0.25 mg twice daily) maintained EoE in remission (<5 eos/hpf) in 36% of patients compared to 0% placebo group [133]. Currently in steroid-responsive patients, long-term therapy with topical corticosteroids may be considered with tapering at the discretion of a gastroenterologist. Data supports the use of both fluticasone and budesonide [126, 132]. Overall, topical steroids are well tolerated with no serious adverse events. Esophageal candidiasis is the most common side effect, effecting between 5% and 26% of patients [124]. Adrenal suppression has been a concern, but studies have not shown evidence of adrenal suppression after an 8–12 week course of topical corticosteroids [134, 135].

Systemic Corticosteroids Systemic steroids have shown efficacy in achieving remission in EoE [136], however they do not appear to have a benefit over swallowed corticosteroids. Given the greater side effect profile of systemic steroids, they are not recommended routinely for treatment in EoE (grade of evidence 1D). A randomized, controlled trial comparing oral prednisone (1 mg/kg/dose twice a day) to topical fluticasone (2 puffs 4 times/day; 110 mg per puff for ages 1–10 years and 220 mg per puff for ages 11 years or older) for 12 weeks demonstrated a greater degree of histologic improvement in the oral agent arm but no significant difference in clinical improvement. Despite starting to taper at week 4, 40% of patients in the oral prednisone group experienced systemic adverse effects (hyperphagia, weight gain, and/or cushingoid features) while the topical steroid group only reported esophageal candidiasis in 15% of patients [119]. In practice, systemic corticosteroids are reserved for refractory or severe cases in which a rapid response is needed. Since these medications have potential for significant toxicity, long-term use of systemic steroids is not recommended.

Experimental Pharmacologic Agents Biologic therapy is emerging as an important potential treatment option for EoE. These include anti–IL-5 monoclonal antibodies (mAb), anti–IL-13 antibodies, and an anti–IL-4 receptor blocker. IL-5 is involved in the maturation, recruitment, and activation of eosinophils. RCTs examining the efficacy of Reslizumab and Mepolizumab, antibodies against IL-5, have shown significant reduction in peak esophageal eosinophil counts although most patients studied did not achieve <5 cells/hpf (grade of evidence 1C, 1D, respectively) [137–139]. Overexpression of IL-13 has been linked to esophageal eosinophilia and tissue remodeling [51]. A mAb against IL-13, QAX576, has been evaluated in a preliminary phase II study of 23 patients with EoE refractory to PPI therapy. The study demonstrated that mean eosinophil counts significantly decreased by 60% with QAX576 treatment as compared with 23% with placebo and the effect was sustained for an additional 6 months in a majority of responders. It also showed improvement in the expression of genetic markers for tissue remodeling, esophageal barrier function, and eosinophil chemotaxis (grade of evidence 1D) [140]. More recently, Hirano et al. conducted a phase II trial with 99 patients to evaluate the efficacy and safety of RPC4046, another mAb against IL-13 (grade of evidence 1D). This study found 25% of EoE patients in the 180 mg RPC4046 group and 20% in the 360 mg RPC4046 group had <6 peak eos/hpf after 16 weeks of treatment compared with 0% in the placebo group. The study also reported statistically significant reduction in the total EREFS score between treatment and placebo arms. It is also noteworthy that approximately half of the enrolled patients were categorized as being steroid refractory and a subgroup analysis found greater reduction in dysphagia symptoms in this subset of patients [141]. IL-4 is another cytokine that has been observed at increased levels in patients with EoE. It shares a common receptor with IL-13 and is a well-described Th2 cytokine that facilitates B-cell class switching to IgE [50]. An anti–IL-4 receptor mAb, Dupilumab, recently approved for the treatment of adults with moderate to severe atopic dermatitis, is being studied for treatment in EoE. In a phase 2, multicenter trial in adults with EoE, preliminary results showed significant improvement in symptoms of dysphagia, esophageal eosinophil counts, and endoscopic features (grade of evidence 1D) [142]. A phase 3 clinical trial is currently being conducted. Overall, promising results from clinical trials are emerging for biologic agents, however their place in the treatment algorithm for EoE has yet to be determined.

Dietary Therapies

Food antigens are primary mediators of the pathogenesis of EoE, and because of this the systematic elimination of particular foods can be an efficacious treatment for EoE. Dietary therapy can be a particularly attractive treatment option for young patients who may have a long disease duration and may want to avoid potential medication side effects. When undergoing EoE treatment via an elimination diet, patients first undergo a baseline endoscopy with biopsies. This is followed by an induction phase consisting of a strict diet for a set period of time. The endoscopy and biopsies are then repeated to assess if histologic remission has been achieved. If the patient is in histologic remission, they then begin a systematic reintroduction of foods over weeks to months, with multiple repeat endoscopies at each stage to determine the trigger antigens. The goal of dietary treatment is to therefore identify possible triggers, eliminate them from the diet permanently, and induce remission of EoE without the need for pharmacologic agents. A meta-analysis of all published retrospective and prospective studies on all dietary therapies for EoE in adult and pediatric patients showed a histologic remission rate of about 65% [143].

Elemental Diet The role of an elemental diet has also been studied in EoE. This is a liquid diet composed of soluble basic nutrient such as amino acids, fats, sugars, vitamins, and minerals. It does not contain intact proteins, since these are thought to be common antigen triggers. In an initial small study of 10 pediatric patients who were refractory to PPI therapy, it was found to be efficacious. An exclusively elemental formula diet for 6 weeks resulted in significant histologic and clinical improvement [144]. Numerous subsequent studies in pediatric patients [83, 145–147] and two studies in adults [148, 149] have supported these findings (grade of evidence 1B). Taken together, these studies showed partial or complete histologic response rates between 83% and 97% for pediatric patients and between 72% and 96% for adult patients. Despite good histologic outcomes, symptomatic improvement was variable and there was a high patient drop-out/noncompliance rate (38%). While no significant weight loss, electrolyte abnormalities, or adverse outcomes have been noted, the inability to intake solid foods has a marked negative impact on quality of life. The elemental diet is reported to be superior to other types of dietary treatments for EoE [143, 147]. However, major drawbacks of this therapy include poor patient adherence due to poor palatability and high cost of elemental formulas. Additionally, a greater number of endoscopies are required during the lengthy food reintroduction process to identify specific triggers. Oral reintroduction starts with the least allergenic foods (vegetables, fruits) to most allergenic foods (milk, wheat, and egg) and typically requires several months to years. Due to the practical limitations of elemental diets, experts recommend consideration of elemental diets only after failure of properly performed medical treatment and/or elimination diet [6, 68].

Allergy Testing-Directed Elimination Diet An elimination diet guided by allergy testing has also been of interest in EoE treatment. In a directed elimination diet, patients who are found to have allergies to certain foods by SPT and/or APT are instructed to eliminate those foods only. This strategy was initially described in 2002 by Spergel et al. in a study of 24 pediatric patients which resulted in 49% histologic remission and significant symptom improvement [150]. The same group conducted similar analyses in subsequent years, finding efficacy in about 50% of patients [41, 151]. However, other studies have found lower response rates (24–40%) in pediatric patients [152, 153]. For adults, the data is limited but shows low response rates, little clinical benefit, and poor correlation between allergy testing treatment results [111, 143, 154–156] (grade of evidence 3). Overall, food allergy testing-based elimination diet induces histologic remission in less than one-third of adult patients. The first study to investigate the efficacy of directed diets in adult EoE patients was conducted in 2006 that included only six patients. The investigators found no change in symptoms for EoE patients undergoing a 6-week allergen-specific elimination diet of wheat, rye, and barley [111]. Subsequent studies assessed histologic response in adult patients with EoE and found response rates of 22–36% [143, 154, 155]. Furthermore, several studies showed that food elimination diets were equally effective in patients with EoE despite negative skin prick results [39, 156]. These studies demonstrated extremely low concordance between SPT results and offending foods causing EoE symptoms. The inability of skin testing to identify specific food hypersensitivities may suggest that the antigenic response is localized to the esophagus and skin is not an appropriate surrogate.

In addition to skin testing, investigators have also noted that most EoE patients have high levels of food-specific IgE levels [157]. Studies have therefore attempted to understand the applicability of using serum allergen-specific IgE levels to help targeted diets. A small case series and one prospective study have shown histologic response with specific IgE- directed diets, but the response result was similar to the traditional 6-food elimination diet [158, 159]. Given the low level of evidence and heterogenous results, allergy testing has limited application in the current management of EoE patients.

Empiric Elimination Diet

In an empiric elimination diet, foods most commonly associated with allergies and esophageal mucosal injury are removed from diet without relying on allergy testing. Because the majority of table foods are allowed, this diet is more practical and palatable for patients. The six-food elimination diet (SFED) and the four-food elimination diet (FFED) are the most common forms of this diet and are recommended for a duration of 4–8 weeks [68]. The SFED removes common dietary antigens including cow's milk, egg, soy, wheat, peanuts/tree nuts, and fish/shellfish [144, 160–162]. SFED was originally studied in children as an alternative to the elemental diet. Kagalwalla et al. first demonstrated that 74% of pediatric subjects who complied with SFED achieved histologic remission (defined as ≤10 eos/HPF) compared to the 88% in the elemental diet arm of the study [161]. SFED has since been corroborated by several other pediatric studies [143, 147, 162, 163] and shown efficacy in adults with EoE [39, 143, 156] (grade of evidence 1C). A prospective study found similar response rates (70%) to SFED in adults using the same histologic criteria and also reported that dysphagia symptom scores decreased in 94% of patients after SFED [156]. A recent meta-analysis showed a combined effectiveness of SFED of 72% with good homogeneity regardless of the patient's age [143]. Additionally, a prospective study found that during the reintroduction challenge, one or two food triggers were identified in 35% and 30% of patients. Cow's milk was the most common food antigen (61.9%), followed by wheat (28.6%), eggs (26.2%), and legumes (23.8%) [39]. In all patients who continued to avoid the offending foods, histopathologic and clinical EoE remission was maintained for up to 3 years [39]. However, one study found that 43% of adult patients who achieved and maintained remission on the elimination diet did eventually stop adhering to the diet [164]. The main reason patients cited for stopping the diet was social/lifestyle barriers. To address this, variations of the SFED with even less dietary restriction has been studied.

Other dietary strategies for EoE include a 4-food elimination diet, elimination of cow's milk, and gluten-free diets. The 4-food group elimination diet removes dairy, wheat, egg, and legumes (the four most common identified triggers). When evaluated in a prospective multicenter study of 52 adult patients, the FFED achieved clinicopathologic remission in 54% of adults [165]. Patients who failed FFED were either rescued with SFED or topical steroids. SFED was effective in one-third of FFED non-responders and fluticasone propionate (400 mg bid for 6 weeks) induced remission in the rest of non-responders [165]. Cow's milk and wheat were again noted to be the most common food triggers. Accordingly, a step-up approach has been hypothesized as another dietary treatment strategy. This involves first eliminating the one or two most common food triggers and subsequently eliminating other common triggers in non-responders. This step-up approach offers more convenience from a lifestyle perspective and may also reduce the number of endoscopic procedures the patient has to undergo. Data on these approaches is still limited. A recent prospective multicenter study conducted in pediatric and adult patients showed that a two-food elimination diet (animal milk and gluten-containing cereals) reported a histologic remission rate of 40% [166].

Currently, there are no controlled comparative studies between dietary therapy and topical steroids. The choice of initial treatment approach should be individualized and based on discussion with the patient. A successful dietary approach requires a highly motivated patient and physician. Collaboration with a registered dietician or allergist to provide patient education and dietary counseling may improve the success of the elimination diet approach.

Endoscopic Treatment

Esophageal dilation can be effective in managing symptoms from EoE complications such as esophageal rings, strictures, and stenoses [74, 167]. Early case reports in the 1990s and 2000s raised concerns of high rates of perforation [168, 169], however subsequent larger studies confirmed that esophageal dilation is a safe and efficacious procedure when performed carefully by an experienced endoscopist (grade of evidence 1C). Three large retrospective studies published in 2010 provided significant data that supported the safety and efficacy of endoscopic dilations in EoE [170–172]. They described a total of 256 EoE patients dilated with either Savary bougies or through-the-scope (TTS) balloons. For clinical improvement, dilations required a mean of 1.2–2.5 sessions to a target esophageal diameter of 16–17 mm (pre-dilation diameter ranging from 4 to 15 mm). The most common postprocedural complaint was retrosternal pain (74%) and no severe post-procedural complications such as perforation were reported. There was a high degree of patient acceptance and all patients were agreeable to repeat dilation if necessary. Impressively, 83–91% of patients experienced dysphagia relief for an average duration of greater than 1 year [170, 171]. A recent meta-analysis published in 2017 included 27 studies and 845 adult and pediatric EoE patients. It showed a clinical improvement in 95% of patients with a minimum target diameter between 15 and 20 mm and a median duration of symptom relief was 12 months [167]. Major complications were rare: perforation (0.38%), hemorrhage (0.05%), and hospitalization (0.67%) and no deaths were reported in the studies. Mucosal tears are expected as the goal of dilation is to disrupt fibrotic remodeling and increase the functional lumen. The improved safety outcomes in more recent studies compared to early reports could be a result of more judicious use of dilation in EoE patients with a strategy of performing less aggressive dilations over more sessions.

While dilation is efficacious in patients with advanced fibrostenotic disease, the optimal time to offer dilation as therapy for EoE patients with dysphagia is still unclear. There has only been one randomized, blinded, controlled trial assessing the role of dilation in adults with EoE [173]. In the study by Kavitt et al., patients with newly diagnosed EoE were randomized to dilation or no dilation at the time of endoscopy. Patients in both the dilation and control arms then received fluticasone and dexlansoprazole for 2 months. To assess outcome, dysphagia score was assessed at 30 and 60 days post-intervention. The authors found that in patients without severe strictures, esophageal dilation followed by pharmacologic treatment was not superior to medical therapy alone. They concluded that in patients with symptomatic EoE with mild to moderate features, dilation may not be necessary as initial strategy and they may do equally well with initiation of pharmacologic management.

Most recent expert consensus and guidelines support a role for conservative dilation as an add-on therapy in symptomatic patients with persistent strictures despite medical or dietary treatment [6, 68]. However, if a critical stricture or history of recurrent food impaction exists then dilation can be considered for first-line therapeutic approach. Currently, a standard esophageal dilation protocol for EoE does not exist, so techniques are based on individual/institutional preference. Both balloon dilators and bougie dilators are used and physician choice is usually guided by the relative benefit each method confers. For example, a benefit of using a through-the-scope balloon dilator is that esophageal mucosa can be inspected between serial dilations without withdrawing and reintroducing the endoscope. On the other hand, a benefit of the bougie dilator is that longer length strictures or multiple sequential strictures can be dilated.

After achieving clinical improvement and optimal esophageal diameter, repeat endoscopic dilatations should be considered only when symptoms begin to recur. The role of dilation as a primary monotherapy in EoE has not been studied. It is important to recognize that dilation of esophageal strictures does not impact the eosinophil burden or inflammatory process of EoE and therefore will not modify the natural course of disease [170]. All EoE patients should therefore receive a treatment targeted to cure esophageal inflammation plus endoscopic dilation if applicable [6].

Conclusion

Eosinophilic esophagitis (EoE) is a benign chronic immune-mediated disorder that carries a significant burden of disease. Current data suggests that the global incidence and prevalence of EoE is rising, particularly in the Western world, and EoE is now recognized as a leading cause of food impaction and dysphagia. As of 2014, the annual health-care burden was estimated to be $1.4 billion in the USA [174]. Recognition of clinical signs, along with laboratory and endoscopic findings, is critical for timely diagnosis and management. We suggest an algorithm for evaluation and treatment (Fig. 6.2). Current treatment options can improve patient quality of life and reduce long-term EoE complications. Significant progress has also been made in understanding the underlying genetic and environmental mechanisms of EoE. Several novel methods to evaluate disease activity and emerging therapies that target inflammatory pathways are under investigation. As diagnostic criteria and treatment endpoints continue to be refined, newer options will undoubtedly play an important role in clinical practice.

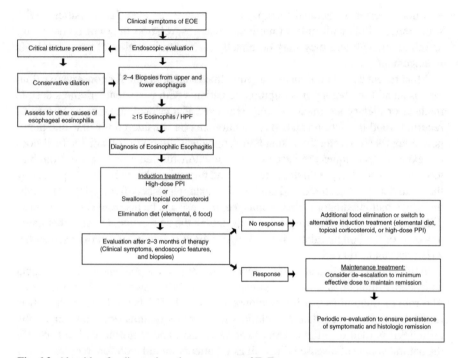

Fig. 6.2 Algorithm for diagnosis and management of EoE

References

1. Dellon ES, Hirano I. Epidemiology and natural history of eosinophilic esophagitis. Gastroenterology. 2018;154(2):319–32. e3
2. Arias A, et al. Systematic review with meta-analysis: the incidence and prevalence of eosinophilic oesophagitis in children and adults in population-based studies. Aliment Pharmacol Ther. 2016;43(1):3–15.
3. Kidambi T, et al. Temporal trends in the relative prevalence of dysphagia etiologies from 1999-2009. World J Gastroenterol. 2012;18(32):4335–41.
4. Dellon ES, et al. The increasing incidence and prevalence of eosinophilic oesophagitis outpaces changes in endoscopic and biopsy practice: national population-based estimates from Denmark. Aliment Pharmacol Ther. 2015;41(7):662–70.
5. Prasad GA, et al. Epidemiology of eosinophilic esophagitis over three decades in Olmsted County, Minnesota. Clin Gastroenterol Hepatol. 2009;7(10):1055–61.
6. Lucendo AJ, et al. Guidelines on eosinophilic esophagitis: evidence-based statements and recommendations for diagnosis and management in children and adults. United European Gastroenterol J. 2017;5(3):335–58.
7. Mansoor E, Cooper GS. The 2010-2015 prevalence of eosinophilic esophagitis in the USA: a population-based study. Dig Dis Sci. 2016;61(10):2928–34.
8. Shaheen NJ, et al. Natural history of eosinophilic esophagitis: a systematic review of epidemiology and disease course. Dis Esophagus. 2018;31(8)
9. Kapel RC, et al. Eosinophilic esophagitis: a prevalent disease in the United States that affects all age groups. Gastroenterology. 2008;134(5):1316–21.

10. Markowitz JE, Clayton SB. Eosinophilic esophagitis in children and adults. Gastrointest Endosc Clin N Am. 2018;28(1):59–75.
11. Maradey-Romero C, et al. The 2011-2014 prevalence of eosinophilic oesophagitis in the elderly amongst 10 million patients in the United States. Aliment Pharmacol Ther. 2015;41(10):1016–22.
12. Furuta GT, et al. Eosinophilic esophagitis in children and adults: a systematic review and consensus recommendations for diagnosis and treatment. Gastroenterology. 2007;133(4):1342–63.
13. Sperry SL, et al. Influence of race and gender on the presentation of eosinophilic esophagitis. Am J Gastroenterol. 2012;107(2):215–21.
14. Franciosi JP, et al. A case-control study of sociodemographic and geographic characteristics of 335 children with eosinophilic esophagitis. Clin Gastroenterol Hepatol. 2009;7(4):415–9.
15. Lipowska AM, Kavitt RT. Demographic features of eosinophilic esophagitis. Gastrointest Endosc Clin N Am. 2018;28(1):27–33.
16. Lynch KL, et al. Gender is a determinative factor in the initial clinical presentation of eosinophilic esophagitis. Dis Esophagus. 2016;29(2):174–8.
17. Moawad FJ, et al. Effects of race and sex on features of eosinophilic esophagitis. Clin Gastroenterol Hepatol. 2016;14(1):23–30.
18. Kim S, Kim S, Sheikh J. Prevalence of eosinophilic esophagitis in a population-based cohort from Southern California. J Allergy Clin Immunol Pract. 2015;3(6):978–9.
19. Yu C, et al. The prevalence of biopsy-proven eosinophilic esophagitis in hispanics undergoing endoscopy is infrequent compared to caucasians: a cross-sectional study. Dig Dis Sci. 2017;62(12):3511–6.
20. Dellon ES. Epidemiology of eosinophilic esophagitis. Gastroenterol Clin N Am. 2014;43(2):201–18.
21. Cherian S, Smith NM, Forbes DA. Rapidly increasing prevalence of eosinophilic oesophagitis in Western Australia. Arch Dis Child. 2006;91(12):1000–4.
22. Kinoshita Y, et al. Systematic review: eosinophilic esophagitis in Asian countries. World J Gastroenterol. 2015;21(27):8433–40.
23. Ma X, et al. Prevalence of esophageal eosinophilia and eosinophilic esophagitis in adults: a population-based endoscopic study in Shanghai, China. Dig Dis Sci. 2015;60(6):1716–23.
24. Fujiwara Y, et al. A multicenter study on the prevalence of eosinophilic esophagitis and PPI-responsive esophageal eosinophilic infiltration. Intern Med. 2012;51(23):3235–9.
25. Jensen ET, et al. Esophageal eosinophilia is increased in rural areas with low population density: results from a national pathology database. Am J Gastroenterol. 2014;109(5):668–75.
26. Hurrell JM, Genta RM, Dellon ES. Prevalence of esophageal eosinophilia varies by climate zone in the United States. Am J Gastroenterol. 2012;107(5):698–706.
27. Fogg MI, Ruchelli E, Spergel JM. Pollen and eosinophilic esophagitis. J Allergy Clin Immunol. 2003;112(4):796–7.
28. Collins MH, et al. Clinical, pathologic, and molecular characterization of familial eosinophilic esophagitis compared with sporadic cases. Clin Gastroenterol Hepatol. 2008;6(6):621–9.
29. Alexander ES, et al. Twin and family studies reveal strong environmental and weaker genetic cues explaining heritability of eosinophilic esophagitis. J Allergy Clin Immunol. 2014;134(5):1084–1092 e1.
30. Litosh VA, et al. Calpain-14 and its association with eosinophilic esophagitis. J Allergy Clin Immunol. 2017;139(6):1762–1771 e7.
31. Martin LJ, et al. Eosinophilic esophagitis (EoE) genetic susceptibility is mediated by synergistic interactions between EoE-specific and general atopic disease loci. J Allergy Clin Immunol. 2018;141(5):1690–8.
32. Blanchard C, et al. Eotaxin-3 and a uniquely conserved gene-expression profile in eosinophilic esophagitis. J Clin Invest. 2006;116(2):536–47.
33. Lim EJ, et al. Epigenetic regulation of the IL-13-induced human eotaxin-3 gene by CREB-binding protein-mediated histone 3 acetylation. J Biol Chem. 2011;286(15):13193–204.

34. Kottyan LC, et al. Genome-wide association analysis of eosinophilic esophagitis provides insight into the tissue specificity of this allergic disease. Nat Genet. 2014;46(8):895–900.
35. Swoger JM, Weiler CR, Arora AS. Eosinophilic esophagitis: is it all allergies? Mayo Clin Proc. 2007;82(12):1541–9.
36. Rayapudi M, et al. Indoor insect allergens are potent inducers of experimental eosinophilic esophagitis in mice. J Leukoc Biol. 2010;88(2):337–46.
37. Attwood SE, et al. Esophageal eosinophilia with dysphagia. A distinct clinicopathologic syndrome. Dig Dis Sci. 1993;38(1):109–16.
38. Assa'ad AH, et al. Pediatric patients with eosinophilic esophagitis: an 8-year follow-up. J Allergy Clin Immunol. 2007;119(3):731–8.
39. Lucendo AJ, et al. Empiric 6-food elimination diet induced and maintained prolonged remission in patients with adult eosinophilic esophagitis: a prospective study on the food cause of the disease. J Allergy Clin Immunol. 2013;131(3):797–804.
40. Vicario M, et al. Local B cells and IgE production in the oesophageal mucosa in eosinophilic oesophagitis. Gut. 2010;59(1):12–20.
41. Spergel JM, et al. Treatment of eosinophilic esophagitis with specific food elimination diet directed by a combination of skin prick and patch tests. Ann Allergy Asthma Immunol. 2005;95(4):336–43.
42. Loizou D, et al. A pilot study of omalizumab in eosinophilic esophagitis. PLoS One. 2015;10(3):e0113483.
43. Clayton F, et al. Eosinophilic esophagitis in adults is associated with IgG4 and not mediated by IgE. Gastroenterology. 2014;147(3):602–9.
44. Mishra A, et al. Critical role for adaptive T cell immunity in experimental eosinophilic esophagitis in mice. J Leukoc Biol. 2007;81(4):916–24.
45. Mishra A, et al. An etiological role for aeroallergens and eosinophils in experimental esophagitis. J Clin Invest. 2001;107(1):83–90.
46. Blanchard C, et al. IL-13 involvement in eosinophilic esophagitis: transcriptome analysis and reversibility with glucocorticoids. J Allergy Clin Immunol. 2007;120(6):1292–300.
47. Kc K, Rothenberg ME, Sherrill JD. In vitro model for studying esophageal epithelial differentiation and allergic inflammatory responses identifies keratin involvement in eosinophilic esophagitis. PLoS One. 2015;10(6):e0127755.
48. Rothenberg ME, et al. Common variants at 5q22 associate with pediatric eosinophilic esophagitis. Nat Genet. 2010;42(4):289–91.
49. Davis BP, et al. Eosinophilic esophagitis-linked calpain 14 is an IL-13-induced protease that mediates esophageal epithelial barrier impairment. JCI Insight. 2016;1(4):e86355.
50. Blanchard C, et al. A striking local esophageal cytokine expression profile in eosinophilic esophagitis. J Allergy Clin Immunol. 2011;127(1):208–17, 217 e1–7.
51. Zuo L, et al. IL-13 induces esophageal remodeling and gene expression by an eosinophil-independent, IL-13R alpha 2-inhibited pathway. J Immunol. 2010;185(1):660–9.
52. Kavitt RT, Hirano I, Vaezi MF. Diagnosis and treatment of eosinophilic esophagitis in adults. Am J Med. 2016;129(9):924–34.
53. Dellon ES, Liacouras CA. Advances in clinical management of eosinophilic esophagitis. Gastroenterology. 2014;147(6):1238–54.
54. Dellon ES, et al. A phenotypic analysis shows that eosinophilic esophagitis is a progressive fibrostenotic disease. Gastrointest Endosc. 2014;79(4):577–85 e4.
55. Safroneeva E, et al. Symptoms have modest accuracy in detecting endoscopic and histologic remission in adults with eosinophilic esophagitis. Gastroenterology. 2016;150(3):581–590 e4.
56. DeBrosse CW, et al. Long-term outcomes in pediatric-onset esophageal eosinophilia. J Allergy Clin Immunol. 2011;128(1):132–8.
57. Menard-Katcher P, et al. The natural history of eosinophilic oesophagitis in the transition from childhood to adulthood. Aliment Pharmacol Ther. 2013;37(1):114–21.

58. Warners MJ, et al. Systematic review: disease activity indices in eosinophilic esophagitis. Am J Gastroenterol. 2017;112(11):1658–69.
59. Dellon ES, et al. Development and field testing of a novel patient-reported outcome measure of dysphagia in patients with eosinophilic esophagitis. Aliment Pharmacol Ther. 2013;38(6):634–42.
60. Schoepfer AM, et al. Development and validation of a symptom-based activity index for adults with eosinophilic esophagitis. Gastroenterology. 2014;147(6):1255–66 e21.
61. Gonzalez-Cervera J, et al. Association between atopic manifestations and eosinophilic esophagitis: a systematic review and meta-analysis. Ann Allergy Asthma Immunol. 2017;118(5):582–590 e2.
62. Dellon ES. Diagnosis and management of eosinophilic esophagitis. Clin Gastroenterol Hepatol. 2012;10(10):1066–78.
63. Abonia JP, et al. High prevalence of eosinophilic esophagitis in patients with inherited connective tissue disorders. J Allergy Clin Immunol. 2013;132(2):378–86.
64. Jensen ET, et al. Increased risk of esophageal eosinophilia and eosinophilic esophagitis in patients with active celiac disease on biopsy. Clin Gastroenterol Hepatol. 2015;13(8):1426–31.
65. Johnsson M, et al. Distinctive blood eosinophilic phenotypes and cytokine patterns in eosinophilic esophagitis, inflammatory bowel disease and airway allergy. J Innate Immun. 2011;3(6):594–604.
66. Dellon ES, et al. Updated international consensus diagnostic criteria for eosinophilic esophagitis: proceedings of the AGREE conference. Gastroenterology. 2018;155(4):1022–1033 e10.
67. Spechler SJ, Genta RM, Souza RF. Thoughts on the complex relationship between gastroesophageal reflux disease and eosinophilic esophagitis. Am J Gastroenterol. 2007;102(6):1301–6.
68. Dellon ES, et al. ACG clinical guideline: Evidenced based approach to the diagnosis and management of esophageal eosinophilia and eosinophilic esophagitis (EoE). Am J Gastroenterol. 2013;108(5):679–92; quiz 693.
69. Eluri S, Dellon ES. Proton pump inhibitor-responsive oesophageal eosinophilia and eosinophilic oesophagitis: more similarities than differences. Curr Opin Gastroenterol. 2015;31(4):309–15.
70. Warners MJ, et al. PPI-responsive esophageal eosinophilia cannot be distinguished from eosinophilic esophagitis by endoscopic signs. Eur J Gastroenterol Hepatol. 2015;27(5):506–11.
71. Dellon ES, et al. Markers of eosinophilic inflammation for diagnosis of eosinophilic esophagitis and proton pump inhibitor-responsive esophageal eosinophilia: a prospective study. Clin Gastroenterol Hepatol. 2014;12(12):2015–22.
72. Lucendo AJ, et al. Dual response to dietary/topical steroid and proton pump inhibitor therapy in adult patients with eosinophilic esophagitis. J Allergy Clin Immunol. 2016;137(3):931–4 e2.
73. Kim HP, et al. The prevalence and diagnostic utility of endoscopic features of eosinophilic esophagitis: a meta-analysis. Clin Gastroenterol Hepatol. 2012;10(9):988–96 e5.
74. Liacouras CA, et al. Eosinophilic esophagitis: updated consensus recommendations for children and adults. J Allergy Clin Immunol. 2011;128(1):3–20 e6; quiz 21–2.
75. Dellon ES, et al. Variability in diagnostic criteria for eosinophilic esophagitis: a systematic review. Am J Gastroenterol. 2007;102(10):2300–13.
76. Hirano I, et al. Endoscopic assessment of the oesophageal features of cosinophilic ocsophagitis: validation of a novel classification and grading system. Gut. 2013;62(4):489–95.
77. Lucendo AJ, et al. Endoscopic, bioptic, and manometric findings in eosinophilic esophagitis before and after steroid therapy: a case series. Endoscopy. 2007;39(9):765–71.
78. Dellon ES, et al. Accuracy of the eosinophilic esophagitis endoscopic reference score in diagnosis and determining response to treatment. Clin Gastroenterol Hepatol. 2016;14(1):31–9.
79. Rodriguez-Sanchez J, et al. The endoscopic reference score shows modest accuracy to predict either clinical or histological activity in adult patients with eosinophilic oesophagitis. Aliment Pharmacol Ther. 2017;45(2):300–9.

80. van Rhijn BD, et al. The endoscopic reference score shows modest accuracy to predict histologic remission in adult patients with eosinophilic esophagitis. Neurogastroenterol Motil. 2016;28(11):1714–22.

81. Nielsen JA, et al. The optimal number of biopsy fragments to establish a morphologic diagnosis of eosinophilic esophagitis. Am J Gastroenterol. 2014;109(4):515–20.

82. Dellon ES, et al. Distribution and variability of esophageal eosinophilia in patients undergoing upper endoscopy. Mod Pathol. 2015;28(3):383–90.

83. Liacouras CA, et al. Eosinophilic esophagitis: a 10-year experience in 381 children. Clin Gastroenterol Hepatol. 2005;3(12):1198–206.

84. Saffari H, et al. Patchy eosinophil distributions in an esophagectomy specimen from a patient with eosinophilic esophagitis: implications for endoscopic biopsy. J Allergy Clin Immunol. 2012;130(3):798–800.

85. Gonsalves N, et al. Histopathologic variability and endoscopic correlates in adults with eosinophilic esophagitis. Gastrointest Endosc. 2006;64(3):313–9.

86. Shah A, et al. Histopathologic variability in children with eosinophilic esophagitis. Am J Gastroenterol. 2009;104(3):716–21.

87. Collins MH. Histopathologic features of eosinophilic esophagitis and eosinophilic gastrointestinal diseases. Gastroenterol Clin N Am. 2014;43(2):257–68.

88. Reed CC, Dellon ES. Eosinophilic esophagitis. Med Clin North Am. 2019;103(1):29–42.

89. Aceves SS. Tissue remodeling in patients with eosinophilic esophagitis: what lies beneath the surface? J Allergy Clin Immunol. 2011;128(5):1047–9.

90. Ates F, et al. Mucosal impedance discriminates GERD from non-GERD conditions. Gastroenterology. 2015;148(2):334–43.

91. van Rhijn BD, et al. Oesophageal baseline impedance values are decreased in patients with eosinophilic oesophagitis. United European Gastroenterol J. 2013;1(4):242–8.

92. van Rhijn BD, et al. Proton pump inhibitors partially restore mucosal integrity in patients with proton pump inhibitor-responsive esophageal eosinophilia but not eosinophilic esophagitis. Clin Gastroenterol Hepatol. 2014;12(11):1815–23 e2.

93. Katzka DA, et al. Endoscopic mucosal impedance measurements correlate with eosinophilia and dilation of intercellular spaces in patients with eosinophilic esophagitis. Clin Gastroenterol Hepatol. 2015;13(7):1242–1248 e1.

94. Carlson DA. Functional lumen imaging probe: the FLIP side of esophageal disease. Curr Opin Gastroenterol. 2016;32(4):310–8.

95. Kwiatek MA, et al. Mechanical properties of the esophagus in eosinophilic esophagitis. Gastroenterology. 2011;140(1):82–90.

96. Nicodeme F, et al. Esophageal distensibility as a measure of disease severity in patients with eosinophilic esophagitis. Clin Gastroenterol Hepatol. 2013;11(9):1101–1107 e1.

97. Hirano I, Pandolfino JE, Boeckxstaens GE. Functional lumen imaging probe for the management of esophageal disorders: expert review from the clinical practice updates committee of the AGA Institute. Clin Gastroenterol Hepatol. 2017;15(3):325–34.

98. Kephart GM, et al. Marked deposition of eosinophil-derived neurotoxin in adult patients with eosinophilic esophagitis. Am J Gastroenterol. 2010;105(2):298–307.

99. Mueller S, et al. Eosinophil infiltration and degranulation in oesophageal mucosa from adult patients with eosinophilic oesophagitis: a retrospective and comparative study on pathological biopsy. J Clin Pathol. 2006;59(11):1175–80.

100. Furuta GT, et al. The oesophageal string test: a novel, minimally invasive method measures mucosal inflammation in eosinophilic oesophagitis. Gut. 2013;62(10):1395–405.

101. Ross-Innes CS, et al. Evaluation of a minimally invasive cell sampling device coupled with assessment of trefoil factor 3 expression for diagnosing Barrett's esophagus: a multi-center case-control study. PLoS Med. 2015;12(1):e1001780.

102. Katzka DA, et al. Accuracy and safety of the cytosponge for assessing histologic activity in eosinophilic esophagitis: a two-center study. Am J Gastroenterol. 2017;112(10):1538–44.

103. Boyce JA, et al. Guidelines for the diagnosis and management of food allergy in the United States: summary of the NIAID-sponsored expert panel report. J Allergy Clin Immunol. 2010;126(6):1105–18.
104. Heine RG, et al. Proposal for a standardized interpretation of the atopy patch test in children with atopic dermatitis and suspected food allergy. Pediatr Allergy Immunol. 2006;17(3):213–7.
105. Warners MJ, et al. Abnormal responses to local esophageal food allergen injections in adult patients with eosinophilic esophagitis. Gastroenterology. 2018;154(1):57–60 e2.
106. Hines BT, et al. Minimally invasive biomarker studies in eosinophilic esophagitis: a systematic review. Ann Allergy Asthma Immunol. 2018;121(2):218–28.
107. Straumann A, et al. Pediatric and adult eosinophilic esophagitis: similarities and differences. Allergy. 2012;67(4):477–90.
108. Baxi S, et al. Clinical presentation of patients with eosinophilic inflammation of the esophagus. Gastrointest Endosc. 2006;64(4):473–8.
109. Rodriguez-Sanchez J, et al. Effectiveness of serological markers of eosinophil activity in monitoring eosinophilic esophagitis. Rev Esp Enferm Dig. 2013;105(8):462–7.
110. Simon D, et al. Eosinophilic esophagitis is characterized by a non-IgE-mediated food hypersensitivity. Allergy. 2016;71(5):611–20.
111. Simon D, et al. Eosinophilic esophagitis in adults--no clinical relevance of wheat and rye sensitizations. Allergy. 2006;61(12):1480–3.
112. Konikoff MR, et al. Potential of blood eosinophils, eosinophil-derived neurotoxin, and eotaxin-3 as biomarkers of eosinophilic esophagitis. Clin Gastroenterol Hepatol. 2006;4(11):1328–36.
113. Bullock JZ, et al. Interplay of adaptive th2 immunity with eotaxin-3/c-C chemokine receptor 3 in eosinophilic esophagitis. J Pediatr Gastroenterol Nutr. 2007;45(1):22–31.
114. Schlag C, et al. Peripheral blood eosinophils and other non-invasive biomarkers can monitor treatment response in eosinophilic oesophagitis. Aliment Pharmacol Ther. 2015;42(9):1122–30.
115. Min SB, et al. Longitudinal evaluation of noninvasive biomarkers for eosinophilic esophagitis. J Clin Gastroenterol. 2017;51(2):127–35.
116. Dellon ES, et al. Utility of a noninvasive serum biomarker panel for diagnosis and monitoring of eosinophilic esophagitis: a prospective study. Am J Gastroenterol. 2015;110(6):821–7.
117. Subbarao G, et al. Exploring potential noninvasive biomarkers in eosinophilic esophagitis in children. J Pediatr Gastroenterol Nutr. 2011;53(6):651–8.
118. Kagalwalla AF, et al. Eosinophilic esophagitis: epithelial mesenchymal transition contributes to esophageal remodeling and reverses with treatment. J Allergy Clin Immunol. 2012;129(5):1387–1396 e7.
119. Schaefer ET, et al. Comparison of oral prednisone and topical fluticasone in the treatment of eosinophilic esophagitis: a randomized trial in children. Clin Gastroenterol Hepatol. 2008;6(2):165–73.
120. Kedika RR, Souza RF, Spechler SJ. Potential anti-inflammatory effects of proton pump inhibitors: a review and discussion of the clinical implications. Dig Dis Sci. 2009;54(11):2312–7.
121. Cortes JR, et al. Omeprazole inhibits IL-4 and IL-13 signaling signal transducer and activator of transcription 6 activation and reduces lung inflammation in murine asthma. J Allergy Clin Immunol. 2009;124(3):607–10, 610 e1.
122. Lucendo AJ, Arias A, Molina-Infante J. Efficacy of proton pump inhibitor drugs for inducing clinical and histologic remission in patients with symptomatic esophageal eosinophilia: a systematic review and meta-analysis. Clin Gastroenterol Hepatol. 2016;14(1):13–22. e1
123. Molina-Infante J, et al. Long-term loss of response in proton pump inhibitor-responsive esophageal eosinophilia is uncommon and influenced by CYP2C19 genotype and rhinoconjunctivitis. Am J Gastroenterol. 2015;110(11):1567–75.

124. Murali AR, et al. Topical steroids in eosinophilic esophagitis: systematic review and meta-analysis of placebo-controlled randomized clinical trials. J Gastroenterol Hepatol. 2016;31(6):1111–9.
125. Chuang MY, et al. Topical steroid therapy for the treatment of eosinophilic esophagitis (EoE): a systematic review and meta-analysis. Clin Transl Gastroenterol. 2015;6:e82.
126. Rawla P, et al. Efficacy and safety of budesonide in the treatment of eosinophilic esophagitis: updated systematic review and meta-analysis of randomized and non-randomized studies. Drugs R D. 2018;18(4):259–69.
127. Lipka S, et al. Systematic review with network meta-analysis: comparative effectiveness of topical steroids vs. PPIs for the treatment of the spectrum of eosinophilic oesophagitis. Aliment Pharmacol Ther. 2016;43(6):663–73.
128. Peterson KA, et al. Comparison of esomeprazole to aerosolized, swallowed fluticasone for eosinophilic esophagitis. Dig Dis Sci. 2010;55(5):1313–9.
129. Moawad FJ, et al. Randomized controlled trial comparing aerosolized swallowed fluticasone to esomeprazole for esophageal eosinophilia. Am J Gastroenterol. 2013;108(3):366–72.
130. Molina-Infante J, et al. Proton pump inhibitor-responsive oesophageal eosinophilia: an entity challenging current diagnostic criteria for eosinophilic oesophagitis. Gut. 2016;65(3):524–31.
131. Dellon ES, et al. Viscous topical is more effective than nebulized steroid therapy for patients with eosinophilic esophagitis. Gastroenterology. 2012;143(2):321–4 e1.
132. Dellon ES, et al. Budesonide oral suspension improves symptomatic, endoscopic, and histologic parameters compared with placebo in patients with eosinophilic esophagitis. Gastroenterology. 2017;152(4):776–786 e5.
133. Straumann A, et al. Long-term budesonide maintenance treatment is partially effective for patients with eosinophilic esophagitis. Clin Gastroenterol Hepatol. 2011;9(5):400–9 e1.
134. Dohil R, et al. Oral viscous budesonide is effective in children with eosinophilic esophagitis in a randomized, placebo-controlled trial. Gastroenterology. 2010;139(2):418–29.
135. Alexander JA, et al. Swallowed fluticasone improves histologic but not symptomatic response of adults with eosinophilic esophagitis. Clin Gastroenterol Hepatol. 2012;10(7):742–749 e1.
136. Liacouras CA, et al. Primary eosinophilic esophagitis in children: successful treatment with oral corticosteroids. J Pediatr Gastroenterol Nutr. 1998;26(4):380–5.
137. Assa'ad AH, et al. An antibody against IL-5 reduces numbers of esophageal intraepithelial eosinophils in children with eosinophilic esophagitis. Gastroenterology. 2011;141(5):1593–604.
138. Spergel JM, et al. Reslizumab in children and adolescents with eosinophilic esophagitis: results of a double-blind, randomized, placebo-controlled trial. J Allergy Clin Immunol. 2012;129(2):456–63, 463 e1–3.
139. Straumann A, et al. Anti-interleukin-5 antibody treatment (mepolizumab) in active eosinophilic oesophagitis: a randomised, placebo-controlled, double-blind trial. Gut. 2010;59(1):21–30.
140. Rothenberg ME, et al. Intravenous anti-IL-13 mAb QAX576 for the treatment of eosinophilic esophagitis. J Allergy Clin Immunol. 2015;135(2):500–7.
141. Hirano I, et al. RPC4046, a monoclonal antibody against IL13, reduces histologic and endoscopic activity in patients with eosinophilic esophagitis. Gastroenterology. 2019;156(3):592–603 e10.
142. Hirano I, Dellon ES, Hamilton JD, Collins MH, Peterson KA, Chehade M, et al., Dupilumab efficacy and safety in adult patients with active eosinophilic esophagitis: a randomized double-blind placebo-controlled phase 2 trial. Presented at: American College of Gastroenterology National Meeting. 2017.
143. Arias A, et al. Efficacy of dietary interventions for inducing histologic remission in patients with eosinophilic esophagitis: a systematic review and meta-analysis. Gastroenterology. 2014;146(7):1639–48.
144. Kelly KJ, et al. Eosinophilic esophagitis attributed to gastroesophageal reflux: improvement with an amino acid-based formula. Gastroenterology. 1995;109(5):1503–12.

145. Markowitz JE, et al. Elemental diet is an effective treatment for eosinophilic esophagitis in children and adolescents. Am J Gastroenterol. 2003;98(4):777–82.
146. Kagalwalla AF, et al. Cow's milk elimination: a novel dietary approach to treat eosinophilic esophagitis. J Pediatr Gastroenterol Nutr. 2012;55(6):711–6.
147. Henderson CJ, et al. Comparative dietary therapy effectiveness in remission of pediatric eosinophilic esophagitis. J Allergy Clin Immunol. 2012;129(6):1570–8.
148. Peterson KA, et al. Elemental diet induces histologic response in adult eosinophilic esophagitis. Am J Gastroenterol. 2013;108(5):759–66.
149. Warners MJ, et al. Elemental diet decreases inflammation and improves symptoms in adult eosinophilic oesophagitis patients. Aliment Pharmacol Ther. 2017;45(6):777–87.
150. Spergel JM, et al. The use of skin prick tests and patch tests to identify causative foods in eosinophilic esophagitis. J Allergy Clin Immunol. 2002;109(2):363–8.
151. Spergel JM, et al. Identification of causative foods in children with eosinophilic esophagitis treated with an elimination diet. J Allergy Clin Immunol. 2012;130(2):461–7 e5.
152. Al-Hussaini A, Al-Idressi E, Al-Zahrani M. The role of allergy evaluation in children with eosinophilic esophagitis. J Gastroenterol. 2013;48(11):1205–12.
153. Rizo Pascual JM, et al. Allergy assessment in children with eosinophilic esophagitis. J Investig Allergol Clin Immunol. 2011;21(1):59–65.
154. Molina-Infante J, et al. Selective elimination diet based on skin testing has suboptimal efficacy for adult eosinophilic esophagitis. J Allergy Clin Immunol. 2012;130(5):1200–2.
155. Wolf WA, et al. Dietary elimination therapy is an effective option for adults with eosinophilic esophagitis. Clin Gastroenterol Hepatol. 2014;12(8):1272–9.
156. Gonsalves N, et al. Elimination diet effectively treats eosinophilic esophagitis in adults; food reintroduction identifies causative factors. Gastroenterology. 2012;142(7):1451–9 e1; quiz e14-5.
157. Erwin EA, et al. Serum IgE measurement and detection of food allergy in pediatric patients with eosinophilic esophagitis. Ann Allergy Asthma Immunol. 2010;104(6):496–502.
158. Rodriguez-Sanchez J, et al. Efficacy of IgE-targeted vs empiric six-food elimination diets for adult eosinophilic oesophagitis. Allergy. 2014;69(7):936–42.
159. Gonzalez-Cervera J, et al. Successful food elimination therapy in adult eosinophilic esophagitis: not all patients are the same. J Clin Gastroenterol. 2012;46(10):855–8.
160. Sampson HA. Update on food allergy. J Allergy Clin Immunol. 2004;113(5):805–19; quiz 820.
161. Kagalwalla AF, et al. Effect of six-food elimination diet on clinical and histologic outcomes in eosinophilic esophagitis. Clin Gastroenterol Hepatol. 2006;4(9):1097–102.
162. Kagalwalla AF, et al. Identification of specific foods responsible for inflammation in children with eosinophilic esophagitis successfully treated with empiric elimination diet. J Pediatr Gastroenterol Nutr. 2011;53(2):145–9.
163. Colson D, et al. The impact of dietary therapy on clinical and biologic parameters of pediatric patients with eosinophilic esophagitis. J Allergy Clin Immunol Pract. 2014;2(5):587–93.
164. Wang R, et al. Assessing adherence and barriers to long-term elimination diet therapy in adults with eosinophilic esophagitis. Dig Dis Sci. 2018;63(7):1756–62.
165. Molina-Infante J, et al. Four-food group elimination diet for adult eosinophilic esophagitis: a prospective multicenter study. J Allergy Clin Immunol. 2014;134(5):1093–9 e1.
166. Molina-Infante J, et al. Step-up empiric elimination diet for pediatric and adult eosinophilic esophagitis: the 2-4-6 study. J Allergy Clin Immunol. 2018;141(4):1365–72.
167. Moawad FJ, et al. Systematic review with meta-analysis: endoscopic dilation is highly effective and safe in children and adults with eosinophilic oesophagitis. Aliment Pharmacol Ther. 2017;46(2):96–105.
168. Cohen MS, et al. An audit of endoscopic complications in adult eosinophilic esophagitis. Clin Gastroenterol Hepatol. 2007;5(10):1149–53.
169. Kaplan M, et al. Endoscopy in eosinophilic esophagitis: "feline" esophagus and perforation risk. Clin Gastroenterol Hepatol. 2003;1(6):433–7.

170. Schoepfer AM, et al. Esophageal dilation in eosinophilic esophagitis: effectiveness, safety, and impact on the underlying inflammation. Am J Gastroenterol. 2010;105(5):1062–70.
171. Bohm M, et al. Esophageal dilation: simple and effective treatment for adults with eosinophilic esophagitis and esophageal rings and narrowing. Dis Esophagus. 2010;23(5):377–85.
172. Dellon ES, et al. Esophageal dilation in eosinophilic esophagitis: safety and predictors of clinical response and complications. Gastrointest Endosc. 2010;71(4):706–12.
173. Kavitt RT, et al. Randomized controlled trial comparing esophageal dilation to no dilation among adults with esophageal eosinophilia and dysphagia. Dis Esophagus. 2016;29(8):983–91.
174. Jensen ET, et al. Health-care utilization, costs, and the burden of disease related to eosinophilic esophagitis in the United States. Am J Gastroenterol. 2015;110(5):626–32.

Chapter 7
Achalasia

Rishi D. Naik and Dhyanesh A. Patel

Introduction

Achalasia is a primary esophageal motility disorder that results from loss of intrinsic inhibitory innervation of the lower esophageal sphincter (LES) and the smooth muscle segment of the esophageal body. Classic symptoms include dysphagia to solids and liquids associated with regurgitation of undigested food. The etiology of achalasia is unclear with several proposed theories including immune-mediated response of neuronal degeneration. Histologically, there has been evidence of inflammation of the myenteric inhibitory ganglion cells with some studies showing loss of inhibitory neurons via inflammation with subsequent neuronal destruction and fibrosis [1, 2]. Improvement in diagnostic modalities with esophageal pressure topography (EPT) has identified subgroups of achalasia patients based on carefully validated metrics to quantify LES relaxation and esophageal peristaltic function. Currently, the Chicago Classification is used to determine the subtype of achalasia (type I, II, or III) based on high-resolution manometry (HRM). Along with the improvement in diagnostic tools, treatment options including endoscopic and surgical options have advanced management for achalasia. As the etiology of achalasia is still undefined, our treatment options are aimed at mechanical disruption of the LES, but a cure for achalasia is still not available.

R. D. Naik (✉) · D. A. Patel
Section of Gastroenterology, Hepatology, and Nutrition, Center for Swallowing and Esophageal Disorders, Digestive Disease Center, Vanderbilt University Medical Center, Nashville, TN, USA
e-mail: Rishi.D.Naik@vumc.org; Dhyanesh.A.Patel@vumc.org

© Springer Nature Switzerland AG 2020 141
D. A. Patel et al. (eds.), *Evaluation and Management of Dysphagia*,
https://doi.org/10.1007/978-3-030-26554-0_7

Epidemiology

Incidence and Prevalence

The incidence of achalasia is 1/100,000, and due to the chronicity of symptoms, the prevalence is around 10/100,000 [3–6]. Achalasia has no age nor gender preference, and its chronicity affects patient's health-related quality of life, work productivity, and functional status [7]. In Iceland, 62 cases of achalasia were diagnosed over a 51-year surveillance (overall incidence 0.6/100,000 per year) [4]. In the United States, hospitalization for achalasia ranged from 0.25/100,000 (<18 years old) to 37/100,000 (>85 years old) [8, 9].

Age

The peak incidence is between 30 and 60 years old [10, 11].

Gender and Race

Achalasia occurs equally among women and men and is without racial predilection.

Genetics

Utilizing research from twin and sibling studies, genetic underpinnings of achalasia show an association with other diseases, such as Parkinson's, Allgrove syndrome, and Down syndrome [12–14]. The most well-known genetic syndrome is Allgrove syndrome, also known as "triple A" syndrome, which included achalasia, alacrima, and adrenal insufficiency due to a defect in the AAAS gene (chromosome 12q13) with defective tryptophan-aspartic acid repeat protein [15–17]. Familial cases of achalasia combined with abnormal polymorphisms of nitric oxide or interleukin expression (IL-23 and IL-10) have added support for a genetic etiology [18–20].

Case-control studies and a genetic association study have shown the contribution of human leukocyte antigen (HLA) class II genes in to susceptibility to achalasia [21–23]. A genetic association study in achalasia and controls mapped a strong major histocompatibility complex association signal by imputing classical HLA haplotypes and amino acid polymorphism. To date, the only known achalasia risk factor is an eight-residue insertion located in the cytoplasmic tail of HLA-DQβ1 receptor [24]. Data are otherwise sparse on genetic and/or phenomic association in achalasia. Studies of molecular pathology have also suggested the consideration of achalasia as an autoimmune inflammatory disorder [25, 26]. This is supported by the presence of anti-myenteric antibodies in the circulation and inflammatory T-cell infiltrates in the myenteric plexus in achalasia. Patients with achalasia are 3.6× more likely to have other autoimmune diseases including uveitis, Type I diabetes, rheumatoid arthritis, systemic lupus erythematous, and Sjögren's syndrome [27]. However, at this time, there is no role for genetic testing in routine clinical practice.

Pathogenesis

Esophageal peristalsis is a result of complicated contractile and relaxation forces. One of the keys to understanding the pathogenesis of achalasia is to better characterize the role of autonomic ganglia in controlling distal esophageal and LES contractility. Esophageal contraction is predominately orchestrated by the postganglionic neurons which are the neurons targeted in achalasia (Fig. 7.1) [28].

Precise balance of the contractions and inhibitions is responsible for the manometric observation of a normal esophageal peristalsis post deglutition [29–32]. In achalasia, the selective destruction of the neuroinhibitory fibers lead to loss of peristalsis and inability of the LES to relax leading to the classic manometry findings of achalasia (Fig. 7.2). The causes of an initial reduction of inhibitory neu-

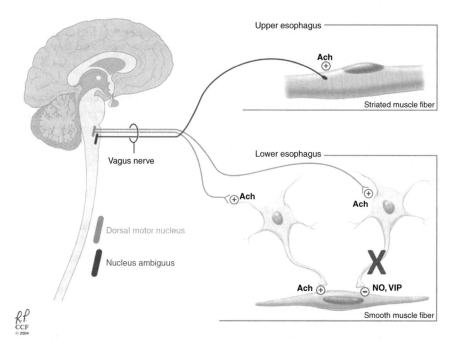

Fig. 7.1 Neuronal injury that secretes VIP and NO leads to unopposed excitatory activity and failure of LES relaxation. (Adapted from: Patel et al. [28])

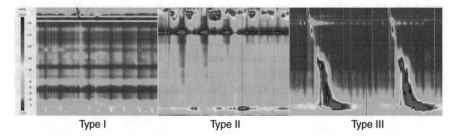

Type I   Type II   Type III

Fig. 7.2 High-resolution manometry showing the three subtypes of achalasia. Type I is character-ized by absent contractility; type II shows pan-esophageal pressurization; and type III shows simultaneous contractions. (Adapted from: Patel et al. [28])

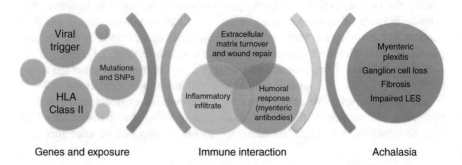

Genes and exposure   Immune interaction   Achalasia

Fig. 7.3 Possible mechanisms for the development of achalasia ranging from viral triggers, geno-type susceptibility, and genetic changes interacting with immune changes which can lead to esoph-ageal neuronal changes. (Adapted from: Patel et al. [28])

rons is unknown with theories including a possible autoimmune etiology (herpes, measles) which may trigger neuronal degeneration in a genetically predisposed host [33]. Achalasia patients are more likely to have concomitant autoimmune diseases and higher prevalence of serum neural antibodies [27, 34]. However, infectious eti-ologies should also be kept in the differential as seen in Chagas disease by the para-site *Trypanosoma cruzi*, which can cause achalasia [35].

The exact cause of the alterations in the myenteric plexus, including progres-sive degeneration and destruction of myenteric neurons, in patients with achalasia remains to be determined. However, studies have suggested a significant decrease or absent NO innervation in the myenteric plexus of patients with achalasia [29, 36]. The current hypothesis is that an initiating event, probably an environmental insult such as a viral infection, creates a cascade of inflammatory changes and damage to the myenteric plexus [33, 37, 38]. This inflammation triggers an autoimmune response, leading to chronic inflammation with subsequent complete destruction of the inhibitory neurons in the myenteric plexus (Fig. 7.3) [1]. A recent study evaluated 26 specimens in patients with achalasia and found inflammatory changes including capillaritis (51%), plexitis (23%), nerve hypertrophy (16%), venulitis (7%), and fibrosis (3%) [26].

Opioids

Detrimental effects of opioids on esophageal motility has been known since the 1980s where repeated dosing of morphine in healthy individuals led to an increase in LES pressure and decreased sphincter relaxation [39]. However, recently multiple studies have shown increased rate of esophagogastric junction outflow obstruction (EGJOO), type III achalasia, and esophageal spasm in patients on chronic opiates suggesting possible opioid-induced esophageal dysfunction [40–43]. The largest retrospective cohort included 2342 patients (224 on chronic daily opioids) and found that patients on opioids were more likely to report dysphagia (62% vs. 43%, $P < 0.01$) and were more likely to have type III achalasia (13% vs 1%, $P < 0.01$), EGJOO (13% vs. 3%, $P < 0.01$), and esophageal spasm (3% vs. 0.5%, $P < 0.01$) [44].

Management of patients with narcotics is difficult, but in the case of achalasia-like symptoms, reduction of narcotics to the lowest dose tolerated or transitioning to non-opioid analgesia is preferred. Manometric abnormalities in patients with opioid-induced esophageal dysfunction can normalize when patients are studied off opiates [45]. In one small case series, three out of five patients using pneumatic dilation for opioid-mediated esophageal dysfunction had little improvement in symptoms [43]. If the opioid cannot be stopped, injection with botulinum toxin can be considered. More invasive procedures, such as pneumatic dilation, surgical myotomy, and peroral endoscopic myotomy (POEM), should be approached with significant caution and reserved for refractory cases after discussion about the risks, benefits, and potential failure given the lower than average response rate in patients on chronic opioids [46, 47].

Diagnosis

Clinical Manifestations

The diagnosis of achalasia starts with symptom presentation of dysphagia, typically to solid and liquids. Patients can also present with associated regurgitation of undigested food or chest pain. Occasionally, patients report having reflux symptoms and are nonresponsive to acid suppression. A high index of suspicion for achalasia should be present for patients with reflux symptoms and regurgitation without symptom improvement despite acid suppression. Younger patients are more likely to report heartburn and chest pain compared to older patients [48]. Obese patients (body mass index >30) present frequently with choking and vomiting [49]. Despite their symptoms of dysphagia, the degree of weight loss varies with a recent study showing the correlation of achalasia with phenotype, where type II achalasia patients were most likely and type III achalasia least likely to have weight loss compared to type I achalasia [50].

Respiratory symptoms are also common due to the increased risk of aspiration secondary to retained food and saliva in the esophagus. Of 110 patients with achalasia, 40% of patients reported at least 1 respiratory symptom daily, which improved after therapy directed at the LES [51, 52]. In a retrospective study, the symptoms of dysphagia preceded respiratory symptoms by an average of 24 months, supporting the retention hypothesis as the etiology for aspiration and respiratory complaints [53]. However, there are several other etiologies of respiratory causes and dysphagia, including oropharyngeal dysphagia, connective tissues diseases (i.e., scleroderma), or extraesophageal gastroesophageal reflux disease (GERD) which should be on the differential.

Subtypes

EPT is a major advancement in the field of esophageal physiology [54]. With the innovative advent of EPT and HRM, achalasia is now recognized to present with three distinct manometric subtypes (Fig. 7.2) [55].All three phenotypes have impaired EGJ relaxation and absent esophageal peristalsis, but the distinguishing features are in the pattern of esophageal pressurization. Type I achalasia is characterized by absence of esophageal pressurization to more than 30 mmHg and has 100% failed peristalsis (aperistalsis), type II is associated with panesophageal pressurization to greater than 30 mm Hg, and type III has spastic contractions due to abnormal lumen obliterating contractions with or without periods of panesophageal pressurization [56].

Manometric subtypes have been shown to have prognostic and treatment implications. Success rates for both pneumatic dilation (PD) and Heller myotomy (HM) are significantly higher in subtypes I and II than type III. The latter subtype (type III) responds the least to reducing the LES pressure, as the segment affected by the spastic motility extends well above the LES [57]. This subtype of achalasia is characterized by chest pain due to lumen obliterating spastic contractions in the distal esophagus. It is proposed that type III achalasia may represent early disease with progression to type II followed by type I over time. However, pathophysiologic basis of this proposed progression is lacking. Recent studies also suggest that type I achalasia may represent decompensated esophagus to outflow obstructions caused by a dysfunctional LES accompanied with a complete aganglionosis [58].

Esophagogastric Junction Outflow Obstruction (EGJOO)

When the IRP is greater than 15 mmHg but there is peristalsis that does not meet criteria for type I, II, or III achalasia, the Chicago Classification labels this as EGJOO. This potential phenotype of achalasia is an important but heterogenous group [59]. There are multiple etiologies of EGJOO including incompletely expressed or early achalasia, esophageal wall stiffness, infiltrative cancer, hiatal hernia, obesity, or opiate-induced [45]. Further evaluation with endoscopic ultrasound, CT, or functional luminal imaging probe (FLIP) can be done to better elucidate the etiology of EGJOO. In some studies, patients with EGJOO were monitored conservatively, and their "disorder" resolved spontaneously [60, 61]. To increase the yield of EGJOO, provocative maneuvers during HRM can help, including rapid drink challenge or solid meal challenge [62, 63]. The mechanism of these maneuvers is that increasing the volume or viscosity of the bolus increases esophageal pressurization and thus IRP increases [47].

Esophagogastroduodenoscopy

Symptoms of dysphagia should prompt an esophagogastroduodenoscopy (EGD) with mucosal biopsies. These findings can help rule out GERD, eosinophilic esophagitis (EoE), or structural causes, such as rings or webs. On EGD, a "puckered" gastroesophageal (GE) junction with retention of solid or liquid material proximal to GE junction is commonly seen (Fig. 7.4). In more advanced cases, the esophagus can be dilated or tortuous due to chronic stasis. There can be resistance with passage of the endoscope through the GE junction due to failure of the LES to relax. When achalasia is suspected, a thorough retroflexion should be completed to fully evaluate the GE junction and cardia to rule out malignancy, which can cause pseudo-achalasia. Due to the stasis from the failure of the LES to relax, there can be esophageal candidiasis, which in the context of an intact immune function should prompt concern for esophageal dysmotility. Endoscopy can be helpful for its ability to rule out other causes of dysphagia and help support a diagnosis of achalasia, but other testing is often needed to confirm the diagnosis of achalasia.

Histological Features

Though biopsies are more helpful to rule out other causes of dysphagia, such as EoE, histopathological analysis has been performed on achalasia patients. Prior studies have shown predominantly capillaritis with varying amounts of plexitis, nerve hypertrophy, venulitis, and fibrosis with identified presence of HSV-1 antibodies supporting a possible neurotropic viral infection leading to an autoimmune inflammatory cascade [25]. In a concentrated histopathological examination, subtypes of achalasia showed greater degree of myenteric ganglion cell loss in type I achalasia compared to type II proposing that type I achalasia may represent disease progression from type II achalasia [58]. In all types of achalasia, there was a spectrum from complete neuronal loss to lymphocytic inflammation to apparently normal tissue suggesting a pathogenically heterogeneous patient group with a common esophagogastric junction outflow obstruction.

Fig. 7.4 Endoscopic evaluation of achalasia showing (**a**) puckered GE junction and (**b**) retained saliva. (Adapted from: Patel et al. [28])

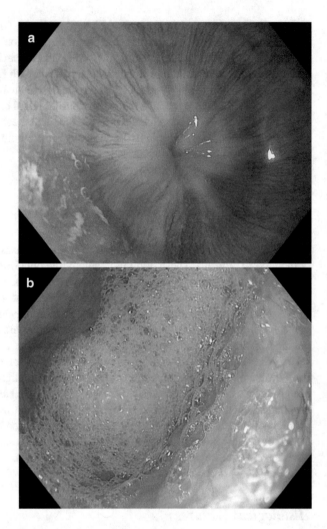

Barium Esophagram

A noninvasive method to help with the diagnosis of achalasia is to perform a barium esophagram, which can show the classic "bird beak's" appearance due to the narrowing of the GE junction. Other findings include aperistalsis, dilated esophagus, or a "cork appearance" of the esophagus (Fig. 7.5). However, this method is not sensitive for diagnosis of achalasia, and other modalities such as manometry are essential to confirm the diagnosis.

Fig. 7.5 Barium
esophagram showing
retained contents in the
proximal esophagus and
"bird beak's" appearance
due to incomplete
relaxation of the lower
esophageal sphincter.
(Adapted from: Patel
et al. [28])

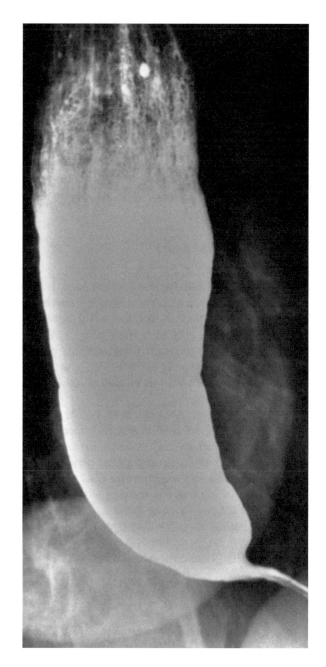

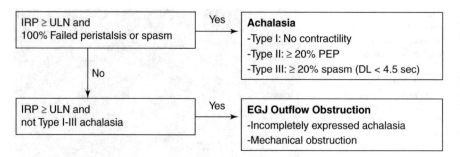

Fig. 7.6 Manometric diagnosis of achalasia and EGJOO. The Chicago Classification v3.0, hierarchical classification. (Modified from Kahrilas et al. [55])

Esophageal Manometry

The gold standard for diagnosis of achalasia is esophageal manometry, which involves transnasal placement of a flexible catheter into the esophagus to measure esophageal pressures and contractions along the length of the esophagus. Prior line tracings from water-perfused or strain gauge systems have now been replacement with high-resolution manometry systems that present pressure tracings in EPT plots [64, 65]. Building on the work of Clouse and plots of contractile activity, the Chicago Classification was created to define and diagnose motility disorders (Fig. 7.6) [55].

By using EPT, achalasia has been further characterized into three clinically important subtypes that have shown differences in response to therapy (Fig. 7.2). The diagnosis of achalasia is made by demonstrating impaired relaxation of the lower esophageal sphincter and absent peristalsis in the absence of esophageal obstruction due to a secondary cause (i.e., pseudo-achalasia from a GE junction tumor). Manometric analysis showing an elevated integrated relaxation pressure and 100% failed peristalsis or spasm meets criteria for achalasia. The phenotype depends if there is no contractility (type I), greater than 20% pan-esophageal pressurization (type II), or greater than 20% spasm [a distal latency less than 4.5 seconds] (type III). These three subtypes of achalasia have prognostic and therapeutic implications [56].

Functional Lumen Imaging Probe (FLIP)

Per Chicago Classification version 3.0, the IRP must be greater than 15 mmHg which means the EGJ pressure is greater than 15 mmHg, which is not always the case, particularly in type I achalasia. The etiology for this may be due to in part for those with advanced disease having very low LES pressures. Prior attempts to decrease the IRP cutoff have been rejected as there are some diagnosis of achalasia with IRP values of 3 mmHg and 5 mmHg, which were seen with the use of functional luminal imaging probe (FLIP) technology and stasis on esophagram [66, 67]. FLIP has aimed to better assess this group of patients with being able to measure a distensibility index, which is a metric relating EGJ opening diameter to intraluminal distensible pressure. Using this index, a threshold of 2.8 mm^2 per mmHg has been the most helpful in diagnosing abnormal EGJ function [68]. Alternatively, one can use minimal bolus flow time during HRM, a timed barium esophagram, or rapid drink challenge to also obtain this diagnosis [63, 69–71]. Intraoperative use of FLIP during laparoscopic HM or POEM might also offer the ability to assess the efficacy of LES myotomy in real-time and predict postoperative symptomatic outcomes [72–74].

Treatment Options

There is no curative option for achalasia; all treatment options are directed toward improving quality of life and attempting to preserve esophageal function and preventing esophageal stasis. Current treatment options aim to reduce the hypertonicity of the LES to improve esophageal emptying by gravity.

Therapeutic options are divided into oral pharmacological, endoscopic (pharmacological, pneumatic dilation, myotomy), and surgical (myotomy or esophagectomy) (Fig. 7.7). The choice of treatment is based on surgical candidacy, age, comorbidities, dilation of esophagus, patient preference, local expertise, and manometric subtype. The most effective therapies to help preserve esophageal function include pneumatic dilation, surgical myotomy, and POEM. Pharmacological therapy, whether oral or endoscopically injected, has decreased efficacy as compared to the three aforementioned techniques. In patients who have end-stage achalasia with severely dilated "sigmoid"-shaped esophagus and nonresponsive to other options, esophagectomy can be considered.

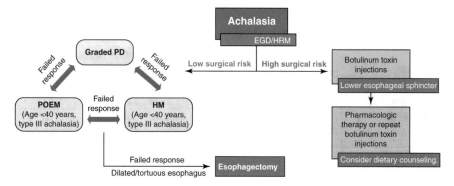

Fig. 7.7 Proposed mechanism of treatment for achalasia based on low and high surgical risk. (Adapted from: Patel et al. [28])

Pharmacological Therapies

Pharmacological therapy is the least effective treatment modality for achalasia. The response to these agents is short lived, and their side-effect profile often limits compliance or dose escalation. Oral therapies are reserved for those patients who are not candidate for more definitive endoscopic or surgical options due to comorbidities. Options for therapy are varied, but the most common include calcium channel blockers (i.e., nifedipine, 10–30 mg given 30–45 minutes prior to meals) or long-acting nitrates (isosorbide dinitrate, 5–10 mg given 15 minutes prior to meals) [75–81]. Both calcium channel blockers and long-acting nitrates cause a rapid reduction in lower esophageal sphincter of up to 47–64%, but unfortunately this translates poorly to symptom improvement with modest dysphagia improvement [76]. An alternative option includes the use of off-label phosphodiesterase-5 inhibitors (i.e., sildenafil) which lowers esophagogastric junction pressure, but symptom improvement is also modest, and long-term studies are lacking [80, 82]. Given the limited efficacy of oral pharmacological therapy, this option is reserved for patients who cannot undergo a more definitive therapeutic approach (Table 7.1).

Endoscopic Options

Botulinum Toxin

For patients who cannot tolerate a more invasive approach, botulinum toxin injection (BTI), a potent inhibitor of acetylcholine release from the presynaptic terminals, is a useful treatment strategy. BTI blocks unopposed cholinergic stimulation caused by the selective loss of inhibitory interneurons. This is injected during endoscopy where under direct visualization, 100 units of toxin are injected in 25 units aliquots in 4 quadrants via a sclero-needle just proximal to the squamo-columnar junction. Issues with the use of BTI are the transitory effect of the injection which often needs

Table 7.1 Nitrates and calcium channel blockers in the treatment of achalasia

Authors	Citation	No. of patients	Treatment	% Symptom improvement	Grade
Gelfond et al.	[76]	15	Nifedipine	53	2
Gelfond et al.	[76]	15	Isosorbide dinitrate	87	2
Rozen et al.	[77]	15	Isosorbide dinitrate	58	2
Gelfond et al.	[78]	24	Isosorbide dinitrate	83	2
Traube et al.	[79]	10	Nifedipine	53	1c
Bortolotti and Labo	[80]	20	Nifedipine	70	2
Coccia et al.	[81]	14	Nifedipine	77	2
Eherer et al.	[82]	3	Sildenafil	0	1d

Modified from Vaezi and Richter [75]

Table 7.2 Botox in the treatment of achalasia

Authors	Citation	No. of patients	<1 mo	6 mo	12 mo	24 mo	Responding to repeat injections	Grade
Vaezi et al.	[83]	22	63	36	32	–	–	1a
Pasricha et al.	[84, 85]	31	90	55	–	–	27	2
Annese et al.	[87]	118	82	–	64	–	100	1a
Cuillere et al.	[88]	55	75	50	–	–	33	2
Rollan et al.	[89]	3	100	66	–	–	–	2
Fishman et al.	[90]	60	70	–	36	–	86	2
Annese et al.	[91]	8	100	13	–	–	100	1d
Gordon and Eaker	[92]	16	75	44	–	–	–	2
Muehldorfer et al.	[93]	12	75	50	25	10	–	1d
Kolbasnik et al.	[94]	30	77	57	39	25	100	2
Mikaeli et al.	[95]	20	65	25	15	–	60	1a
Allescher et al.	[96]	23	74	–	45	30	–	2
Neubrand et al.	[97]	25	65	–	–	36	0	2

Modified from Hoogerwerf et al. [206]

repeat procedures typically every 6–12 months. Complications with the procedure include chest pain (16–25%) and rarely more serious complications of mediastinitis and allergy to an egg-based protein.

The immediate response to BTI is as high as 80–90%, but over half of patients are symptomatic at 1 year (Table 7.2) [83–97]. Predictive factors for response to BTI include older age (over 40 years old), type II phenotype, and decreased basal LES pressure following treatment [84]. Repeated BTI can make surgical myotomy more difficult due to the creation of fibrosis; hence BTI should not be first line for patients who are eligible for more definite endoscopic or surgical options [98]. Though more effective than oral pharmacological therapy, BTI is not as effective as PD, POEM, or surgical myotomy. As discussed previously, for patients with achalasia-like phenotype from opioids who cannot stop their opioid, BTI might be a better alternative.

Pneumatic Dilation (PD)

PD is performed using an noncompliant balloon that employs air pressures to disrupt or fracture the LES circular muscle fibers and is an effective nonsurgical option in the treatment of achalasia [10, 99]. Currently, the most widely used balloon dilator for PD is the Rigiflex, a nonradiopaque graded size polyethylene balloon. The Rigiflex dilators can be performed under direct visualization or under radiological guidance (fluoroscopy) [100, 101]. The dilators are available in three diameters (3.0, 3.5, and 4.0 cm), which allow a graded dilated approach. When employing this graded approach, relief of symptoms is possible in 50–93% of patients (Table 7.3) [100, 102–127].

Table 7.3 Rigiflex balloon dilatation for the treatment of achalasia

Authors	Citation	No. of patients	Study design	% with excl goodresponse	Follow-up in months(mean)	Perforation rate (%)	Grade
Lambroza and Schuman	[100]	27	P	89	21	0	2
Vela et al.	[102]	106	R	44	36	1.9	2
Cox et al.	[104]	7	P	86	9	0	2
Gelfand and Kozarek	[105]	24	P	93	NR	0	2
Barkin et al.	[106]	50	P	90	20	2	2
Stark et al.	[107]	10	P	74	6	0	1d
Makela et al.	[108]	17	R	75	6	5.9	2
Levine et al.	[109]	62	R	85	NR	0	2
Kim et al.	[110]	14	P	75	4	0	2
Lee et al.	[111]	28	P	87	NR	0	2
Abid et al.	[112]	36	P	88	27	6.6	2
Wehrmann et al.	[113]	40	R	87	NR	2.5	2
Muehldorfer et al.	[114]	12	R	83	18	8.3	1d
Bhatnager et al.	[115]	15	R	84	14	0	2
Gideon et al.	[116]	24	R	NR	6	4	1d
Khan et al.	[117]	9	P	85	NR	0	2
Kadakia and Wong	[118]	56	P	88	59	0	2
Chan et al.	[119]	66	R	62	55	4.5	2
Dobrucali et al.	[120]	43	P	54	29	2.3	2
Kostic et al.	[121]	26	P	87	12	NR	2
Mikaeli et al.	[122]	62	P	55	71	3.7	2
Mikaeli et al.	[122]	200	P	65	36	0	2
Ghoshal et al.	[123]	126	R	78	15	0.8	2
Guardino et al.	[124]	96	R	74	7	1.7	2
Guardino et al.	[124]	12	R	50	11	0	2
Boztas et al.	[125]	50	R	67	38	0	2
Karamanolis et al.	[126]	153	R	51	192	0.5	2
Katsinelos et al.	[127]	39	R	58	108	5.4	2

Modified and updated from Vaezi and Richter [75], Gelfand and Kozarek [105]
P prospective, *R* retrospective

Graded PD is performed by an initial dilation at 3.0 cm, then 3.5 cm, and finishing at 4.0 cm with 4–6 weeks in between dilations. Reassessment of symptoms and LES pressure can be performed between each session to determine the necessity of subsequent treatments. It is estimated that a third of patients treated with PD will experience symptom relapse within 4–6 years.

Predictive factors of a poor clinical response to treatment include age less than 40 years, male sex, LES pressure after dilation greater than 10–15 mmHg, and continued symptoms after one or two treatments [128–131]. Additionally, males younger than 45 years of age may not be as responsive to the serial approach possibly due to thicker LES musculature. In these patients, it is recommended to either start with PD at 3.5 cm or proceed straight to surgical myotomy as the initial step in management.

Of the manometric subtypes, type II achalasia has better outcomes with PD [132]. Surgical myotomy has a greater response than a single pneumatic dilation, but a graded approach with PD is a reasonable alternative to surgery as it has similar efficacy. Given the risk of perforation, which is around 2%, all patients who undergo PD must be surgical candidates in case a perforation were to occur [133]. Depending on the length and extent of the perforation, the complication can be managed conservatively with stent placement, antibiotics, and parenteral nutrition; however, larger perforations with mediastinal contamination will need a surgical repair via thoracostomy. Post-dilation, there is an increased risk of GERD, seen in 15–35% of patients post PD due to the disruption of the LES. Hence, initiation of acid suppression is recommended for patients with pre-existing GERD or new symptoms of heartburn or reflux [134]. It is important to note that dysphagia after PD can be due to the underlying achalasia or could be due to a reflux stricture; endoscopy can help separate these two etiologies.

Peroral Endoscopic Myotomy (POEM)

Peroral endoscopic myotomy (POEM) is a minimally invasive endoscopic technique and is one of the most recent advances in the treatment of achalasia (Table 7.4). The procedure is performed endoscopically with a small mucosal incision in the mid-esophagus and creating a submucosal tunnel to the gastric cardia. This technique allows careful and selective myotomy of the circular muscle.

In 2010, Inoue and investigators published a prospective trial of 17 patients undergoing endoscopic myotomy that revealed significant reduction in the index of dysphagia symptoms (10 to 1.3, $P = 0.01$) as well as resting LES pressure (52.4 to 19.9 mmHg, $P = 0.01$) [135]. Given the safety profile of this procedure, POEM entered into clinical practice and has been studied since its inception. In 2014, Bhayani conducted a prospective observational study that compared 64 patients treated by LHM and 37 by POEM, which showed that mean operative time and

Table 7.4 Peroral endoscopic myotomy for the treatment of achalasia

Authors	Citation	No. of patients	Study design	% with excellent/ goodresponse	Follow-up in months(mean)	Notes	Grade
Inoue et al.	[135]	17	P	100	5	Showed safety profile of POEM	2
Bhayani et al.	[136]	101	P	100	1	Comparison of HM and POEM	2
Tan et al.	[140]	63	P	100	15.5	Anterior vs. Posterior Approach	1c
Tyberg et al.	[141]	51	P	94	12	POEM for salvage post-HM	1c
Yao et al.	[142]	66	P	95	5.6	11 patients with prior PD or botox	2
Hu et al.	[143]	32	P	96	24	Advanced achalasia	2
Teitelbaum et al.	[144]	41	P	90	15	Improvement of esophagram and HRM	2
Zhou et al.	[145]	12	P	90	10.4	POEM for salvage post-HM	2
Swanstrom et al.	[146]	18	P	100	11.4	GERD in 46% patients postoperatively	2
Shiwaku et al.	[147]	1346	R	95.1	12	Multicenter study, 28% with prior PD	1b
Grimes et al.	[148]	100	P	95	2	Double-scope POEM	1c
Liu et al.	[149]	82	P	96.3	18	open POEM	4
Chandan et al.	[150]	210	R	89.6	2.7–27	Meta-analysis	1a
Kim et al.	[151]	83	R	90.9	16	Two-center study	2
Kane et al.	[152]	40	R	87.5	8.1	Longer myotomy length with POEM	2
Zhang et al.	[153]	32	R	90.6	27	Type III achalasia only	2
Chen et al.	[154]	45	P	100	24	Increased postop GERD in type I	2

P prospective, *R* retrospective

length of stay were significantly higher in the LHM cohort, but complication rates were similar [136]. Moreover, patient symptoms, manometry, and postoperative esophageal acid exposure revealed similar outcomes among the two groups.

The preparation for POEM begins with a liquid diet 1–5 days prior to the procedure to minimize residual food in the esophagus [137]. The first step in the procedure involves injection of 10 mL of saline solution with contrast (methylene blue or indigo carmine) to the central esophagus 10–16 cm proximal to the squamocolumnar junction [138]. Following this, a 2 cm incision is made to gain access into the submucosal space. Then, a submucosal tunnel is dissected through the EGJ and 2–3 cm into the gastric cardia [139]. Once access is made to the circular muscle layer of the LES, the myotomy is usually extended to 6 cm into the esophagus and 2 cm below the EGJ. Since its inception, there have been multiple studies showing its efficacy in improvement of dysphagia scores and manometric or imaging modalities, with ranges of 87.5–100% efficacy [135, 136, 140–154]. Patients with type III achalasia have a greater than 90% response rate to POEM, possibly owing to the longer myotomy length [155].

Serious adverse events are rare with POEM. They occur at a rate of less than 0.1% with the most common serious event being perforation [156]. Another, albeit less serious, complication following POEM is GERD. Although initial studies showed significantly higher prevalence of GERD post-POEM up to 58%, recent studies in carefully selected patients have shown short-term postoperative clinical symptoms of GERD following POEM is 10.9% and might be comparable to that of LHM [157, 158]. However, given the high potential risk of reflux post-POEM, a recent clinical practice update from expert review and best practice advice from the American Gastroenterological Association recommended that this should be discussed with patients undergoing POEM including potential ramifications of indefinite need for proton pump inhibitor therapy and/or surveillance endoscopy after POEM [159].

Surgical Options

Laparoscopic Heller Myotomy

Surgical myotomy, a technique involving the division of the circular muscle fibers of the LES, was initially performed via an open thoracotomy and laparotomy approach. Studies at the time revealed good response with 60–94% of patients achieving symptomatic improvement when followed over 1–36 years, and this approach has since been replaced with laparoscopic Heller myotomy (LHM) which resulted in less morbidity and faster recovery time (Table 7.5) [75, 102, 121, 160–186]. A systematic review analyzing surgical techniques in 4871 patients reported patient symptom improvement after all surgical myotomies, which included 84.5% of those who underwent the open transabdominal approach, 83.3% of those with the

Table 7.5 Laparoscopic myotomy for the treatment of achalasia

Authors	Citation	No. of patients	Antireflux procedure	% symptom improvement good/excellent	Follow-up in months(mean)	% complication GERD	Grade
Vela et al.	[102]	73	Yes (D/T)	57	72	56	2
Kostic et al.	[121]	25	Yes (T)	96	12	NR	1d
Rosati et al.	[160]	25	Yes	96	12	NR	2
Ancona et al.	[161]	17	Yes (Dᵃ)	100	8	6	2
Mitchell et al.	[162]	14	Yes (D)	86	NR	7	4
Swanstrom and Pennings	[163]	12	Yes (Tᵇ)	100	16	16	4
Raiser et al.	[164]	39	Yes (D/T)	63	26	27	2
Morino et al.	[165]	18	Yes (D)	100	8	6	4
Robertson et al.	[166]	10	No	88	14	13	4
Bonovina et al.	[167]	33	Yes (D)	97	12	NR	4
Delgado et al.	[168]	12	Yes (D)	83	4	NR	2
Hunter et al.	[169]	40	Yes (D/T)	90	13	18	2
Kjellin et al.	[170]	21	No	52	22	38	4
Ackroyd et al.	[171]	82	Yes (D)	87	24	5	2
Yamamura et al.	[172]	24	Yes (D)	88	17	0	4
Patti et al.	[173]	102	Yes (D)	89	25	NR	2
Pechlivanides et al.	[174]	29	Yes (D)	90	12	10	4
Sharp et al.	[175]	100	No	87	10	14	4
Donahue et al.	[176]	81	Yes (D)	84	45	26	4
Zaninotto et al.	[177]	113	Yes (D)	92	12	5	4
Luketich et al.	[178]	62	Yes (D/T)	92	19	9	3
Decker et al.	[179]	73	Yes (D/T)	83	31	11	2
Mineo et al.	[180]	14	Yes (D)	NR	85	14	4
Gockel et al.	[181]	108	Yes (D)	97	55	22	4
Wright et al.	[182]	52	Yes (D)	83	45	19	2
Wright et al.	[182]	63	Yes (T)	95	46	50	2
Khajanchee et al.	[183]	121	Yes (T)	84	9	33	2
Zaninotto et al.	[184]	40	Yes (D/Fᶜ)	88	38	3	1d
Csendes et al.	[185]	67	Yes (D)	73	190	33	2
Ramacciato et al.	[186]	17	Yes (D)	94	18	6	2

Modified from Vaezi and Richter [75]

ᵃ*D* Dor

ᵇ*T* Toupet

ᶜ*F* Floppy

P prospective, *R* retrospective, *NR* not reported

open transthoracic approach, 77.6% of those with the thoracoscopic approach, and 89.3% of those who had a LHM [103]. A subset of the analysis comparing studies with LHM (3086), and the thoracoscopic approach (211) showed better symptomatic improvement with the laparoscopic approach compared to the thoracoscopic approach (89.3 vs 77.6%, $P = 0.048$) [103].

A complication of any myotomy is GERD, and given the surgical approach, a fundoplication at time of myotomy has helped to decrease postoperative GERD. Reflux may be less if fundoplication is added to myotomy (41.5% without fundoplication vs 14.5% with fundoplication, $P = 001$) [103]. A randomized controlled trial comparing myotomy with or without fundoplication reported that performing intraoperative fundoplication was associated with a lower incidence of postoperative reflux [187]. Rawlings and investigators demonstrated in a randomized control trial comparing anterior Dor with posterior Toupet fundoplication that both provide similar outcomes in terms of postoperative reflux following LHM [188].

Furthermore, LHM and POEM have been shown to have similar efficacy with a recent systematic review and meta-analysis comparing the two interventions noting improvement in dysphagia at 24 months were 92.7% for POEM and 90.0% for LHM, but patients undergoing POEM were more likely to develop GERD symptoms (OR 1.69, 95% CI 1.33–2.14) and erosive esophagitis (9.31, 95% CI 4.71–18.85) [189].

Prognosis

Despite no curative therapies for achalasia, current management allows an improved quality of life. With the advent of HRM, achalasia phenotypes have also shown prognostic implications with type II achalasia having the best prognosis after myotomy or pneumatic dilation (96% success rate) compared to type I which has 81% success rate and type III which has a 66% success rate [57]. However, success rate for type I and type III are also now >90% with the advent of POEM. Post-intervention, a timed barium esophagram by taking radiographs at 1, 2, and 5 minutes post-barium to evaluate esophageal emptying can also be considered to predict the effectiveness of treatment [190].

Achalasia is a lifelong disease and these patients need continued follow-up. These evaluations are based on determining esophageal symptoms, nutritional status, and imaging when indicated, including a timed barium esophagram [99]. For the patient who is willing to repeat a manometry, HRM can be completed to evaluate for return of esophageal contractile activity [191]. The decision for repeat treatment is based on a combination of symptoms, fitness for repeat treatment, and signs of retention on either a timed barium esophagram, EGD, or continued absence peristalsis on manometry.

Long-term complications of achalasia include an increased risk of squamous cell carcinoma (SCC) with a prevalence of 26 cases in 1000 achalasia patients [192]. The etiology of SCC is felt to be due to persistent esophageal stasis [193]. There is insufficient evidence to support routine screening for SCC; however, this decision for surveillance should be discussed with the patient and provider on a personalized approach [194]. In addition to SCC, patients with achalasia have an increased incidence of aspiration pneumonia, lower respiratory tract infections, and higher mortality [195].

Treatment Failures

Currently there is no curative treatment for achalasia. Up to 20% of patients will need additional treatment within 5 years [196–199]. Achalasia can progress to mega-esophagus or end-stage disease in around 6–20% of patients [200]. Options for these patients include botulinum toxin injection, repeat pneumatic dilation, or repeat myotomy. A recent multicenter retrospective cohort study assessing both technical and clinical efficacy of POEM in treating achalasia after a failed HM showed technical success of 98% with clinical response up to 81% in patients who had previously failed HM with median follow-up of 9 months [201]. Similarly, in an intention-to-treat analysis at 12 months, clinical success of PD after HM was also comparable to POEM at 89% [158, 202]. Lastly, redo HM also has similar clinical success rate in this group at 73–89% with median follow-up of 2–3.6 years [203, 204]. Thus, all these options can be considered in patients who have lack of response to initial therapy [205]. For patients with severe esophageal dilation with symptoms not responsive to repeat endoscopic options or myotomy, a surgical esophagectomy can be considered (Fig. 7.7).

Conclusion

Achalasia is characterized by impairment in nitrergic inhibitory neurotransmission resulting in non-relaxing LES and aperistalsis of the esophageal body. Patients often present with dysphagia to solids and/or liquid with varying degree of weight loss. Endoscopy is essential to rule out causes of pseudo-achalasia, and high-resolution manometry is the gold standard test for diagnosis. Current treatment options provide excellent palliation of symptoms in patients with achalasia (Table 7.6).

Table 7.6 Quality of evidence for GRADE system	Level 1A: Large RCTs or systematic reviews/meta-analysis
	Level 1B: High-quality cohort study
	Level 1C: Moderate-sized RCT or meta-analysis of small trials
	Level 1D: At least one RCT
	Level 2: One high-quality of nonrandomized cohort
	Level 3: At least one high-quality case-control study
	Level 4: High-quality case series
	Level 5: Opinions from experts

References

1. Goldblum JR, Rice TW, Richter JE. Histopathologic features in esophagomyotomy specimens from patients with achalasia. Gastroenterology. 1996;111:648–54.
2. Frieling T, et al. Family occurrence of achalasia and diffuse spasm of the oesophagus. Gut. 1988;29:1595–602. https://doi.org/10.1136/gut.29.11.1595.
3. Farrukh A, DeCaestecker J, Mayberry JF. An epidemiological study of achalasia among the South Asian population of Leicester, 1986–2005. Dysphagia. 2008;23:161–4. https://doi.org/10.1007/s00455-007-9116-1.
4. Birgisson S, Richter JE. Achalasia in Iceland, 1952–2002: an epidemiologic study. Dig Dis Sci. 2007;52:1855–60. https://doi.org/10.1007/s10620-006-9286-y.
5. Sadowski DC, Ackah F, Jiang B, Svenson LW. Achalasia: incidence, prevalence and survival. A population-based study. Neurogastroenterol Motil. 2010;22:e256–61. https://doi.org/10.1111/j.1365-2982.2010.01511.x.
6. Enestvedt BK, Williams JL, Sonnenberg A. Epidemiology and practice patterns of achalasia in a large multi-centre database. Aliment Pharmacol Ther. 2011;33:1209–14. https://doi.org/10.1111/j.1365-2036.2011.04655.x.
7. Nenshi R, et al. The cost of achalasia: quantifying the effect of symptomatic disease on patient cost burden, treatment time, and work productivity. Surg Innov. 2010;17:291–4. https://doi.org/10.1177/1553350610376392.
8. Sonnenberg A. Hospitalization for achalasia in the United States 1997–2006. Dig Dis Sci. 2009;54:1680–5. https://doi.org/10.1007/s10620-009-0863-8.
9. Sonnenberg A, Massey BT, McCarty DJ, Jacobsen SJ. Epidemiology of hospitalization for achalasia in the United States. Dig Dis Sci. 1993;38:233–44.
10. Vaezi MF, Richter JE. Diagnosis and management of achalasia. American College of Gastroenterology Practice Parameter Committee. Am J Gastroenterol. 1999;94:3406–12. https://doi.org/10.1111/j.1572-0241.1999.01639.x.
11. Francis DL, Katzka DA. Achalasia: update on the disease and its treatment. Gastroenterology. 2010;139:369–74. https://doi.org/10.1053/j.gastro.2010.06.024.
12. Johnston BT, et al. Repetitive proximal esophageal contractions: a new manometric finding and a possible further link between Parkinson's disease and achalasia. Dysphagia. 2001;16:186–9.
13. Viegelmann G, Low Y, Sriram B, Chu HP. Achalasia and Down syndrome: a unique association not to be missed. Singapore Med J. 2014;55:e107–8. https://doi.org/10.11622/smedj.2013260.
14. Jung KW, et al. Genetic evaluation of ALADIN gene in early-onset achalasia and alacrima patients. J Neurogastroenterol Motil. 2011;17:169–73. https://doi.org/10.5056/jnm.2011.17.2.169.
15. Stuckey BG, Mastaglia FL, Reed WD, Pullan PT. Glucocorticoid insufficiency, achalasia, alacrima with autonomic motor neuropathy. Ann Intern Med. 1987;106:61–3.
16. Sarathi V, Shah NS. Triple-A syndrome. Adv Exp Med Biol. 2010;685:1–8.
17. Gordillo-Gonzalez G, et al. Achalasia familiar: report of a family with an autosomal dominant pattern of inherence. Dis Esophagus. 2011;24:E1–4. https://doi.org/10.1111/j.1442-2050.2010.01124.x.
18. Vigo AG, Martinez A, de la Concha EG, Urcelay E, Ruiz de Leon A. Suggested association of NOS2A polymorphism in idiopathic achalasia: no evidence in a large case-control study. Am J Gastroenterol. 2009;104:1326–7. https://doi.org/10.1038/ajg.2009.72.

19. de Leon AR, et al. Association between idiopathic achalasia and IL23R gene. Neurogastroenterol Motil. 2010;22:734–738, e218. https://doi.org/10.1111/j.1365-2982.2010.01497.x.

20. Nunez C, et al. Association of IL10 promoter polymorphisms with idiopathic achalasia. Hum Immunol. 2011;72:749–52. https://doi.org/10.1016/j.humimm.2011.05.017.

21. Wong RK, Maydonovitch CL, Metz SJ, Baker JR Jr. Significant DQw1 association in achalasia. Dig Dis Sci. 1989;34:349–52.

22. De la Concha EG, et al. Contribution of HLA class II genes to susceptibility in achalasia. Tissue Antigens. 1998;52:381–4.

23. Verne GN, et al. Association of HLA-DR and -DQ alleles with idiopathic achalasia. Gastroenterology. 1999;117:26–31.

24. Gockel I, et al. Common variants in the HLA-DQ region confer susceptibility to idiopathic achalasia. Nat Genet. 2014;46:901–4. https://doi.org/10.1038/ng.3029.

25. Furuzawa-Carballeda J, et al. Achalasia--an autoimmune inflammatory disease: a cross-sectional study. J Immunol Res. 2015;2015:729217. https://doi.org/10.1155/2015/729217.

26. Furuzawa-Carballeda J, et al. New insights into the pathophysiology of achalasia and implications for future treatment. World J Gastroenterol: WJG. 2016;22:7892–907. https://doi.org/10.3748/wjg.v22.i35.7892.

27. Booy JD, Takata J, Tomlinson G, Urbach DR. The prevalence of autoimmune disease in patients with esophageal achalasia. Dis Esophagus. 2012;25:209–13. https://doi.org/10.1111/j.1442-2050.2011.01249.x.

28. Patel DA, Lappas BM, Vaezi MF. An overview of achalasia and its subtypes. Gastroenterol Hepatol (NY). 2017;13:411–21.

29. Park W, Vaezi MF. Etiology and pathogenesis of achalasia: the current understanding. Am J Gastroenterol. 2005;100:1404–14. https://doi.org/10.1111/j.1572-0241.2005.41775.x.

30. Kuramoto H, Kadowaki M, Yoshida N. Morphological demonstration of a vagal inhibitory pathway to the lower esophageal sphincter via nitrergic neurons in the rat esophagus. Neurogastroenterol Motil. 2013;25:e485–94. https://doi.org/10.1111/nmo.12146.

31. Murray J, Du C, Ledlow A, Bates JN, Conklin JL. Nitric oxide: mediator of nonadrenergic noncholinergic responses of opossum esophageal muscle. Am J Physiol. 1991;261:G401–6.

32. Guelrud M, et al. The effect of vasoactive intestinal polypeptide on the lower esophageal sphincter in achalasia. Gastroenterology. 1992;103:377–82.

33. Boeckxstaens GE. Achalasia: virus-induced euthanasia of neurons? Am J Gastroenterol. 2008;103:1610–2. https://doi.org/10.1111/j.1572-0241.2008.01967.x.

34. Kraichely RE, Farrugia G, Pittock SJ, Castell DO, Lennon VA. Neural autoantibody profile of primary achalasia. Dig Dis Sci. 2010;55:307–11. https://doi.org/10.1007/s10620-009-0838-9.

35. de Oliveira RB, Rezende Filho J, Dantas RO, Iazigi N. The spectrum of esophageal motor disorders in Chagas' disease. Am J Gastroenterol. 1995;90:1119–24.

36. Mearin F, et al. Patients with achalasia lack nitric oxide synthase in the gastro-oesophageal junction. Eur J Clin Invest. 1993;23:724–8.

37. Kahrilas PJ, Boeckxstaens G. The spectrum of achalasia: lessons from studies of pathophysiology and high-resolution manometry. Gastroenterology. 2013;145:954–65. https://doi.org/10.1053/j.gastro.2013.08.038.

38. Ates F, Vaezi MF. The pathogenesis and management of achalasia: current status and future directions. Gut Liver. 2015;9:449–63. https://doi.org/10.5009/gnl14446.

39. Dowlatshahi K, Evander A, Walther B, Skinner DB. Influence of morphine on the distal oesophagus and the lower oesophageal sphincter--a manometric study. Gut. 1985;26:802–6. https://doi.org/10.1136/gut.26.8.802.

40. Penagini R, Bianchi PA. Effect of morphine on gastroesophageal reflux and transient lower esophageal sphincter relaxation. Gastroenterology. 1997;113:409–14.

41. Penagini R, Picone A, Bianchi PA. Effect of morphine and naloxone on motor response of the human esophagus to swallowing and distension. Am J Physiol. 1996;271:G675–80. https://doi.org/10.1152/ajpgi.1996.271.4.G675.

42. Kraichely RE, Arora AS, Murray JA. Opiate-induced oesophageal dysmotility. Aliment Pharmacol Ther. 2010;31:601–6. https://doi.org/10.1111/j.1365-2036.2009.04212.x.
43. Gonzalez ES, Bellver VO, Jaime FC, Cortes JA, Gil VG. Opioid-induced lower esophageal sphincter dysfunction. J Neurogastroenterol Motil. 2015;21:618–20. https://doi.org/10.5056/jnm15108.
44. Babaei A, Szabo A, Shad S, Massey BT. Chronic daily opioid exposure is associated with dysphagia, esophageal outflow obstruction, and disordered peristalsis. Neurogastroenterol Motil. 2019;31:e13601. https://doi.org/10.1111/nmo.13601.
45. Ratuapli SK, et al. Opioid-induced esophageal dysfunction (OIED) in patients on chronic opioids. Am J Gastroenterol. 2015;110:979–84. https://doi.org/10.1038/ajg.2015.154.
46. Ortiz V, Garcia-Campos M, Saez-Gonzalez E, del Pozo P, Garrigues V. A concise review of opioid-induced esophageal dysfunction: is this a new clinical entity? Dis Esophagus. 2018;31:doy003. https://doi.org/10.1093/dote/doy003.
47. Kahrilas PJ, Bredenoord AJ, Carlson DA, Pandolfino JE. Advances in management of esophageal motility disorders. Clin Gastroenterol Hepatol. 2018;16:1692–700. https://doi.org/10.1016/j.cgh.2018.04.026.
48. Schechter RB, Lemme EM, Novais P, Biccas B. Achalasia in the elderly patient: a comparative study. Arq Gastroenterol. 2011;48:19–23.
49. Rakita SS, Villadolid D, Kalipersad C, Thometz D, Rosemurgy A. BMI affects presenting symptoms of achalasia and outcome after Heller myotomy. Surg Endosc. 2007;21:258–64. https://doi.org/10.1007/s00464-006-0113-5.
50. Patel DA, et al. Weight loss in achalasia is determined by its phenotype. Dis Esophagus. 2018;31:doy046. https://doi.org/10.1093/dote/doy046.
51. Khandelwal S, et al. Improvement of respiratory symptoms following Heller myotomy for achalasia. J Gastrointest Surg. 2011;15:235–9. https://doi.org/10.1007/s11605-010-1397-2.
52. Sinan H, et al. Prevalence of respiratory symptoms in patients with achalasia. Dis Esophagus. 2011;24:224–8. https://doi.org/10.1111/j.1442-2050.2010.01126.x.
53. Gupta M, et al. Respiratory dysfunction is common in patients with achalasia and improves after pneumatic dilation. Dig Dis Sci. 2014;59:744–52. https://doi.org/10.1007/s10620-013-2971-8.
54. Clouse RE, Staiano A. Topography of the esophageal peristaltic pressure wave. Am J Physiol. 1991;261:G677–84.
55. Kahrilas PJ, et al. The Chicago classification of esophageal motility disorders, v3.0. Neurogastroenterol Motil. 2015;27:160–74. https://doi.org/10.1111/nmo.12477.
56. Pandolfino JE, et al. Achalasia: a new clinically relevant classification by high-resolution manometry. Gastroenterology. 2008;135:1526–33. https://doi.org/10.1053/j.gastro.2008.07.022.
57. Rohof WO, et al. Outcomes of treatment for achalasia depend on manometric subtype. Gastroenterology. 2013;144:718–25; quiz e713–714. https://doi.org/10.1053/j.gastro.2012.12.027.
58. Sodikoff JB, et al. Histopathologic patterns among achalasia subtypes. Neurogastroenterol Motil. 2016;28:139–45. https://doi.org/10.1111/nmo.12711.
59. Scherer JR, Kwiatek MA, Soper NJ, Pandolfino JE, Kahrilas PJ. Functional esophagogastric junction obstruction with intact peristalsis: a heterogeneous syndrome sometimes akin to achalasia. J Gastrointest Surg. 2009;13:2219–25. https://doi.org/10.1007/s11605-009-0975-7.
60. van Hoeij FB, Smout AJ, Bredenoord AJ. Characterization of idiopathic esophagogastric junction outflow obstruction. Neurogastroenterol Motil. 2015;27:1310–6. https://doi.org/10.1111/nmo.12625.
61. Perez-Fernandez MT, Santander C, Marinero A, Burgos-Santamaria D, Chavarria-Herbozo C. Characterization and follow-up of esophagogastric junction outflow obstruction detected by high resolution manometry. Neurogastroenterol Motil. 2016;28:116–26. https://doi.org/10.1111/nmo.12708.

62. Sweis R, Anggiansah A, Wong T, Brady G, Fox M. Assessment of esophageal dysfunction and symptoms during and after a standardized test meal: development and clinical validation of a new methodology utilizing high-resolution manometry. Neurogastroenterol Motil. 2014;26:215–28. https://doi.org/10.1111/nmo.12252.

63. Ang D, et al. Rapid Drink Challenge in high-resolution manometry: an adjunctive test for detection of esophageal motility disorders. Neurogastroenterol Motil. 2017;29:e12902. https://doi.org/10.1111/nmo.12902.

64. Bogte A, Bredenoord AJ, Oors J, Siersema PD, Smout AJ. Reproducibility of esophageal high-resolution manometry. Neurogastroenterol Motil. 2011;23:e271–6. https://doi.org/10.1111/j.1365-2982.2011.01713.x.

65. Fox M, et al. High-resolution manometry predicts the success of oesophageal bolus transport and identifies clinically important abnormalities not detected by conventional manometry. Neurogastroenterol Motil. 2004;16:533–42. https://doi.org/10.1111/j.1365-2982.2004.00539.x.

66. Lin Z, et al. Refining the criterion for an abnormal Integrated Relaxation Pressure in esophageal pressure topography based on the pattern of esophageal contractility using a classification and regression tree model. Neurogastroenterol Motil. 2012;24:e356–63. https://doi.org/10.1111/j.1365-2982.2012.01952.x.

67. Ponds FA, Bredenoord AJ, Kessing BF, Smout AJ. Esophagogastric junction distensibility identifies achalasia subgroup with manometrically normal esophagogastric junction relaxation. Neurogastroenterol Motil. 2017;29:e12908. https://doi.org/10.1111/nmo.12908.

68. Pandolfino JE, et al. Distensibility of the esophagogastric junction assessed with the functional lumen imaging probe (FLIP) in achalasia patients. Neurogastroenterol Motil. 2013;25:496–501. https://doi.org/10.1111/nmo.12097.

69. Lin Z, et al. Flow time through esophagogastric junction derived during high-resolution impedance-manometry studies: a novel parameter for assessing esophageal bolus transit. Am J Physiol Gastrointest Liver Physiol. 2014;307:G158–63. https://doi.org/10.1152/ajpgi.00119.2014.

70. Lin Z, et al. High-resolution impedance manometry measurement of bolus flow time in achalasia and its correlation with dysphagia. Neurogastroenterol Motil. 2015;27:1232–8. https://doi.org/10.1111/nmo.12613.

71. Fornari F, Bravi I, Penagini R, Tack J, Sifrim D. Multiple rapid swallowing: a complementary test during standard oesophageal manometry. Neurogastroenterol Motil. 2009;21:718–e741. https://doi.org/10.1111/j.1365-2982.2009.01273.x.

72. Teitelbaum EN, et al. An extended proximal esophageal myotomy is necessary to normalize EGJ distensibility during Heller myotomy for achalasia, but not POEM. Surg Endosc. 2014;28:2840–7. https://doi.org/10.1007/s00464-014-3563-1.

73. Teitelbaum EN, et al. Esophagogastric junction distensibility measurements during Heller myotomy and POEM for achalasia predict postoperative symptomatic outcomes. Surg Endosc. 2015;29:522–8. https://doi.org/10.1007/s00464-014-3733-1.

74. Ngamruengphong S, et al. Intraoperative measurement of esophagogastric junction cross-sectional area by impedance planimetry correlates with clinical outcomes of peroral endoscopic myotomy for achalasia: a multicenter study. Surg Endosc. 2016;30:2886–94. https://doi.org/10.1007/s00464-015-4574-2.

75. Vaezi MF, Richter JE. Current therapies for achalasia: comparison and efficacy. J Clin Gastroenterol. 1998;27:21–35.

76. Gelfond M, Rozen P, Gilat T. Isosorbide dinitrate and nifedipine treatment of achalasia: a clinical, manometric and radionuclide evaluation. Gastroenterology. 1982;83:963–9.

77. Rozen P, Gelfond M, Salzman S, Baron J, Gilat T. Radionuclide confirmation of the therapeutic value of isosorbide dinitrate in relieving the dysphagia in achalasia. J Clin Gastroenterol. 1982;4:17–22.

78. Gelfond M, Rozen P, Keren S, Gilat T. Effect of nitrates on LOS pressure in achalasia: a potential therapeutic aid. Gut. 1981;22:312–8. https://doi.org/10.1136/gut.22.4.312.

79. Traube M, Dubovik S, Lange RC, McCallum RW. The role of nifedipine therapy in acha-
    lasia: results of a randomized, double-blind, placebo-controlled study. Am J Gastroenterol.
    1989;84:1259–62.
80. Bortolotti M, Labo G. Clinical and manometric effects of nifedipine in patients with esopha-
    geal achalasia. Gastroenterology. 1981;80:39–44.
81. Coccia G, Bortolotti M, Michetti P, Dodero M. Prospective clinical and manometric study
    comparing pneumatic dilatation and sublingual nifedipine in the treatment of oesophageal
    achalasia. Gut. 1991;32:604–6. https://doi.org/10.1136/gut.32.6.604.
82. Eherer AJ, et al. Effect of sildenafil on oesophageal motor function in healthy subjects and
    patients with oesophageal motor disorders. Gut. 2002;50:758–64. https://doi.org/10.1136/
    gut.50.6.758.
83. Vaezi MF, et al. Botulinum toxin versus pneumatic dilatation in the treatment of achalasia: a
    randomised trial. Gut. 1999;44:231–9. https://doi.org/10.1136/gut.44.2.231.
84. Pasricha PJ, Rai R, Ravich WJ, Hendrix TR, Kalloo AN. Botulinum toxin for achalasia: long-
    term outcome and predictors of response. Gastroenterology. 1996;110:1410–5.
85. Pasricha PJ, et al. Intrasphincteric botulinum toxin for the treatment of achalasia. N Engl J
    Med. 1995;332:774–8. https://doi.org/10.1056/NEJM199503233321203.
86. Pasricha PJ, Ravich WJ, Kalloo AN. Botulinum toxin for achalasia. Lancet. 1993;341:244–5.
87. Annese V, et al. A multicentre randomised study of intrasphincteric botulinum toxin in
    patients with oesophageal achalasia. GISMAD Achalasia Study Group. Gut. 2000;46:597–
    600. https://doi.org/10.1136/gut.46.5.597.
88. Cuilliere C, et al. Achalasia: outcome of patients treated with intrasphincteric injection of
    botulinum toxin. Gut. 1997;41:87–92. https://doi.org/10.1136/gut.41.1.87.
89. Rollan A, Gonzalez R, Carvajal S, Chianale J. Endoscopic intrasphincteric injection of botu-
    linum toxin for the treatment of achalasia. J Clin Gastroenterol. 1995;20:189–91.
90. Fishman VM, et al. Symptomatic improvement in achalasia after botulinum toxin injection of
    the lower esophageal sphincter. Am J Gastroenterol. 1996;91:1724–30.
91. Annese V, et al. Controlled trial of botulinum toxin injection versus placebo and pneumatic
    dilation in achalasia. Gastroenterology. 1996;111:1418–24.
92. Gordon JM, Eaker EY. Prospective study of esophageal botulinum toxin injection in high-risk
    achalasia patients. Am J Gastroenterol. 1997;92:1812–7.
93. Muehldorfer SM, et al. Esophageal achalasia: intrasphincteric injection of botulinum toxin A
    versus balloon dilation. Endoscopy. 1999;31:517–21. https://doi.org/10.1055/s-1999-56.
94. Kolbasnik J, Waterfall WE, Fachnie B, Chen Y, Tougas G. Long-term efficacy of Botulinum
    toxin in classical achalasia: a prospective study. Am J Gastroenterol. 1999;94:3434–9. https://
    doi.org/10.1111/j.1572-0241.1999.01605.x.
95. Mikaeli J, Fazel A, Montazeri G, Yaghoobi M, Malekzadeh R. Randomized controlled trial
    comparing botulinum toxin injection to pneumatic dilatation for the treatment of achalasia.
    Aliment Pharmacol Ther. 2001;15:1389–96.
96. Allescher HD, et al. Treatment of achalasia: botulinum toxin injection vs. pneumatic bal-
    loon dilation. A prospective study with long-term follow-up. Endoscopy. 2001;33:1007–17.
    https://doi.org/10.1055/s-2001-18935.
97. Neubrand M, Scheurlen C, Schepke M, Sauerbruch T. Long-term results and prognostic fac-
    tors in the treatment of achalasia with botulinum toxin. Endoscopy. 2002;34:519–23. https://
    doi.org/10.1055/s-2002-33225.
98. Smith CD, Stival A, Howell DL, Swafford V. Endoscopic therapy for achalasia before Heller
    myotomy results in worse outcomes than heller myotomy alone. Ann Surg. 2006;243:579–
    84; discussion 584–576. https://doi.org/10.1097/01.sla.0000217524.75529.2d.
99. Vaezi MF, Pandolfino JE, Vela MF. ACG clinical guideline: diagnosis and management
    of achalasia. Am J Gastroenterol. 2013;108:1238–49; quiz 1250. https://doi.org/10.1038/
    ajg.2013.196.
100. Lambroza A, Schuman RW. Pneumatic dilation for achalasia without fluoroscopic guidance:
    safety and efficacy. Am J Gastroenterol. 1995;90:1226–9.

101. Thomas V, Harish K, Sunilkumar K. Pneumatic dilation of achalasia cardia under direct endoscopy: the debate continues. Gastrointest Endosc. 2006;63:734. https://doi.org/10.1016/j.gie.2005.11.023.
102. Vela MF, et al. The long-term efficacy of pneumatic dilatation and Heller myotomy for the treatment of achalasia. Clin Gastroenterol Hepatol. 2006;4:580–7.
103. Campos GM, et al. Endoscopic and surgical treatments for achalasia: a systematic review and meta-analysis. Ann Surg. 2009;249:45–57. https://doi.org/10.1097/SLA.0b013e31818e43ab.
104. Cox J, Buckton GK, Bennett JR. Balloon dilatation in achalasia: a new dilator. Gut. 1986;27:986–9. https://doi.org/10.1136/gut.27.8.986.
105. Gelfand MD, Kozarek RA. An experience with polyethylene balloons for pneumatic dilation in achalasia. Am J Gastroenterol. 1989;84:924–7.
106. Barkin JS, Guelrud M, Reiner DK, Goldberg RI, Phillips RS. Forceful balloon dilation: an outpatient procedure for achalasia. Gastrointest Endosc. 1990;36:123–6.
107. Stark GA, Castell DO, Richter JE, Wu WC. Prospective randomized comparison of Brown-McHardy and microvasive balloon dilators in treatment of achalasia. Am J Gastroenterol. 1990;85:1322–6.
108. Makela J, Kiviniemi H, Laitinen S. Heller's cardiomyotomy compared with pneumatic dilatation for treatment of oesophageal achalasia. Eur J Surg. 1991;157:411–4.
109. Levine ML, Moskowitz GW, Dorf BS, Bank S. Pneumatic dilation in patients with achalasia with a modified Gruntzig dilator (Levine) under direct endoscopic control: results after 5 years. Am J Gastroenterol. 1991;86:1581–4.
110. Kim CH, et al. Achalasia: prospective evaluation of relationship between lower esophageal sphincter pressure, esophageal transit, and esophageal diameter and symptoms in response to pneumatic dilation. Mayo Clin Proc. 1993;68:1067–73. https://doi.org/10.1016/s0025-6196(12)60900-8.
111. Lee JD, Cecil BD, Brown PE, Wright RA. The Cohen test does not predict outcome in achalasia after pneumatic dilation. Gastrointest Endosc. 1993;39:157–60.
112. Abid S, et al. Treatment of achalasia: the best of both worlds. Am J Gastroenterol. 1994;89:979–85.
113. Wehrmann T, Jacobi V, Jung M, Lembcke B, Caspary WF. Pneumatic dilation in achalasia with a low-compliance balloon: results of a 5-year prospective evaluation. Gastrointest Endosc. 1995;42:31–6.
114. Muehldorfer SM, Hahn EG, Ell C. High- and low-compliance balloon dilators in patients with achalasia: a randomized prospective comparative trial. Gastrointest Endosc. 1996;44:398–403.
115. Bhatnagar MS, Nanivadekar SA, Sawant P, Rathi PM. Achalasia cardia dilatation using polyethylene balloon (Rigiflex) dilators. Indian J Gastroenterol. 1996;15:49–51.
116. Gideon RM, Castell DO, Yarze J. Prospective randomized comparison of pneumatic dilatation technique in patients with idiopathic achalasia. Dig Dis Sci. 1999;44:1853–7.
117. Khan AA, et al. Massively dilated esophagus in achalasia: response to pneumatic balloon dilation. Am J Gastroenterol. 1999;94:2363–6. https://doi.org/10.1111/j.1572-0241.1999.01358.x.
118. Kadakia SC, Wong RK. Graded pneumatic dilation using Rigiflex achalasia dilators in patients with primary esophageal achalasia. Am J Gastroenterol. 1993;88:34–8.
119. Chan KC, et al. Short-term and long-term results of endoscopic balloon dilation for achalasia: 12 years' experience. Endoscopy. 2004;36:690–4. https://doi.org/10.1055/s-2004-825659.
120. Dobrucali A, Erzin Y, Tuncer M, Dirican A. Long-term results of graded pneumatic dilatation under endoscopic guidance in patients with primary esophageal achalasia. World J Gastroenterol. 2004;10:3322–7. https://doi.org/10.3748/wjg.v10.i22.3322.
121. Kostic S, et al. Pneumatic dilatation or laparoscopic cardiomyotomy in the management of newly diagnosed idiopathic achalasia. Results of a randomized controlled trial. World J Surg. 2007;31:470–8. https://doi.org/10.1007/s00268-006-0600-9.
122. Mikaeli J, Bishehsari F, Montazeri G, Yaghoobi M, Malekzadeh R. Pneumatic balloon dilatation in achalasia: a prospective comparison of safety and efficacy with different balloon diameters. Aliment Pharmacol Ther. 2004;20:431–6. https://doi.org/10.1111/j.1365-2036.2004.02080.x.

123. Ghoshal UC, et al. Long-term follow-up after pneumatic dilation for achalasia cardia: factors associated with treatment failure and recurrence. Am J Gastroenterol. 2004;99:2304–10. https://doi.org/10.1111/j.1572-0241.2004.40099.x.
124. Guardino JM, Vela MF, Connor JT, Richter JE. Pneumatic dilation for the treatment of achalasia in untreated patients and patients with failed Heller myotomy. J Clin Gastroenterol. 2004;38:855–60.
125. Boztas G, et al. Pneumatic balloon dilatation in primary achalasia: the long-term follow-up results. Hepatogastroenterology. 2005;52:475–80.
126. Karamanolis G, et al. Long-term outcome of pneumatic dilation in the treatment of achalasia. Am J Gastroenterol. 2005;100:270–4. https://doi.org/10.1111/j.1572-0241.2005.40093.x.
127. Katsinelos P, et al. Long-term results of pneumatic dilation for achalasia: a 15 years' experience. World J Gastroenterol. 2005;11:5701–5. https://doi.org/10.3748/wjg.v11.i36.5701.
128. Tuset JA, Lujan M, Huguet JM, Canelles P, Medina E. Endoscopic pneumatic balloon dilation in primary achalasia: predictive factors, complications, and long-term follow-up. Dis Esophagus. 2009;22:74–9. https://doi.org/10.1111/j.1442-2050.2008.00874.x.
129. Eckardt VF, Aignherr C, Bernhard G. Predictors of outcome in patients with achalasia treated by pneumatic dilation. Gastroenterology. 1992;103:1732–8.
130. Gockel I, Junginger T, Bernhard G, Eckardt VF. Heller myotomy for failed pneumatic dilation in achalasia: how effective is it? Ann Surg. 2004;239:371–7. https://doi.org/10.1097/01.sla.0000114228.34809.01.
131. Farhoomand K, Connor JT, Richter JE, Achkar E, Vaezi MF. Predictors of outcome of pneumatic dilation in achalasia. Clin Gastroenterol Hepatol. 2004;2:389–94.
132. Salvador R, et al. The preoperative manometric pattern predicts the outcome of surgical treatment for esophageal achalasia. J Gastrointest Surg. 2010;14:1635–45. https://doi.org/10.1007/s11605-010-1318-4.
133. Eckardt VF, Kanzler G, Westermeier T. Complications and their impact after pneumatic dilation for achalasia: prospective long-term follow-up study. Gastrointest Endosc. 1997;45:349–53.
134. Vanuytsel T, et al. Conservative management of esophageal perforations during pneumatic dilation for idiopathic esophageal achalasia. Clin Gastroenterol Hepatol. 2012;10:142–9. https://doi.org/10.1016/j.cgh.2011.10.032.
135. Inoue H, et al. Peroral endoscopic myotomy (POEM) for esophageal achalasia. Endoscopy. 2010;42:265–71. https://doi.org/10.1055/s-0029-1244080.
136. Bhayani NH, et al. A comparative study on comprehensive, objective outcomes of laparoscopic Heller myotomy with per-oral endoscopic myotomy (POEM) for achalasia. Ann Surg. 2014;259:1098–103. https://doi.org/10.1097/SLA.0000000000000268.
137. Stavropoulos SN, Modayil RJ, Friedel D, Savides T. The international per oral endoscopic myotomy survey (IPOEMS): a snapshot of the global POEM experience. Surg Endosc. 2013;27:3322–38. https://doi.org/10.1007/s00464-013-2913-8.
138. Lujan-Sanchis M, et al. Management of primary achalasia: the role of endoscopy. World J Gastrointest Endosc. 2015;7:593–605. https://doi.org/10.4253/wjge.v7.i6.593.
139. Bechara R, Ikeda H, Inoue H. Peroral endoscopic myotomy: an evolving treatment for achalasia. Nat Rev Gastroenterol Hepatol. 2015;12:410–26. https://doi.org/10.1038/nrgastro.2015.87.
140. Tan Y, et al. Efficacy of anterior versus posterior per-oral endoscopic myotomy for treating achalasia: a randomized, prospective study. Gastrointest Endosc. 2018;88:46–54. https://doi.org/10.1016/j.gie.2018.03.009.
141. Tyberg A, et al. Peroral endoscopic myotomy as salvation technique post-Heller: international experience. Dig Endosc. 2018;30:52–6. https://doi.org/10.1111/den.12918.
142. Yao S, Linghu E. Peroral endoscopic myotomy can improve esophageal motility in patients with achalasia from a large sample self-control research (66 patients). PLoS One. 2015;10:e0125942. https://doi.org/10.1371/journal.pone.0125942.
143. Hu JW, et al. Peroral endoscopic myotomy for advanced achalasia with sigmoid-shaped esophagus: long-term outcomes from a prospective, single-center study. Surg Endosc. 2015;29:2841–50. https://doi.org/10.1007/s00464-014-4013-9.

144. Teitelbaum EN, et al. Symptomatic and physiologic outcomes one year after peroral esophageal myotomy (POEM) for treatment of achalasia. Surg Endosc. 2014;28:3359–65. https://doi.org/10.1007/s00464-014-3628-1.
145. Zhou PH, et al. Peroral endoscopic remyotomy for failed Heller myotomy: a prospective single-center study. Endoscopy. 2013;45:161–6. https://doi.org/10.1055/s-0032-1326203.
146. Swanstrom LL, et al. Long-term outcomes of an endoscopic myotomy for achalasia: the POEM procedure. Ann Surg. 2012;256:659–67. https://doi.org/10.1097/SLA.0b013e31826b5212.
147. Shiwaku H. et al. Multicenter collaborative retrospective evaluation of peroral endoscopic myotomy for esophageal achalasia: analysis of data from more than 1300 patients at eight facilities in Japan. Surg Endosc. 2019. https://doi.org/10.1007/s00464-019-06833-8.
148. Grimes KL, et al. Double-scope per oral endoscopic myotomy (POEM): a prospective randomized controlled trial. Surg Endosc. 2016;30:1344–51. https://doi.org/10.1007/s00464-015-4396-2.
149. Liu W. et al. Open peroral endoscopic myotomy for the treatment of achalasia: a case series of 82 cases. Dis Esophagus. 2019. https://doi.org/10.1093/dote/doz052.
150. Chandan S. et al. Clinical efficacy of per-oral endoscopic myotomy (POEM) for spastic esophageal disorders: a systematic review and meta-analysis. Surg Endosc. 2019. https://doi.org/10.1007/s00464-019-06819-6.
151. Kim WH, et al. Comparison of the outcomes of peroral endoscopic myotomy for achalasia according to manometric subtype. Gut Liver. 2017;11:642–7. https://doi.org/10.5009/gnl16545.
152. Kane ED, Budhraja V, Desilets DJ, Romanelli JR. Myotomy length informed by high-resolution esophageal manometry (HREM) results in improved per-oral endoscopic myotomy (POEM) outcomes for type III achalasia. Surg Endosc. 2019;33:886–94. https://doi.org/10.1007/s00464-018-6356-0.
153. Zhang W, Linghu EQ. Peroral endoscopic myotomy for type III achalasia of Chicago classification: outcomes with a minimum follow-up of 24 months. J Gastrointest Surg. 2017;21:785–91. https://doi.org/10.1007/s11605-017-3398-x.
154. Chen X, et al. Two-year follow-up for 45 patients with achalasia who underwent peroral endoscopic myotomy. Eur J Cardiothorac Surg. 2015;47:890–6. https://doi.org/10.1093/ejcts/ezu320.
155. Khashab MA, et al. International multicenter experience with peroral endoscopic myotomy for the treatment of spastic esophageal disorders refractory to medical therapy (with video). Gastrointest Endosc. 2015;81:1170–7. https://doi.org/10.1016/j.gie.2014.10.011.
156. Stavropoulos SN, et al. Per-oral endoscopic myotomy white paper summary. Surg Endosc. 2014;28:2005–19. https://doi.org/10.1007/s00464-014-3630-7.
157. Talukdar R, Inoue H, Nageshwar Reddy D. Efficacy of peroral endoscopic myotomy (POEM) in the treatment of achalasia: a systematic review and meta-analysis. Surg Endosc. 2015;29:3030–46. https://doi.org/10.1007/s00464-014-4040-6.
158. Kumbhari V, et al. Gastroesophageal reflux after peroral endoscopic myotomy: a multicenter case-control study. Endoscopy. 2017;49:634–42. https://doi.org/10.1055/s-0043-105485.
159. Kahrilas PJ, Katzka D, Richter JE. Clinical practice update: the use of per-oral endoscopic myotomy in achalasia: expert review and best practice advice from the AGA Institute. Gastroenterology. 2017;153:1205–11. https://doi.org/10.1053/j.gastro.2017.10.001.
160. Rosati R, et al. Laparoscopic approach to esophageal achalasia. Am J Surg. 1995;169:424–7.
161. Ancona E, et al. Esophageal achalasia: laparoscopic versus conventional open Heller-Dor operation. Am J Surg. 1995;170:265–70.
162. Mitchell PC, et al. Laparoscopic cardiomyotomy with a Dor patch for achalasia. Can J Surg. 1995;38:445–8.
163. Swanstrom LL, Pennings J. Laparoscopic esophagomyotomy for achalasia. Surg Endosc. 1995;9:286–90; discussion 290–282.
164. Raiser F, et al. Heller myotomy via minimal-access surgery. An evaluation of antireflux procedures. Arch Surg. 1996;131:593–7; discussion 597–598.

165. Morino M, Rebecchi F, Festa V, Garrone C. Laparoscopic Heller cardiomyotomy with intra-operative manometry in the management of oesophageal achalasia. Int Surg. 1995;80:332–5.
166. Robertson GS, Lloyd DM, Wicks AC, de Caestecker J, Veitch PS. Laparoscopic Heller's cardiomyotomy without an antireflux procedure. Br J Surg. 1995;82:957–9.
167. Bonavina L, Rosati R, Segalin A, Peracchia A. Laparoscopic Heller-Dor operation for the treatment of oesophageal achalasia: technique and early results. Ann Chir Gynaecol. 1995;84:165–8.
168. Delgado F, et al. Laparoscopic treatment of esophageal achalasia. Surg Laparosc Endosc. 1996;6:83–90.
169. Hunter JG, Trus TL, Branum GD, Waring JP. Laparoscopic Heller myotomy and fundoplication for achalasia. Ann Surg. 1997;225:655–64; discussion 664–655. https://doi.org/10.1097/00000658-199706000-00003.
170. Kjellin AP, Granqvist S, Ramel S, Thor KB. Laparoscopic myotomy without fundoplication in patients with achalasia. Eur J Surg. 1999;165:1162–6. https://doi.org/10.1080/110241599750007702.
171. Ackroyd R, Watson DI, Devitt PG, Jamieson GG. Laparoscopic cardiomyotomy and anterior partial fundoplication for achalasia. Surg Endosc. 2001;15:683–6. https://doi.org/10.1007/s004640080037.
172. Yamamura MS, Gilster JC, Myers BS, Deveney CW, Sheppard BC. Laparoscopic heller myotomy and anterior fundoplication for achalasia results in a high degree of patient satisfaction. Arch Surg. 2000;135:902–6.
173. Patti MG, et al. Laparoscopic Heller myotomy and Dor fundoplication for achalasia: analysis of successes and failures. Arch Surg. 2001;136:870–7.
174. Pechlivanides G, et al. Laparoscopic Heller cardiomyotomy and Dor fundoplication for esophageal achalasia: possible factors predicting outcome. Arch Surg. 2001;136:1240–3.
175. Sharp KW, Khaitan L, Scholz S, Holzman MD, Richards WO. 100 consecutive minimally invasive Heller myotomies: lessons learned. Ann Surg. 2002;235:631–8; discussion 638–639. https://doi.org/10.1097/00000658-200205000-00004.
176. Donahue PE, Horgan S, Liu KJ, Madura JA. Floppy Dor fundoplication after esophagocardiomyotomy for achalasia. Surgery. 2002;132:716–22; discussion 722–713.
177. Zaninotto G, et al. Etiology, diagnosis, and treatment of failures after laparoscopic Heller myotomy for achalasia. Ann Surg. 2002;235:186–92. https://doi.org/10.1097/00000658-200202000-00005.
178. Luketich JD, et al. Outcomes after minimally invasive esophagomyotomy. Ann Thorac Surg. 2001;72:1909–12; discussion 1912–1903.
179. Decker G, et al. Gastrointestinal quality of life before and after laparoscopic heller myotomy with partial posterior fundoplication. Ann Surg. 2002;236:750–8; discussion 758. https://doi.org/10.1097/00000658-200212000-00007.
180. Mineo TC, Ambrogi V. Long-term results and quality of life after surgery for oesophageal achalasia: one surgeon's experience. Eur J Cardiothorac Surg. 2004;25:1089–96. https://doi.org/10.1016/j.ejcts.2004.01.043.
181. Gockel I, Junginger T, Eckardt VF. Long-term results of conventional myotomy in patients with achalasia: a prospective 20-year analysis. J Gastrointest Surg. 2006;10:1400–8. https://doi.org/10.1016/j.gassur.2006.07.006.
182. Wright AS, Williams CW, Pellegrini CA, Oelschlager BK. Long-term outcomes confirm the superior efficacy of extended Heller myotomy with Toupet fundoplication for achalasia. Surg Endosc. 2007;21:713–8. https://doi.org/10.1007/s00464-006-9165-9.
183. Khajanchee YS, Kanneganti S, Leatherwood AE, Hansen PD, Swanstrom LL. Laparoscopic Heller myotomy with Toupet fundoplication: outcomes predictors in 121 consecutive patients. Arch Surg. 2005;140:827–33; discussion 833–824. https://doi.org/10.1001/archsurg.140.9.827.
184. Zaninotto G, et al. Randomized controlled trial of botulinum toxin versus laparoscopic heller myotomy for esophageal achalasia. Ann Surg. 2004;239:364–70. https://doi.org/10.1097/01.sla.0000114217.52941.c5.

185. Csendes A, et al. Very late results of esophagomyotomy for patients with achalasia: clinical, endoscopic, histologic, manometric, and acid reflux studies in 67 patients for a mean follow-up of 190 months. Ann Surg. 2006;243:196–203. https://doi.org/10.1097/01.sla.0000197469.12632.e0.

186. Ramacciato G, et al. The laparoscopic approach with antireflux surgery is superior to the thoracoscopic approach for the treatment of esophageal achalasia. Experience of a single surgical unit. Surg Endosc. 2002;16:1431–7. https://doi.org/10.1007/s00464-001-9215-2.

187. Richards WO, et al. Heller myotomy versus Heller myotomy with Dor fundoplication for achalasia: a prospective randomized double-blind clinical trial. Ann Surg. 2004;240:405–12; discussion 412–405. https://doi.org/10.1097/01.sla.0000136940.32255.51.

188. Rawlings A, et al. Laparoscopic Dor versus Toupet fundoplication following Heller myotomy for achalasia: results of a multicenter, prospective, randomized-controlled trial. Surg Endosc. 2012;26:18–26. https://doi.org/10.1007/s00464-011-1822-y.

189. Schlottmann F, Luckett DJ, Fine J, Shaheen NJ, Patti MG. Laparoscopic Heller myotomy versus peroral endoscopic myotomy (POEM) for achalasia: a systematic review and meta-analysis. Ann Surg. 2018;267:451–60. https://doi.org/10.1097/SLA.0000000000002311.

190. Vaezi MF, Baker ME, Achkar E, Richter JE. Timed barium oesophagram: better predictor of long term success after pneumatic dilation in achalasia than symptom assessment. Gut. 2002;50:765–70. https://doi.org/10.1136/gut.50.6.765.

191. Roman S, et al. Partial recovery of peristalsis after myotomy for achalasia: more the rule than the exception. JAMA Surg. 2013;148:157–64. https://doi.org/10.1001/2013.jamasurg.38.

192. Tustumi F, et al. Esophageal achalasia: a risk factor for carcinoma. A systematic review and meta-analysis. Dis Esophagus. 2017;30:1–8. https://doi.org/10.1093/dote/dox072.

193. Leeuwenburgh I, et al. Long-term esophageal cancer risk in patients with primary achalasia: a prospective study. Am J Gastroenterol. 2010;105:2144–9. https://doi.org/10.1038/ajg.2010.263.

194. Ravi K, Geno DM, Katzka DA. Esophageal cancer screening in achalasia: is there a consensus? Dis Esophagus. 2015;28:299–304. https://doi.org/10.1111/dote.12196.

195. Harvey PR, et al. Incidence, morbidity and mortality of patients with achalasia in England: findings from a study of nationwide hospital and primary care data. Gut. 2019;68:790–5. https://doi.org/10.1136/gutjnl-2018-316089.

196. Zaninotto G, et al. Long-term results (6–10 years) of laparoscopic fundoplication. J Gastrointest Surg. 2007;11:1138–45. https://doi.org/10.1007/s11605-007-0195-y.

197. Zaninotto G, et al. Four hundred laparoscopic myotomies for esophageal achalasia: a single centre experience. Ann Surg. 2008;248:986–93. https://doi.org/10.1097/SLA.0b013e3181907bdd.

198. Bonatti H, et al. Long-term results of laparoscopic Heller myotomy with partial fundoplication for the treatment of achalasia. Am J Surg. 2005;190:874–8. https://doi.org/10.1016/j.amjsurg.2005.08.012.

199. Costantini M, et al. The laparoscopic Heller-Dor operation remains an effective treatment for esophageal achalasia at a minimum 6-year follow-up. Surg Endosc. 2005;19:345–51. https://doi.org/10.1007/s00464-004-8941-7.

200. Eckardt VF, Hoischen T, Bernhard G. Life expectancy, complications, and causes of death in patients with achalasia: results of a 33-year follow-up investigation. Eur J Gastroenterol Hepatol. 2008;20:956–60. https://doi.org/10.1097/MEG.0b013e3282fbf5e5.

201. Ngamruengphong S, et al. Efficacy and safety of peroral endoscopic myotomy for treatment of achalasia after failed Heller myotomy. Clin Gastroenterol Hepatol. 2017;15:1531–1537. e1533. https://doi.org/10.1016/j.cgh.2017.01.031.

202. Legros L, et al. Long-term results of pneumatic dilatation for relapsing symptoms of achalasia after Heller myotomy. Neurogastroenterol Motil. 2014;26:1248–55. https://doi.org/10.1111/nmo.12380.

203. Rakita S, Villadolid D, Kalipersad C, Thometz D, Rosemurgy A. Outcomes promote reoperative Heller myotomy for symptoms of achalasia. Surg Endosc. 2007;21:1709–14. https://doi.org/10.1007/s00464-007-9226-8.
204. Grotenhuis BA, et al. Reoperation for dysphagia after cardiomyotomy for achalasia. Am J Surg. 2007;194:678–82. https://doi.org/10.1016/j.amjsurg.2007.01.035.
205. Patel DA, Vaezi MF. Refractory achalasia: is POEM changing the paradigm? Clin Gastroenterol Hepatol. 2017;15:1504–6. https://doi.org/10.1016/j.cgh.2017.04.032.
206. Hoogerwerf WA, et al. Pharmacologic therapy in treating achalasia. Gastrointest Endosc Clin N Am. 2001;11:311–23.

Chapter 8
Spastic Motor Disorders

Jennifer X. Cai and Walter W. Chan

Introduction

Spastic esophageal disorders are currently comprised of three main clinical entities, distal esophageal spasm (DES), hypercontractile or jackhammer esophagus, and type III (spastic) achalasia, as defined by high-resolution esophageal manometry. While no population-based studies exist for non-achalasia esophageal motility disorders, the prevalence of DES is thought be similar to that of achalasia, approximating 1 in 100,000 in the USA [1]. Recent studies also estimated that 1–4% of patients undergoing esophageal manometry for dysphagia and/or chest pain demonstrate findings suggestive of a spastic disorder [2–5].

Generally, spastic esophageal disorders are characterized by increased contractile vigor or premature propagation of swallow-induced esophageal body contractions. Despite similarities in symptomatology among patients with these disorders, the heterogeneity of this population (with respect to clinical outcomes) may signal mechanistically distinct esophageal pathologies. In addition, the evolution from conventional to high-resolution esophageal manometry (HRM) and the development of new diagnostic parameters by the Chicago Classification (CC) have shifted the notion of how spastic disorders should be defined [6]. Nutcracker esophagus was originally characterized on conventional manometry by an average contraction amplitude of greater than 180 mmHg in the distal esophagus, a cutoff that was subsequently increased to 220 mmHg to improve diagnostic specificity. When HRM became available and the initial versions of CC were established, this diagnosis was redefined using the new metric distal contractile integral (DCI). While a mean DCI

J. X. Cai · W. W. Chan (✉)
Division of Gastroenterology, Hepatology and Endoscopy, Brigham and Women's Hospital, Boston, MA, USA

Harvard Medical School, Boston, MA, USA
e-mail: wwchan@bwh.harvard.edu

© Springer Nature Switzerland AG 2020
D. A. Patel et al. (eds.), *Evaluation and Management of Dysphagia*,
https://doi.org/10.1007/978-3-030-26554-0_8

value between 5000 and 8000 mmHg·s·cm was identified as hypertensive peristalsis or nutcracker esophagus, conditions with significantly increased contractile vigor (DCI greater than 8000 mmHg.s.cm) were further classified as hypercontractile or jackhammer esophagus. Most recently, nutcracker esophagus has been eliminated entirely from the latest iteration of CC (version 3.0) published in 2015, given that up to 5% of normal, healthy subjects may achieve mean DCI values within that range (5000–8000) [7]. Instead, hypercontractile or jackhammer esophagus is now defined in CC version 3.0 as DCI greater than 8000 mmHg·s·cm in at least 20% of liquid test swallows (which has not been observed in control subjects and thought to represent a more homogeneous phenotype) [6]. Hypertensive lower esophageal sphincter (LES), traditionally defined as a basal LES pressure of greater than 45 mmHg, is associated with high-amplitude peristaltic contractions in the distal esophagus in approximately 50% of patients who present with chest pain and may also be correlated with incomplete relaxation of the LES after a liquid swallow. However, the relationship between clinical symptoms and elevated basal LES pressure alone has not been clearly established. Hypertensive LES, therefore, is not currently a diagnostic entity in CC version 3.0. Hypercontractile LES, defined as a post-glutitive LES contraction with excessive duration or amplitude, has been previously described and associated with symptoms. A recent study found that including the hypercontractile LES to the DCI measurement of the esophageal body infrequently results in reclassification of diagnosis among patients presenting with dysphagia or chest pain. Hypercontractile LES, therefore, is now included as part of the evaluation of esophageal body hypercontractility in CC v3.0. The same manometric classification system defines DES as ≥20% premature contractions with a distal latency (DL) of less than 4.5 seconds. While both DES and spastic achalasia are characterized by premature propagation of contractions and diminished DL, insufficient LES relaxation is only a feature of the latter.

In this chapter, we will focus on the pathophysiology, clinical presentation, diagnosis, and management of DES and jackhammer esophagus, given the discussion of achalasia in the preceding chapter.

Pathophysiology

The pathophysiology of spastic esophageal disorders is not fully elucidated. Biopsies of the esophageal muscularis propria and myenteric plexus are rarely endoscopically accessible for clinicopathologic investigation, and patients with spastic disorders typically do not require esophageal surgery [1]. In the absence of more definitive histopathologic evidence, the prevailing theory for the mechanism underlying spastic esophageal disorders centers on the delicate balance between inhibitory and excitatory neuronal regulation of the esophageal smooth muscles [8]. The myenteric plexus located between the longitudinal and circular muscle layers of the esophagus contains the inhibitory and excitatory innervations responsible for motor function control of both muscular layers. At baseline, the esophagus is in a contractile state mediated by excitatory cholinergic neurons. During deglutition, activation of inhibitory neurons and the resultant release of transmitters such as nitric oxide and vasoactive intestinal peptide lead to relaxation of both the lower esophageal sphincter and the esophageal body. Normal peristalsis then follows when coordinated actions of the inhibitory and excitatory neurons lead to sequential contraction and relaxation of the esophageal body smooth muscle, progressing aborally toward the lower esophageal sphincter. This is facilitated by a neural gradient of increasing inhibitory ganglionic neurons when progressing distally to the lower esophageal sphincter [9]. Thus, the inhibitory innervation generally controls the relaxation of the lower esophageal sphincter and the peristaltic pattern of the esophageal body during a normal swallow, while the excitatory innervation is primarily responsible for the basal tone of the lower esophageal sphincter and the contractile force of esophageal body smooth muscles. Spastic disorders may, therefore, result from disturbances in the inhibitory system, excitatory system, or both (Fig. 8.1).

The pathology of DES is thought to be related to impaired inhibition, leading to a reduction in contractile latency and inappropriate premature contraction of the distal esophagus [8]. Prior research has shown a dose-dependent elongation of the latency period after swallowing, decrease in mean duration of contractions, and alleviation of clinical symptoms in DES patients following infusion of glyceryl trinitrate, which may enhance the nitric oxide-mediated inhibitory drive [10]. In a study of healthy, asymptomatic patients, administration of recombinant human hemoglobin, a nitric oxide scavenger, precipitated esophageal spasm, characterized

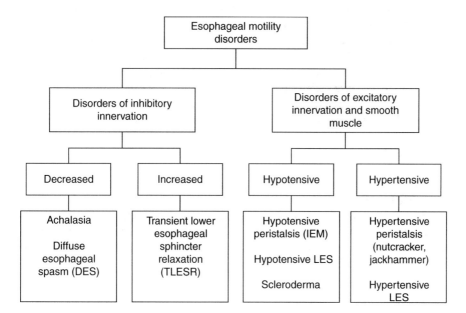

Fig. 8.1 Esophageal motility disorders

by increased velocity of peristaltic contraction and spontaneous, simultaneous high-pressure contractions, in eight out of nine subjects [11].

In contrast, the pathology in jackhammer esophagus is felt to be due to increased excitatory cholinergic drive, resulting in myocyte hypertrophy and amplified contractions [1]. The administration of an acetylcholinesterase inhibitor (edrophonium) has been shown to induce an increase in circular and longitudinal muscle contraction amplitude, duration, and asynchrony during peristalsis, whereas administration of an acetylcholine receptor antagonist (atropine) reversed those same effects in a dose-dependent manner [12, 13]. Other studies have postulated that an obstructive physiology at the esophagogastric junction (EGJ) may also yield a compensatory esophageal hypercontractility [14, 15].

Clinical Presentation

Distal Esophageal Spasm

The predominant symptoms of DES are dysphagia and chest pain. Dysphagia can be from solid or liquid ingestion and may be accompanied by regurgitation, heartburn, odynophagia, as well as intermittent retention of swallowed bolus that may be relieved by emesis. Notably, patients' ability to localize the site of their bolus retention to the distal esophagus is notoriously inaccurate, with a success rate of only 60% [1]. Esophageal chest pain may be similar in quality and location to cardiac angina, often characterized by a crushing pressure radiating to the shoulder, jaw, or back. DES patients with chest pain may have higher distal esophageal contraction amplitudes compared to DES patients who experience primarily dysphagia or regurgitation [16]. Regardless, a high level of suspicion should be employed in patients with other risk factors for cardiovascular disease, which must be ruled out. Furthermore, because esophageal motility disorders (and especially spastic disorders) are rare compared to other etiologies of dysphagia, it is important to consider a broad differential including more commonly seen anatomic, inflammatory, infectious, neoplastic, and iatrogenic causes of dysphagia. Other esophageal diseases which can lead to dysphagia, such as gastroesophageal reflux disease (GERD), may also coexist with spastic disorders. In a study of 108 patients with DES, 41 (34%) had pathologic acid reflux diagnosed on pH testing or endoscopy [17]. In fact, GERD is also considered a possible etiologic contributor to DES. Epiphrenic diverticula may also occur as a consequence of spastic esophageal disorders, particularly in those with an underlying connection tissue disorder – in a series of 21 cases of epiphrenic diverticulosis, DES was found in 24%, nutcracker esophagus in 24%, and achalasia in 9% of patients [18].

Jackhammer Esophagus

Similar to DES, the most common presenting symptoms of hypercontractile esophagus are also dysphagia and chest discomfort. In a recent European cohort study of 34 patients with jackhammer esophagus, 23 patients (67.6%) suffered from dysphagia, and 16 patients (47.1%) reported having chest pain [19]. It has been suggested that bolus transit is less affected because the distal latency is preserved in a jackhammer pattern; however, the natural history of hypercontractile esophagus remains unknown.

Diagnosis

Upper Endoscopy

The evaluation of esophageal dysphagia often starts with an upper endoscopy to exclude structural causes including mechanical obstruction, stricture, ring, and esophagitis. In addition, endoscopy offers the ability to obtain multiple biopsies to rule out eosinophilic esophagitis in otherwise normal-appearing mucosa [20]. While no specific endoscopic findings are diagnostic of esophageal spastic disorders, the presence of epiphrenic diverticulosis should raise clinical suspicion. Abnormal and disorderly esophageal contractions may also be seen during endoscopy, although these findings are neither sensitive nor specific.

Esophageal Manometry

HRM with esophageal pressure topography has largely replaced conventional manometry in recent years, and measurements of integrated relaxation pressure (IRP), DL, and DCI form the very basis of categorization used to define esophageal motility disorders, making manometry indispensable in the diagnosis of spastic esophageal diseases. Under the most updated version of CC, DES and jackhammer esophagus are diagnosed based on the proportion of test swallows on HRM that are premature (short DL <4.5 sec) or hypercontractile (high DCI >8000 mmHg.s.cm), respectively, with ≥20% being the cutoff for both conditions (Fig. 8.2). More recently, other novel metrics have emerged that may further improve the interpretation of DCI to better characterize spastic disorders. One such technique separates the pre- and postpeak phases of the

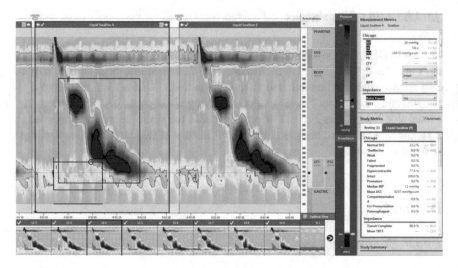

Fig. 8.2 Diagnosis of DES and jackhammer esophagus (Chicago Classification)

contractile pressure wave. The traditional DCI measurement appears to have a greater contribution from postpeak contractile activity in a study of 71 healthy subjects [21]. When asymptomatic controls were compared to 38 patients with jackhammer esophagus, those with jackhammer had greater contractile integral in both phases, as well as a higher postpeak to prepeak ratio. In addition, there was a correlation between this ratio and dysphagia symptom scores, suggesting that postpeak contractile integral (and abnormality in the postpeak phase of peristalsis) may play a greater role in dysphagia severity among patients with jackhammer esophagus [22].

Barium Swallow

Barium esophagram is often used as an adjunct to endoscopy and manometry, providing valuable information regarding peristalsis, esophageal sphincters function, and bolus transit and clearance through the EGJ [1]. The study is best performed in the prone position to obviate any contribution from gravity to esophageal clearance. However, in a study of 100 patients with complaints of esophageal symptoms who were evaluated by barium swallow and gold standard HRM, barium esophagram had a sensitivity of only 77% and specificity of 35% for detecting non-achalasia esophageal dysmotility, thereby limiting its role as a stand-alone test for spastic motility disorders [23].

The classic finding of corkscrew or rosary bead appearance on barium swallow (Fig. 8.3), corresponding to the simultaneous smooth muscle contractions of DES, is also rare. In 1 study of 14 patients with DES diagnosed on barium study

Fig. 8.3 Classic finding of corkscrew or rosary bead appearance on barium swallow

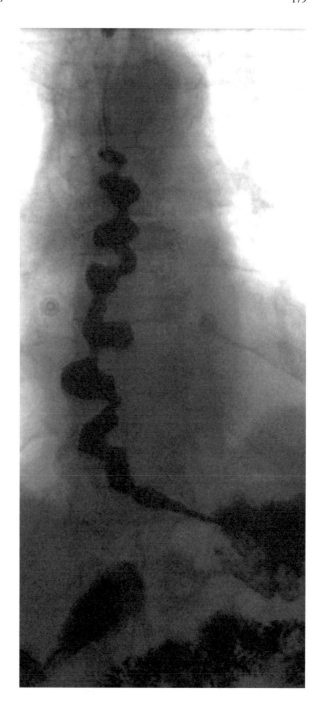

and confirmed by HRM, only 2 patients had a corkscrew appearance, whereas the rest demonstrated nonperistaltic contractions that did not fully obliterate the lumen [24]. Another study of 108 DES patients, of which 76 had esophagrams, noted 46 patients (61%) with abnormal peristalsis, although only 3 (4%) exhibited a corkscrew appearance [17]. Similarly, jackhammer esophagus may be associated with both normal and nonspecific barium swallow findings, including uncoordinated primary peristalsis and tertiary contractions [25].

Computed Tomography (CT) Scan and Endoscopic Ultrasound (EUS)

Spastic disorders may be associated with esophageal wall thickening which can be detected on cross-sectional CT imaging. In a series of 33 patients with evidence of DES on barium swallow, 7 (21%) were found to have esophageal muscle thickening on CT, up to 11.9 mm just proximal to the gastroesophageal junction, whereas normal thickness typically does not exceed 3 mm [26]. This thickening is more likely to be smooth and circumferential as opposed to nodular and asymmetric, which may raise the possibility of tumor involvement. EUS is another imaging modality which can quantify esophageal thickening as well as identify any intramural or extrinsically compressing masses that could lead to abnormal contraction.

Intraluminal Impedance Measurement

Multichannel intraluminal impedance measurement allows for an evaluation of bolus transit without subjecting patients to the radiation exposure intrinsic to barium esophagrams, with 97% concordance with videofluoroscopy in determining bolus transit among asymptomatic patients [27]. Among patients with dysphagia, concordance was similarly high for severe barium stasis and incomplete bolus transit (97%) [28]. HRM with concurrent intraluminal impedance measurement has also been employed to assess bolus transit as a function of distal esophageal amplitude, where contractions <30 mmHg corresponded to 85% sensitivity and 66% specificity in identifying incomplete bolus transit [1, 29]. Additional studies are needed to determine how these complementary technologies may be best utilized in further characterizing spastic esophageal disorders.

Functional Lumen Imaging Probe (FLIP)

FLIP utilizes high-resolution impedance planimetry, which measures esophageal wall and EGJ compliance by assessing how distension pressure of the esophagus reacts to volumetric expansion. FLIP offers an adjunctive method, primarily in conjunction with manometry, to objectively evaluate esophageal motility disorders. As FLIP is performed during upper endoscopy, it also minimizes patient discomfort, as it does not require trans-nasal catheter insertion while awake. The primary, and most validated, metric obtained on FLIP is the EGJ-distensibility index (DI), considered abnormal if <2.8 mm²/mmHg. The newer FLIP topography identifies patterns of esophageal body contractile response to esophageal distention that may correspond to esophageal motility disorders. While repetitive antegrade contractions is the normal esophageal response on FLIP, repetitive retrograde contractions have been associated with spastic esophageal dysmotility. In a recent study of 145 patients with dysphagia, FLIP was able to identify patterns suggestive of dysmotility in 50% of those with normal HRM. In addition, in some patients diagnosed with jackhammer esophagus on HRM, FLIP findings were more indicative of spastic achalasia, highlighting the fact that this method may be particularly useful in cases where a manometric diagnosis is unclear [30, 31].

Treatment

Management Approach

Despite proposed differences in the pathophysiology underlying each spastic disorder, the management approach to both DES and hypercontractile esophagus is similar. Initially, an assessment for and treatment of GERD should be undertaken – not only because GERD is a common culprit of dysphagia as well as chest pain and has significant symptom overlap with spastic esophageal disease but also because GERD itself may induce or worsen esophageal dysmotility. Appropriate treatment of reflux may, therefore, reduce esophageal symptoms related to dysmotility. Moreover, many medications used to treat spasticity are smooth muscle relaxants, which may worsen any underlying reflux that may be present. In fact, prior studies have found GERD to be significantly more common than primary esophageal motility disorders in noncardiac chest pain. Treatment targeting esophageal spasm without first ruling out or controlling underlying GERD may worsen the patients' symptoms.

In patients with no pathologic acid reflux or well-controlled GERD, primary efforts should be focused on symptom relief of dysphagia and noncardiac chest pain. In the following discussion of the pharmacotherapeutic, endoscopic, and surgical modalities of treatment of spastic esophageal disorders, much of the experience is anecdotal, and more large, prospective, randomized, controlled trials (Table 8.1) are needed to further validate the value of these therapies.

Table 8.1 Trials of treatment therapies for spastic esophageal disorders

Therapy	Intervention (alternative intervention for clinical use)	Study design	Study size (N)	Level of evidence
Pharmacologic				
Smooth muscle relaxants				
Peppermint oil	Five drops in 10 mL of water (2 Altoid mints sublingually qac)	Case series	8	4 [32]
Calcium channel blockers	Diltiazem 60–90 mg qid (Nifedipine 10 mg qac)	Double-blind crossover, per protocol analysis	14	1D [33]
Nitrates	IV glyceryl trinitrate 100–200mcg/kg/h (sublingual nitroglycerin, isosorbide dinitrate 10 mg during or after meals)	Case series	5	4 [10]
Neuromodulators				
Tricyclic antidepressants	Imipramine 50 mg qhs vs clonidine 0.1 mg bid vs placebo bid (nortriptyline/ amitriptyline 10–25 mg qhs)	Double-blind, placebo-controlled crossover	60	1C [34]
Trazodone	Trazodone 100–150 mg daily vs placebo	Double-blind, placebo-controlled	29	3 [35]
Selective serotonin reuptake inhibitors	IV citalopram 20 mg (fluoxetine 10–20 mg/day, paroxetine 10–20 mg/day, sertraline 25–50 mg/day)	Double-blind crossover	10	3 [36]
Phosphodiesterase-5 inhibitors	Sildenafil 50 mg vs placebo	Double-blind, placebo-controlled	17	1D [37]
Theophylline	Theophylline SR 200 mg bid vs placebo	Double-blind, placebo-controlled	25	1D [38]
Endoscopic				
Botulinum toxin injection	Botulinum toxin injection 8 × 12.5 U vs saline 8 × 0.5 mL in 4 quadrants at 2 and 7 cm above EGJ	Double-blind, placebo-controlled crossover	22	1D [39]

Table 8.1 (continued)

Therapy	Intervention (alternative intervention for clinical use)	Study design	Study size (N)	Level of evidence
Esophageal dilation	Mercury bougienage 54Fr therapeutic vs 24Fr placebo (pneumatic dilation)	Double-blind, placebo-controlled crossover	8	1D [40]
Peroral endoscopic myotomy	Peroral endoscopic myotomy	Systematic review, meta-analysis	179	1A [41]
Surgical				
Heller myotomy	Extended myotomy (14 cm in esophagus, 2 cm below EGJ) with anterior fundoplication	Case series	20	4 [42]
Adjunctive				
Biofeedback	Sipping while viewing motility tracings, double swallows	Case report	1	5 [43]

Abbreviations: *qac* before each meal, *qid* four times daily, IV intravenous, *qhs* before bedtime, *bid* twice daily, *EGJ* esophagogastric junction

Pharmacotherapy

Current medical therapies for spastic disorders of the esophagus can be divided into two main categories based on treatment targets, namely, the abnormal motor function and the sensitivity of the esophagus. Smooth muscle relaxants decrease the amplitude and restore the peristaltic pattern of esophageal smooth muscle contractions, while neuromodulators aim to reduce the afferent input and hypersensitivity of the esophagus to control symptoms.

Smooth Muscle Relaxants

Peppermint oil has been shown to act as a smooth muscle relaxant in the gastrointestinal tract of animal models and has had some success in the treatment of colonic spasm, dyspepsia, and irritable bowel syndrome [44–47]. In a series of eight patients with DES, peppermint oil, administered as five drops in 10 mL of water, completely eliminated simultaneous esophageal contractions in all patients with decreased variability of amplitude and duration of contractions, although chest pain was relieved in only two patients [32].

Other dedicated smooth muscle relaxants, such as calcium channel blockers and nitrates, aim to decrease esophageal body contraction amplitude as well as LES pressure. In a small randomized, double-blind, crossover prospective trial of 14 patients with high-amplitude esophageal contractions, diltiazem was found to have a positive impact on chest pain symptoms as well as peristaltic pressure on manometry compared to placebo [33]. Effective doses have been suggested in the range of diltiazem 60–90 mg four times daily and nifedipine 10 mg given 30 minutes prior to meals. Nitrates were shown to significantly decrease the mean duration of esophageal contractions and alleviate symptoms during swallows in a small case series of five DES patients with no reported adverse side effects of headache, flushing, or hypotension [10]. No controlled trials on the effect of nitrates on DES or jackhammer esophagus have been conducted to date.

An alternative to nitrates is phosphodiesterase-5 inhibitor, which blocks the degradation of nitric oxide, thereby prolonging smooth muscle relaxation in symptomatic DES and jackhammer esophagus [9]. Sildenafil, a commonly used phosphodiesterase-5 inhibitor, was found to lower LES pressure and contraction amplitudes in a randomized double-blind study of 6 healthy subjects and 11 patients with hypercontractile esophagus [37]. In a case report of two patients with refractory DES, sildenafil 25–50 mg twice daily relieved dysphagia and chest pain and suppressed esophageal contraction completely for liquid swallows and reduced frequency of spasm for solid swallows [48]. Limitations include side effects of headache and dizziness as well as lack of insurance coverage for a medication which is mainly approved for erectile dysfunction [9].

Neuromodulators

Patients with chest pain refractory to calcium channel blockers or nitrates may benefit from neuromodulators which primarily target a reduction in visceral hypersensitivity rather than an improvement in the underlying esophageal motility. Low-dose tricyclic antidepressants (TCA) have been the best studied neuromodulators thus far. Imipramine 50 mg at nighttime was shown in a randomized, double-blind, placebo-controlled trial of 60 patients with normal coronary angiograms to significantly reduce chest pain [34]. Other commonly used TCA include amitriptyline and nortriptyline, starting at doses of 10–25 mg with escalation to 50–75 mg over weeks to months with minimal mood-altering effect [49]. Due to the variable effect of tricyclics on respective acetylcholine, histamine, and adrenergic receptors, failure of one drug in this class to modulate pain is not necessarily predictive of future failure with another TCA. Possible side effects of TCA should be discussed with patients including drowsiness (therefore medication is optimally taken at bedtime), orthostatic hypotension, constipation, dry mouth, urinary retention, and blurred vision due to its anticholinergic effect. If improvement is achieved with TCA, the medication should be continued for 6–12 months before initiating a slow taper to the lowest effective dose for symptom control. The anxiolytic, trazodone, has also been shown in a double-blind, placebo-controlled trial of 29 patients to improve the sense of global well-being as well as distress over esophageal symptoms. However, both the placebo and trazodone (100–150 mg) groups reported significant reduction in chest pain, highlighting the importance of reassurance and multidisciplinary anxiety and hypervigilance-reducing strategies in this population [1, 35]. Selective serotonin reuptake inhibitors (SSRI) have a more targeted pharmacologic effect than TCA [50]. Intravenous citalopram 20 mg was investigated in a double-blind, crossover study of ten healthy volunteers and found to increase the threshold of first perception as well as discomfort related to both mechanical balloon distention and chemical acid perfusion in the esophagus [36]. Recommended initial doses of SSRIs include fluoxetine 10–20 mg/day, paroxetine 10–20 mg/day, and sertraline 25–50 mg/day [50]. Due to their selective 5-HT activity, SSRIs are typically better tolerated than TCAs, although nausea, vomiting, diarrhea, and stomach upset may occur [51].

Theophylline also acts both as a smooth muscle relaxant and a visceral analgesic by blocking adenosine receptors [52]. Following an open-label pilot study, a subsequent randomized placebo-controlled study of 25 patients with esophageal chest pain found that theophylline 200 mg twice daily improved chest pain in 58% of patients compared to 6% in the placebo group [38, 53].

Endoscopic Therapy

Patients with spastic esophageal disorders who are refractory to pharmacologic therapies may be candidates for endoscopic treatment, including botulinum toxin injection. While primarily studied and utilized in the treatment of achalasia, botulinum toxin injection has demonstrated some symptomatic benefits in non-achalasia spastic motility disorders as well when delivered to multiple levels of the esophageal body (2 and 7 cm above LES). A smaller study of 13 patients reported symptomatic improvement of DES and jackhammer esophagus at 2 months and, to a lesser extent, at 6 months [54]. In a prospective, randomized crossover trial of 22 patients with DES or nutcracker esophagus, botulinum toxin resulted in a 50% response rate at 1 month compared to 10% in placebo saline injection [39].

Esophageal dilation has been suggested in spastic esophageal disorders; however, the rationale and evidence are lacking. In a prospective, double-blind, crossover trial of eight patients with nutcracker esophagus, there were no significant differences in chest pain, dysphagia, LES pressure, or contraction amplitude between placebo dilation with a 24Fr bougie compared to therapeutic dilation with a 54Fr bougie [55]. In a case series of nine patients who were refractory to medical and bougienage dilation, pneumatic dilation produced improvement in dysphagia and regurgitation in eight patients over 37.4 months with associated LES pressure reduction. However, there are no controlled trials to date for this therapy, and the risk of perforation (up to 5% in achalasia patients) may outweigh the benefit [40]. Moreover, it is unclear whether patients who had symptomatic improvement from pneumatic dilation would be more appropriately classified as having spastic achalasia, highlighting the importance (and difficulty) of manometric diagnostic accuracy [9].

Over the past decade, peroral endoscopic myotomy (POEM) has become a promising alternative to surgery by accessing the circular muscle layer at the LES via a submucosal tunnel. While the majority of studies have been dedicated to the treatment of achalasia, a systematic review and meta-analysis of 8 observational studies comprising 179 patients with spastic disorders including 18 patients with DES and 37 with jackhammer esophagus found success rates of 88 and 72%, respectively [41]. More recently, an international multicenter study of POEM in non-achalasia esophageal motility disorders, including 17 DES, 18 jackhammer esophagus, and 15 EGJ outflow obstruction patterns, reported clinical success in 85% of DES and jackhammer patients and 93% of EGJOO patients. Challenges unique to performing POEM in DES include hyperactive spastic contractions complicating the creation of the submucosal tunnel, need for greater length of the myotomy, extended procedure duration, and increased postoperative pain and hospital length of stay [56]. At present, there are no randomized controlled trials comparing POEM to other therapeutic modalities and no longitudinal studies of POEM for spastic disorders.

Surgery

Heller myotomy involves a surgical, rather than endoscopic, incision of the circular muscle layer of the LES and is often accompanied by a partial or full fundoplication as a preventative measure against postsurgical reflux. As with POEM, longer myotomies tend to be performed for DES compared to achalasia, the extent of which is often guided by manometry [9]. In a prospective study evaluating 20 patients with extended myotomy (14 cm in the esophagus and 2 cm below the EGJ) and anterior fundoplication for DES, dysphagia and chest pain were improved in 100 and 90%, respectively, over 50 months of follow-up [42]. There is sparse data available regarding surgical myotomy in jackhammer esophagus. Notably, in both POEM and surgical myotomy techniques, the disruption of the LES alone does not fully address the underlying reduced latency or hypercontractile pathophysiology of DES and jackhammer esophagus, respectively, and should be considered in the overall management of these disorders [25].

Adjunctive Therapy

Biofeedback, consisting of sipping water while viewing a corresponding motility tracing and double swallowing with and without visual feedback, has been shown in a single case study of DES to reduce anxiety regarding esophageal symptoms [43]. Biofeedback using diaphragmatic breathing led to symptom reduction in five of nine patients with functional esophageal chest pain, but not in functional heartburn [57]. Cognitive behavioral therapy (CBT) has also been used for management of noncardiac chest pain. A small randomized, controlled study revealed significant reduction in chest pain, disruption of daily life, autonomic symptoms, as well as psychological morbidity in patients who underwent CBT compared to conventional treatment [52, 58]. To date, no studies evaluating the role of CBT in spastic disorders have yet to be conducted.

Prognosis

The overall prognosis for patients suffering from DES and hypercontractile esophagus is good, with no known increased risk for esophageal malignancy or mortality. Although the above treatments may not always be effective, spastic esophageal conditions typically have a benign course and may even improve with time. A longitudinal study encompassing 3–10 years following the initial manometry diagnosis of 137 patients with DES, nutcracker esophagus, and hypocontractile esophagus revealed that symptoms of dysphagia and chest pain in all three conditions improved significantly over time [59]. In rare cases, patients with DES may progress to develop achalasia, although there are no known manometric or clinical predictors [60].

Conclusion

The spastic esophageal disorders, encompassing distal esophageal spasm, jackhammer esophagus, and spastic achalasia, have evolved in definition over time with the advent of high-resolution manometry and esophageal pressure topography. Although often classified together due to a similarity in clinical presentation characterized by dysphagia and chest pain, their underlying pathophysiology suggests fundamental differences as disorders of decreased inhibitory versus increased excitatory innervation. Emerging technologies such as impedance planimetry and novel manometric parameters complement traditional diagnostic modalities such as endoscopy and contrast radiography, with the hope of clarifying the clinical and physiological distinctions among these spastic disorders. As new techniques such as peroral endoscopic myotomy demonstrate higher success and comparable safety profiles compared to conventional pharmacotherapy or even other endoscopic and surgical therapies, additional longitudinal, randomized controlled studies will be needed to validate the treatment of spastic esophageal disorders.

References

1. Pandolfino JE, Kahrilas PJ. Esophageal neuromuscular function and motility disorders. In: Feldman M, Friedman L, Brandt L, editors. Sleisenger and fordtran's gastrointestinal and liver disease. 10th ed. Philadelphia: Saunders; 2016. p. 733–754.e738.
2. Jia Y, Arenas J, Hejazi RA, Elhanafi S, Saadi M, McCallum RW. Frequency of jackhammer esophagus as the extreme phenotypes of esophageal hypercontractility based on the new Chicago classification. J Clin Gastroenterol. 2016;50(8):615–8.
3. Pandolfino JE, Roman S, Carlson D, et al. Distal esophageal spasm in high-resolution esophageal pressure topography: defining clinical phenotypes. Gastroenterology. 2011;141(2):469–75.
4. Pandolfino JE, Kwiatek MA, Nealis T, Bulsiewicz W, Post J, Kahrilas PJ. Achalasia: a new clinically relevant classification by high-resolution manometry. Gastroenterology. 2008;135(5):1526–33.

5. Pandolfino JE, Ghosh SK, Rice J, Clarke JO, Kwiatek MA, Kahrilas PJ. Classifying esophageal motility by pressure topography characteristics: a study of 400 patients and 75 controls. Am J Gastroenterol. 2008;103(1):27–37.
6. Kahrilas PJ, Bredenoord AJ, Fox M, et al. The Chicago classification of esophageal motility disorders, v3.0. Neurogastroenterol Motil. 2015;27(2):160–74.
7. Roman S, Pandolfino JE, Chen J, Boris L, Luger D, Kahrilas PJ. Phenotypes and clinical context of hypercontractility in high-resolution esophageal pressure topography (EPT). Am J Gastroenterol. 2012;107(1):37–45.
8. Behar J, Biancani P. Pathogenesis of simultaneous esophageal contractions in patients with motility disorders. Gastroenterology. 1993;105(1):111–8.
9. Roman S, Kahrilas PJ. Management of spastic disorders of the esophagus. Gastroenterol Clin North Am. 2013;42(1):27–43.
10. Konturek JW, Gillessen A, Domschke W. Diffuse esophageal spasm: a malfunction that involves nitric oxide? Scand J Gastroenterol. 1995;30(11):1041–5.
11. Murray JA, Ledlow A, Launspach J, Evans D, Loveday M, Conklin JL. The effects of recombinant human hemoglobin on esophageal motor functions in humans. Gastroenterology. 1995;109(4):1241–8.
12. Korsapati H, Babaei A, Bhargava V, Mittal RK. Cholinergic stimulation induces asynchrony between the circular and longitudinal muscle contraction during esophageal peristalsis. Am J Physiol Gastrointest Liver Physiol. 2008;294(3):G694–8.
13. Korsapati H, Bhargava V, Mittal RK. Reversal of asynchrony between circular and longitudinal muscle contraction in nutcracker esophagus by atropine. Gastroenterology. 2008;135(3):796–802.
14. Gyawali CP, Kushnir VM. High-resolution manometric characteristics help differentiate types of distal esophageal obstruction in patients with peristalsis. Neurogastroenterol Motil. 2011;23(6):502–e197.
15. Mittal RK, Ren J, McCallum RW, Shaffer HA Jr, Sluss J. Modulation of feline esophageal contractions by bolus volume and outflow obstruction. Am J Physiol. 1990;258(2 Pt 1):G208–15.
16. Tutuian R, Mainie I, Agrawal A, Gideon RM, Katz PO, Castell DO. Symptom and function heterogenicity among patients with distal esophageal spasm: studies using combined impedance-manometry. Am J Gastroenterol. 2006;101(3):464–9.
17. Almansa C, Heckman MG, DeVault KR, Bouras E, Achem SR. Esophageal spasm: demographic, clinical, radiographic, and manometric features in 108 patients. Dis Esophagus. 2012;25(3):214–21.
18. Tedesco P, Fisichella PM, Way LW, Patti MG. Cause and treatment of epiphrenic diverticula. Am J Surg. 2005;190(6):891–4.
19. Herregods TV, Smout AJ, Ooi JL, Sifrim D, Bredenoord AJ. Jackhammer esophagus: Observations on a European cohort. Neurogastroenterol Motil. 2017;29(4):e12975.
20. Gonsalves N, Policarpio-Nicolas M, Zhang Q, Rao MS, Hirano I. Histopathologic variability and endoscopic correlates in adults with eosinophilic esophagitis. Gastrointest Endosc. 2006;64(3):313–9.
21. Xiao Y, Carlson DA, Lin Z, Rinella N, Sifrim D, Pandolfino JE. Assessing the pre- and postpeak phases in a swallow using esophageal pressure topography. Neurogastroenterol Motil. 2017;29(9):e13099.
22. Xiao Y, Carlson DA, Lin Z, Alhalel N, Pandolfino JE. Jackhammer esophagus: assessing the balance between prepeak and postpeak contractile integral. Neurogastroenterol Motil. 2018;30(5):e13262.
23. Finnerty BM, Aronova A, Cheguevara A, et al. Esophageal dysmotility and the utility of barium swallow: an opaque diagnosis. Gastroenterology. 2015;148(4, Supplement 1):S1131–2.
24. Prabhakar A, Levine MS, Rubesin S, Laufer I, Katzka D. Relationship between diffuse esophageal spasm and lower esophageal sphincter dysfunction on barium studies and manometry in 14 patients. AJR Am J Roentgenol. 2004;183(2):409–13.
25. Clermont MP, Ahuja NK. The relevance of spastic esophageal disorders as a diagnostic category. Curr Gastroenterol Rep. 2018;20(9):42.

26. Goldberg MF, Levine MS, Torigian DA. Diffuse esophageal spasm: CT findings in seven patients. AJR Am J Roentgenol. 2008;191(3):758–63.
27. Imam H, Sanmiguel C, Larive B, Bhat Y, Soffer E. Study of intestinal flow by combined videofluoroscopy, manometry, and multiple intraluminal impedance. Am J Physiol Gastrointest Liver Physiol. 2004;286(2):G263–70.
28. Cho YK, Choi MG, Oh SN, et al. Comparison of bolus transit patterns identified by esophageal impedance to barium esophagram in patients with dysphagia. Dis Esophagus. 2012;25(1):17–25.
29. Tutuian R, Castell DO. Clarification of the esophageal function defect in patients with manometric ineffective esophageal motility: studies using combined impedance-manometry. Clin Gastroenterol Hepatol. 2004;2(3):230–6.
30. Carlson DA, Kahrilas PJ, Lin Z, et al. Evaluation of esophageal motility utilizing the functional lumen imaging probe. Am J Gastroenterol. 2016;111(12):1726–35.
31. Ahuja NK, Clarke JO. The role of impedance planimetry in the evaluation of esophageal disorders. Curr Gastroenterol Rep. 2017;19(2):7.
32. Pimentel M, Bonorris GG, Chow EJ, Lin HC. Peppermint oil improves the manometric findings in diffuse esophageal spasm. J Clin Gastroenterol. 2001;33(1):27–31.
33. Cattau EL Jr, Castell DO, Johnson DA, et al. Diltiazem therapy for symptoms associated with nutcracker esophagus. Am J Gastroenterol. 1991;86(3):272–6.
34. Cannon RO 3rd, Quyyumi AA, Mincemoyer R, et al. Imipramine in patients with chest pain despite normal coronary angiograms. N Engl J Med. 1994;330(20):1411–7.
35. Clouse RE, Lustman PJ, Eckert TC, Ferney DM, Griffith LS. Low-dose trazodone for symptomatic patients with esophageal contraction abnormalities. A double-blind, placebo-controlled trial. Gastroenterology. 1987;92(4):1027–36.
36. Broekaert D, Fischler B, Sifrim D, Janssens J, Tack J. Influence of citalopram, a selective serotonin reuptake inhibitor, on oesophageal hypersensitivity: a double-blind, placebo-controlled study. Aliment Pharmacol Ther. 2006;23(3):365–70.
37. Eherer AJ, Schwetz I, Hammer HF, et al. Effect of sildenafil on oesophageal motor function in healthy subjects and patients with oesophageal motor disorders. Gut. 2002;50(6):758–64.
38. Rao SS, Mudipalli RS, Remes-Troche JM, Utech CL, Zimmerman B. Theophylline improves esophageal chest pain--a randomized, placebo-controlled study. Am J Gastroenterol. 2007;102(5):930–8.
39. Vanuytsel T, Bisschops R, Farre R, et al. Botulinum toxin reduces dysphagia in patients with nonachalasia primary esophageal motility disorders. Clin Gastroenterol Hepatol. 2013;11(9):1115–1121.e1112.
40. Ebert EC, Ouyang A, Wright SH, Cohen S, Lipshutz WH. Pneumatic dilatation in patients with symptomatic diffuse esophageal spasm and lower esophageal sphincter dysfunction. Dig Dis Sci. 1983;28(6):481–5.
41. Khan MA, Kumbhari V, Ngamruengphong S, et al. Is POEM the answer for management of spastic esophageal disorders? A systematic review and meta-analysis. Dig Dis Sci. 2017;62(1):35–44.
42. Leconte M, Douard R, Gaudric M, Dumontier I, Chaussade S, Dousset B. Functional results after extended myotomy for diffuse oesophageal spasm. Br J Surg. 2007;94(9):1113–8.
43. Latimer PR. Biofeedback and self-regulation in the treatment of diffuse esophageal spasm: a single-case study. Biofeedback Self Regul. 1981;6(2):181–9.
44. Hills JM, Aaronson PI. The mechanism of action of peppermint oil on gastrointestinal smooth muscle. An analysis using patch clamp electrophysiology and isolated tissue pharmacology in rabbit and guinea pig. Gastroenterology. 1991;101(1):55–65.
45. Kingham JG. Peppermint oil and colon spasm. Lancet (London, England). 1995;346(8981):986.
46. May B, Kuntz HD, Kieser M, Kohler S. Efficacy of a fixed peppermint oil/caraway oil combination in non-ulcer dyspepsia. Arzneimittelforschung. 1996;46(12):1149–53.
47. Khanna R, MacDonald JK, Levesque BG. Peppermint oil for the treatment of irritable bowel syndrome: a systematic review and meta-analysis. J Clin Gastroenterol. 2014;48(6):505–12.

48. Fox M, Sweis R, Wong T, Anggiansah A. Sildenafil relieves symptoms and normalizes motility in patients with oesophageal spasm: a report of two cases. Neurogastroenterol Motil. 2007;19(10):798–803.
49. Fass R, Dickman R. Non-cardiac chest pain: an update. Neurogastroenterol Motil. 2006;18(6):408–17.
50. Dickman R, Maradey-Romero C, Fass R. The role of pain modulators in esophageal disorders – no pain no gain. Neurogastroenterol Motil. 2014;26(5):603–10.
51. Sindrup SH, Otto M, Finnerup NB, Jensen TS. Antidepressants in the treatment of neuropathic pain. Basic Clin Pharmacol Toxicol. 2005;96(6):399–409.
52. Coss-Adame E, Erdogan A, Rao SS. Treatment of esophageal (noncardiac) chest pain: an expert review. Clin Gastroenterol Hepatol. 2014;12(8):1224–45.
53. Rao SS, Mudipalli RS, Mujica V, Utech CL, Zhao X, Conklin JL. An open-label trial of theophylline for functional chest pain. Dig Dis Sci. 2002;47(12):2763–8.
54. Marjoux S, Brochard C, Roman S, et al. Botulinum toxin injection for hypercontractile or spastic esophageal motility disorders: may high-resolution manometry help to select cases? Dis Esophagus. 2015;28(8):735–41.
55. Winters C, Artnak EJ, Benjamin SB, Castell DO. Esophageal bougienage in symptomatic patients with the nutcracker esophagus. A primary esophageal motility disorder. JAMA. 1984;252(3):363–6.
56. Ponds FA, Smout A, Fockens P, Bredenoord AJ. Challenges of peroral endoscopic myotomy in the treatment of distal esophageal spasm. Scand J Gastroenterol. 2018;53(3):252–5.
57. Shapiro M, Shanani R, Taback H, Abramowich D, Scapa E, Broide E. Functional chest pain responds to biofeedback treatment but functional heartburn does not: what is the difference? Eur J Gastroenterol Hepatol. 2012;24(6):708–14.
58. Klimes I, Mayou RA, Pearce MJ, Coles L, Fagg JR. Psychological treatment for atypical non-cardiac chest pain: a controlled evaluation. Psychol Med. 1990;20(3):605–11.
59. Spencer HL, Smith L, Riley SA. A questionnaire study to assess long-term outcome in patients with abnormal esophageal manometry. Dysphagia. 2006;21(3):149–55.
60. Khatami SS, Khandwala F, Shay SS, Vaezi MF. Does diffuse esophageal spasm progress to achalasia? A prospective cohort study. Dig Dis Sci. 2005;50(9):1605–10.

Chapter 9
Ineffective Motility Disorder

Akinari Sawada, Kornilia Nikaki, and Daniel Sifrim

Definition

Ineffective esophageal motility (IEM) was defined as a distinct esophageal motility disorder for the first time in 1997 by Leite et al. [1] replacing the previously used terminology of nonspecific esophageal motility disorder (NEMD) [2]. Based on conventional manometry, a peristaltic contraction of <30 mmHg at the distal esophagus is associated with ineffective bolus clearance [3], and therefore originally IEM was characterized by ≥30% [1, 4] and later on ≥50% of wet swallows followed by contractions with an amplitude of <30 mmHg or absent/failed peristalsis [5] as the latter was more frequently associated with abnormal bolus transit and symptoms of dysphagia and heartburn [6]. The threshold of 30 mmHg in contractile vigor corresponds to a distal contractile integral (DCI) of 450 mmHg.cm.s in HRM which was adopted by the latest Chicago Classification of esophageal motility disorders (version 3.0) [7]. It is recognized, however, that failed peristalsis (DCI < 100 mmHg. cm.s), rather than weak peristalsis (DCI 100-450 mmHg.cm.s), has a clearer prognostic value in reflux burden [8] and is associated with impaired bolus clearance and symptomatic dysphagia [9]. Apart from the peristaltic pressure measured during esophageal manometry, evaluation of esophageal motility might include assessment of bolus transit using impedance measurements. At present such assessment is not included in the definition of IEM. It is important to acknowledge that IEM can be observed in normal healthy volunteers (in up to 17% of those tested in the supine position and 33% if measured in the upright position) [10].

The definition of IEM is based on expert opinion (Evidence level 5), and it is likely that this may be redefined or further graded and refined. For example,

A. Sawada · K. Nikaki · D. Sifrim (✉)
Wingate Institute of Neurogastroenterology, Barts and the London School of Medicine and Dentistry, Queen Mary University of London, London, UK
e-mail: m1164972@med.osaka-cu.ac.jp; k.nikaki@qmul.ac.uk; d.sifrim@qmul.ac.uk

© Springer Nature Switzerland AG 2020

191

D. A. Patel et al. (eds.), *Evaluation and Management of Dysphagia*,
https://doi.org/10.1007/978-3-030-26554-0_9

Hiestand et al. have proposed the terms of IEM Alternans and IEM Persistens, where in the first group there are one or more normal peristaltic contractions, while in the second, there are none [11]. The clinical implication of this distinction lies in the higher likelihood of severe reflux disease in the second group and poor response to proton-pump inhibitor (PPI) therapy. The use of provocative testing and more specifically the use of multiple rapid swallowing – MRS – as standard during HRM protocols nowadays [12] alongside the introduction of solid test meals for the detection of major esophageal motility disorders [13] may also play role in the distinction of IEM in the future. MRS is performed by administering five 2-ml swallows rapidly and assessing the gastroesophageal junction (GEJ) inhibition and after-MRS contraction. Adequacy of peristaltic reserve is defined as a ratio of MRS DCI over mean single swallow DCI of >1 [14], but as reproducibility in IEM is poor following a single MRS [15], it is proposed that a minimum of three MRS tests should be undertaken [16]. Esophageal peristaltic reserve assessment may be able to guide more effectively the type of anti-reflux surgery performed or inform clinicians and patients of the risk of postoperative dysphagia [17, 18].

Pathophysiology of Esophageal Peristalsis and IEM

There is synchronized onset, peak, and duration of contraction of the circular and longitudinal esophageal muscle layers [19] traveling in a sequential fashion. Relaxation is initiated with swallowing, which happens simultaneously through esophageal peristalsis, and bolus propagation involves esophageal contraction proximal and relaxation distal to the bolus [20] throughout the esophagus but with a gradient that resembles the sequential peristaltic pattern and is longer in duration at the distal esophagus compared to the proximal [21–24]. During primary peristalsis, neuronal control of proximal striated muscle and distal smooth muscle contraction is dependent on brainstem nuclei. Excitatory vagal efferents from the nucleus ambiguus innervate the striated muscle of the upper esophagus whilst the esophageal smooth muscle is innervated through myenteric ganglia from preganglionic neurons in the dorsal motor nucleus of the vagus [25]. Moreover, direct activation of excitatory and inhibitory motor neurons in the myenteric plexus of the LES leads to LES relaxation with an oroaxial esophageal stretch above the level of the LES and LES contraction with a transverse stretch [26]. Also, the esophageal body exhibits a tonic contractile activity mainly controlled by a continuous excitatory input, while a nitric oxide inhibitory pathway may regulate this background contractile tone [24, 27]. Finally, there is an important influence on the vigor of esophageal peristalsis through vagal afferent and efferent innervation with regulation at the central nervous system. These pathways can be significantly affected by extra-esophageal factors including psychological stress [28].

Secondary peristalsis is the end result of esophago-esophageal reflexes, mediated by mucosal and deep mechanoreceptors in the muscularis and cholinergic nerves, which are activated by esophageal distension [29]. The amplitude and velocity of secondary peristalsis are stimulus-specific but independent to site or volume. Clearance of refluxate is dependent on secondary peristalsis, especially during sleep periods where lack of spontaneous swallowing and supine position does not contribute toward esophageal clearance [30, 31].

The variety of factors determining esophageal peristalsis, bolus transit, and clearance can only imply that IEM is multifactorial and the end result of a defect(s) in any of these pathways. In summary, the degree of IEM is dependent on the defects along (A) the preload mechanosensitive arm that is fired off with the initial stretching of the esophageal muscle prior to contraction, (B) the intrinsic esophageal contractility, and (C) the afterload resistance that the contraction should overcome [32].

IEM and Symptoms

IEM is categorized as a minor esophageal motility disorder, found in as many as 30% of patients undergoing HRM [7]. Even asymptomatic healthy subjects may have IEM occasionally. Therefore, there is some controversy about the causal relationship between IEM and symptoms such as dysphagia (Evidence level 2). On the one hand, Roman et al. showed that nonobstructive dysphagia patients had more frequent large (>5 cm) or small (2–5 cm) breaks of esophageal peristalsis compared to asymptomatic subjects [33]. On the other hand, other studies suggested that IEM was unlikely to cause dysphagia. In sildenafil-induced IEM in healthy subjects, there was no correlation between severe smooth muscle hypomotility, bolus transit, and bolus perception [34]. Chen CL et al. reported poor correlation between esophageal motility/bolus transit and symptoms in nonobstructing dysphagia patients [35]. Moreover, Xiao Y et al. showed that abnormal esophageal motility during HRM was not clearly associated with esophageal symptoms [36]. Finally, IEM was found in less than 15% of patients presenting with noncardiac chest pain [37].

IEM and Gastroesophageal Reflux Disease (GERD)

IEM and GERD may have a mutual influence between each other. GERD can contribute to the development of IEM and vice versa (Evidence level 3). The most common esophageal motor disorder in GERD is esophageal body hypomotility; however, most NERD patients (the most frequent GERD phenotype) have normal motility [38]. On the other hand, several studies suggested an association between acid reflux and esophageal body hypomotility. Chan WW et al. showed that hypomotility was more prevalent in patients with high acid exposure time (AET) (≥4.5%) than low AET (<4.5%) [39]. Besides, the prevalence of esophageal hypomotility parallels with severity of GERD from almost absent in NERD to very frequent in erosive reflux disease and Barrett's esophagus [40, 41]. Simrén M et al. showed that only severe IEM prolonged volume and acid clearance in the upright position and acid clearance in the supine position [42]. Finally, Ribolsi M et al. demonstrated that weak peristalsis with large breaks was more relevant to abnormal acid exposure than frequent weak peristalsis without breaks (DCI < 450) [43].

Medical Conditions Related to IEM

Some medical conditions may cause decreased esophageal smooth muscle contractility.

Among patients with systemic sclerosis (SSc) complaining of esophageal symptoms, 64% had hypomotility with either absent contractility (41%) or IEM (23%). Interestingly, none of the patients with absent contractility showed peristaltic reserve (adequate aftercontraction) as assessed using multiple rapid swallows (MRS) [44] (Evidence level 4). Patients with Parkinson's disease complaining of esophageal symptoms often had a pattern of IEM (55%) [45] (Evidence level 4). Medications such as cyclobenzaprine, tizanidine, methocarbamol, and metaxalone may also be associated with IEM [46] (Evidence level 3).

IEM and Anti-reflux Surgery (ARS)

ARS is an important and frequent treatment for GERD patients. There are two main types of ARS techniques, i.e., partial and total (Nissen) fundoplication. The selection of ARS technique, in relation to presence or absence of preoperative IEM and postoperative dysphagia, has been a matter of controversy for many years. Some meta-analyses showed that partial fundoplication causes less postoperative dysphagia, lower risk of reoperation, and similar reflux control compared with total fundoplication [47–49] (Evidence level 1A). However, large case-control studies reported few side effects by Nissen fundoplication [50] (Evidence level 3). Whereas a tailored surgical approach (based on preoperative esophageal motility) prevented postoperative dysphagia in some studies [51] (Evidence level 5), several other studies showed that preoperative esophageal dysmotility was not associated with postoperative dysphagia regardless of type of fundoplication [52–56] (Evidence level 1C). Magnetic sphincter augmentation (MSA) was more recently developed for surgical treatment of GERD. The device mechanically reinforces the function of the lower esophageal sphincter (LES). Normal esophageal body peristalsis is assumed to be required to open the magnetic device when patient swallows [57]. So far, the safety and effectiveness of this device have not been established for GERD patients with significant esophageal motility disorders [58] (Evidence level 5).

Several studies found that fundoplication improved esophageal contractility as 30–50% of patients with preoperative IEM normalized their motility [59–61]. In contrast, other studies showed that fundoplication caused IEM in 30–50% of normal motility patients [18, 56] (Evidence level 3).

Finally, performance of a provocative test, multiple rapid swallows (MRS), during the preoperative HRM allows determination of adequacy of an after-contraction post-MRS. This parameter can predict not only the development of IEM but also late postoperative dysphagia [14, 18] (Evidence level 3).

Management

Treatment of IEM should be considered if there is a clinical suspicion that IEM might be the mechanism behind the patient's symptom (i.e., abnormal reflux clearance or dysphagia). Unfortunately, at present, there is no clearly demonstrated pharmacological agent that can improve both esophageal smooth muscle contractility and related symptoms. Therefore, dietary and lifestyle management to facilitate bolus transit is recommended first [62] (Evidence level 5).

Non-pharmacological Treatment

Patients should have meals in the upright position, chew well, and frequently drink liquid during meal to make bolus transit easier. Thus, gravity, pharyngeal pump, and hydrostatic force seem to play a key role in bolus transit apart from esophageal peristalsis [42, 63] (Evidence level 2).

Spicy food (containing chili) has been suggested to increase amplitude of esophageal contractions. Capsaicin (contained in chili) provoked an increase in the amplitude of esophageal body waves in GERD patients with IEM and healthy subjects [64, 65] (Evidence level 2).

Transcranial direct current stimulation to esophageal cortical area increased amplitude of distal esophageal contraction in patients with nonerosive reflux disease and functional heartburn, [66] (Evidence level 1D); however, so far this intervention is an experimental intervention and is not available for clinical practice.

Pharmacological Treatment

Most well-known prokinetic agents (metoclopramide, domperidone) are not well-established as agents improving esophageal motility in patients with IEM [67, 68] (Evidence level 1D).

Mosapride, a selective 5-HT$_4$ agonist, may increase the amplitude of primary esophageal contraction slightly. The combination therapy with PPI moderately decreased GERD symptoms compared to PPI therapy alone [69–71] (Evidence level 1D). Prucalopride is another 5-HT$_4$ agonist which promotes the release of acetylcholine from neurons of the myenteric plexus. Kessing BF et al. showed that prucalopride reduced esophageal acid exposure and accelerated gastric emptying but did not change esophageal motility in healthy volunteers [72] (Evidence level 1D). In contrast, Lei WY et al. showed that prucalopride increased esophageal contraction amplitude in GERD patients with IEM [73] (Evidence level 1D).

Macrolide antibiotics such as erythromycin and azithromycin have prokinetic effect via motilin receptors. Intravenous administration of erythromycin increased LES pressure and amplitude of esophageal contraction in 15 GERD patients [74] (Evidence level 1D). Azithromycin reduced esophageal acid exposure in GERD patients and following lung transplant [75] (Evidence level 2).

Buspirone developed as an anxiolytic drug is a partial agonist for the serotonin 5-HT_{1A} receptors and an antagonist for the dopamine D2 receptor with weak affinity to the 5-HT_2 receptors. Buspirone increased esophageal contraction in healthy volunteers [76, 77].

A recent randomized double-blind placebo-controlled crossover study showed 30% normalization of esophageal contraction by not only buspirone but placebo in patients with IEM [78] (Evidence level 1D). Additionally, buspirone increased LES resting pressure and decreased esophageal symptoms in systemic sclerosis patients; however, it did not affect the amplitude of distal esophageal contraction [79, 80] (Evidence level 2).

References

1. Leite LP, Johnston BT, Barrett J, Castell JA, Castell DO. Ineffective esophageal motility (IEM): the primary finding in patients with nonspecific esophageal motility disorder. Dig Dis Sci. 1997;42(9):1859–65.
2. Richter JE, Wu WC, Johns DN, Blackwell JN, Nelson JL 3rd, Castell JA, et al. Esophageal manometry in 95 healthy adult volunteers. Variability of pressures with age and frequency of "abnormal" contractions. Dig Dis Sci. 1987;32(6):583–92.
3. Kahrilas PJ, Dodds WJ, Hogan WJ. Effect of peristaltic dysfunction on esophageal volume clearance. Gastroenterology. 1988;94(1):73–80.
4. Spechler SJ, Castell DO. Classification of oesophageal motility abnormalities. Gut. 2001;49(1):145–51.
5. Tutuian R, Castell DO. Clarification of the esophageal function defect in patients with manometric ineffective esophageal motility: studies using combined impedance-manometry. Clin Gastroenterol Hepatol. 2004;2(3):230–6.
6. Blonski W, Vela M, Safder A, Hila A, Castell DO. Revised criterion for diagnosis of ineffective esophageal motility is associated with more frequent dysphagia and greater bolus transit abnormalities. Am J Gastroenterol. 2008;103(3):699–704.
7. Kahrilas PJ, Bredenoord AJ, Fox M, Gyawali CP, Roman S, Smout AJPM, et al. The Chicago classification of esophageal motility disorders, v3.0. Neurogastroenterol Motil. 2015;27(2):160–74.
8. Rengarajan A, Bolkhir A, Gor P, Wang D, Munigala S, Gyawali CP. Esophagogastric junction and esophageal body contraction metrics on high-resolution manometry predict esophageal acid burden. Neurogastroenterol Motil. 2018;30(5):e13267.
9. Jain A, Baker JR, Chen JW. In ineffective esophageal motility, failed swallows are more functionally relevant than weak swallows. Neurogastroenterol Motil. 2018;30(6):e13297.

10. Hollenstein M, Thwaites P, Butikofer S, Heinrich H, Sauter M, Ulmer I, et al. Pharyngeal swallowing and oesophageal motility during a solid meal test: a prospective study in healthy volunteers and patients with major motility disorders. Lancet Gastroenterol Hepatol. 2017;2(9):644–53.

11. Hiestand M, Abdel Jalil A, Castell DO. Manometric subtypes of ineffective esophageal motility. Clin Transl Gastroenterol. 2017;8(3):e78.

12. Sweis R, Heinrich H, Fox M. Variation in esophageal physiology testing in clinical practice: results from an international survey. Neurogastroenterol Motil. 2018;30(3):e13215.

13. Ang D, Misselwitz B, Hollenstein M, Knowles K, Wright J, Tucker E, et al. Diagnostic yield of high-resolution manometry with a solid test meal for clinically relevant, symptomatic oesophageal motility disorders: serial diagnostic study. Lancet Gastroenterol Hepatol. 2017;2(9):654–61.

14. Shaker A, Stoikes N, Drapekin J, Kushnir V, Brunt LM, Gyawali CP. Multiple rapid swallow responses during esophageal high-resolution manometry reflect esophageal body peristaltic reserve. Am J Gastroenterol. 2013;108(11):1706–12.

15. Price LH, Li Y, Patel A, Gyawali CP. Reproducibility patterns of multiple rapid swallows during high resolution esophageal manometry provide insights into esophageal pathophysiology. Neurogastroenterol Motil. 2014;26(5):646–53.

16. Mauro A, Savarino E, De Bortoli N, Tolone S, Pugliese D, Franchina M, et al. Optimal number of multiple rapid swallows needed during high-resolution esophageal manometry for accurate prediction of contraction reserve. Neurogastroenterol Motil. 2018;30(4):e13253.

17. Stoikes N, Drapekin J, Kushnir V, Shaker A, Brunt LM, Gyawali CP. The value of multiple rapid swallows during preoperative esophageal manometry before laparoscopic antireflux surgery. Surg Endosc. 2012;26(12):3401–7.

18. Mello MD, Shriver AR, Li Y, Patel A, Gyawali CP. Ineffective esophageal motility phenotypes following fundoplication in gastroesophageal reflux disease. Neurogastroenterol Motil. 2016;28(2):292–8.

19. Mittal RK, Padda B, Bhalla V, Bhargava V, Liu J. Synchrony between circular and longitudinal muscle contractions during peristalsis in normal subjects. Am J Physiol Gastrointest Liver Physiol. 2006;290(3):G431–8.

20. Bayliss WM, Starling EH. The movements and innervation of the small intestine. J Physiol. 1899;24(2):99–143.

21. Sifrim D, Janssens J, Vantrappen G. Failing deglutitive inhibition in primary esophageal motility disorders. Gastroenterology. 1994;106(4):875–82.

22. Sifrim D, Janssens J, Vantrappen G. A wave of inhibition precedes primary peristaltic contractions in the human esophagus. Gastroenterology. 1992;103(3):876–82.

23. Abrahao L Jr, Bhargava V, Babaei A, Ho A, Mittal RK. Swallow induces a peristaltic wave of distension that marches in front of the peristaltic wave of contraction. Neurogastroenterol Motil. 2011;23(3):201–7, e110.

24. Mittal RK. Regulation and dysregulation of esophageal peristalsis by the integrated function of circular and longitudinal muscle layers in health and disease. Am J Physiol Gastrointest Liver Physiol. 2016;311(3):G431–G43.

25. Paterson WG, Diamant NE. Esophageal motor physiology. In: Shaker R, Belafsky PC, Postma GN, Easterling C, editors. Principles of deglutition: a multidisciplinary text for swallowing and its disorders. New York: Springer New York; 2013. p. 303–18.

26. Jiang Y, Bhargava V, Mittal RK. Mechanism of stretch-activated excitatory and inhibitory responses in the lower esophageal sphincter. Am J Physiol Gastrointest Liver Physiol. 2009;297(2):G397–405.

27. Zhang X, Tack J, Janssens J, Sifrim DA. Neural regulation of tone in the oesophageal body: in vivo barostat assessment of volume–pressure relationships in the feline oesophagus. Neurogastroenterol Motil. 2004;16(1):13–21.

28. Chen J-H. Ineffective esophageal motility and the vagus: current challenges and future prospects. Clin Exp Gastroenterol. 2016;9:291–9.

29. Schoeman MN, Holloway RH. Stimulation and characteristics of secondary oesophageal peristalsis in normal subjects. Gut. 1994;35(2):152–8.
30. Dodds WJ, Kahrilas PJ, Dent J, Hogan WJ, Kern MK, Arndorfer RC. Analysis of spontaneous gastroesophageal reflux and esophageal acid clearance in patients with reflux esophagitis. Neurogastroenterol Motil. 1990;2(2):79–89.
31. Schoeman MN, Holloway RH. Integrity and characteristics of secondary oesophageal peristalsis in patients with gastro-oesophageal reflux disease. Gut. 1995;36(4):499–504.
32. Woodland P, Ooi JL, Grassi F, Nikaki K, Lee C, Evans JA, et al. Superficial esophageal mucosal afferent nerves may contribute to reflux hypersensitivity in non-erosive reflux disease. Gastroenterology. 2017;153:1230–9.
33. Roman S, Lin Z, Kwiatek MA, Pandolfino JE, Kahrilas PJ. Weak peristalsis in esophageal pressure topography: classification and association with dysphagia. Am J Gastroenterol. 2011;106(2):349–56.
34. Lazarescu A, Karamanolis G, Aprile L, De Oliveira RB, Dantas R, Sifrim D. Perception of dysphagia: lack of correlation with objective measurements of esophageal function. Neurogastroenterol Motil. 2010;22(12):1292. 7, e336–7
35. Chen CL, Yi CH. Clinical correlates of dysphagia to oesophageal dysmotility: studies using combined manometry and impedance. Neurogastroenterol Motil. 2008;20(6):611–7.
36. Xiao Y, Kahrilas PJ, Nicodème F, Lin Z, Roman S, Pandolfino JE. Lack of correlation between HRM metrics and symptoms during the manometric protocol. Am J Gastroenterol. 2014;109(4):521–6.
37. Dekel R, Pearson T, Wendel C, De Garmo P, Fennerty MB, Fass R. Assessment of oesophageal motor function in patients with dysphagia or chest pain – the clinical outcomes research initiative experience. Aliment Pharmacol Ther. 2003;18(11–12):1083–9.
38. Savarino E, Bredenoord AJ, Fox M, Pandolfino JE, Roman S, Gyawali CP, et al. Expert consensus document: advances in the physiological assessment and diagnosis of GERD. Nat Rev Gastroenterol Hepatol. 2017;14(11):665–76.
39. Chan WW, Haroian LR, Gyawali CP. Value of preoperative esophageal function studies before laparoscopic antireflux surgery. Surg Endosc. 2011;25(9):2943–9.
40. Savarino E, Gemignani L, Pohl D, Zentilin P, Dulbecco P, Assandri L, et al. Oesophageal motility and bolus transit abnormalities increase in parallel with the severity of gastro-oesophageal reflux disease. Aliment Pharmacol Ther. 2011;34(4):476–86.
41. Kahrilas PJ, Dodds WJ, Hogan WJ, Kern M, Arndorfer RC, Reece A. Esophageal peristaltic dysfunction in peptic esophagitis. Gastroenterology. 1986;91(4):897–904.
42. Simrén M, Silny J, Holloway R, Tack J, Janssens J, Sifrim D. Relevance of ineffective oesophageal motility during oesophageal acid clearance. Gut. 2003;52(6):784–90.
43. Ribolsi M, Balestrieri P, Emerenziani S, Guarino MP, Cicala M. Weak peristalsis with large breaks is associated with higher acid exposure and delayed reflux clearance in the supine position in GERD patients. Am J Gastroenterol. 2014;109(1):46–51.
44. Carlson DA, Crowell MD, Kimmel JN, Patel A, Gyawali CP, Hinchcliff M, et al. Loss of peristaltic reserve, determined by multiple rapid swallows, is the most frequent esophageal motility abnormality in patients with systemic sclerosis. Clin Gastroenterol Hepatol. 2016;14(10):1502–6.
45. Su A, Gandhy R, Barlow C, Triadafilopoulos G. Clinical and manometric characteristics of patients with Parkinson's disease and esophageal symptoms. Dis Esophagus. 2017;30(4):1–6.
46. Rangan V, George NS, Khan F, Geng Z, Gabbard S, Kichler A, et al. Severity of ineffective esophageal motility is associated with utilization of skeletal muscle relaxant medications. Neurogastroenterol Motil. 2018;30(4):e13235.
47. Varin O, Velstra B, De Sutter S, Ceelen W. Total vs partial fundoplication in the treatment of gastroesophageal reflux disease: a meta-analysis. Arch Surg (Chicago, IL: 1960). 2009;144(3):273–8.
48. Amer MA, Smith MD, Khoo CH, Herbison GP, McCall JL. Network meta-analysis of surgical management of gastro-oesophageal reflux disease in adults. Br J Surg. 2018;105(11):1398–407.
49. Catarci M, Gentileschi P, Papi C, Carrara A, Marrese R, Gaspari AL, et al. Evidence-based appraisal of antireflux fundoplication. Ann Surg. 2004;239(3):325–37.

50. Sgromo B, Irvine LA, Cuschieri A, Shimi SM. Long-term comparative outcome between laparoscopic total Nissen and Toupet fundoplication: symptomatic relief, patient satisfaction and quality of life. Surg Endosc. 2008;22(4):1048–53.
51. Hunter JG, Trus TL, Branum GD, Waring JP, Wood WC. A physiologic approach to laparoscopic fundoplication for gastroesophageal reflux disease. Ann Surg. 1996;223(6):673–85; discussion 85–7.
52. Rydberg L, Ruth M, Abrahamsson H, Lundell L. Tailoring antireflux surgery: a randomized clinical trial. World J Surg. 1999;23(6):612–8.
53. Fibbe C, Layer P, Keller J, Strate U, Emmermann A, Zornig C. Esophageal motility in reflux disease before and after fundoplication: a prospective, randomized, clinical, and manometric study. Gastroenterology. 2001;121(1):5–14.
54. Booth M, Stratford J, Dehn TC. Preoperative esophageal body motility does not influence the outcome of laparoscopic Nissen fundoplication for gastroesophageal reflux disease. Dis Esophagus. 2002;15(1):57–60.
55. Strate U, Emmermann A, Fibbe C, Layer P, Zornig C. Laparoscopic fundoplication: Nissen versus Toupet two-year outcome of a prospective randomized study of 200 patients regarding preoperative esophageal motility. Surg Endosc. 2008;22(1):21–30.
56. Booth MI, Stratford J, Jones L, Dehn TC. Randomized clinical trial of laparoscopic total (Nissen) versus posterior partial (Toupet) fundoplication for gastro-oesophageal reflux disease based on preoperative oesophageal manometry. Br J Surg. 2008;95(1):57–63.
57. Smith CD, DeVault KR, Buchanan M. Introduction of mechanical sphincter augmentation for gastroesophageal reflux disease into practice: early clinical outcomes and keys to successful adoption. J Am Coll Surg. 2014;218(4):776–81.
58. Telem DA, Wright AS, Shah PC, Hutter MM. SAGES technology and value assessment committee (TAVAC) safety and effectiveness analysis: LINX. Surg Endosc. 2017;31(10):3811–26.
59. Munitiz V, Ortiz A, Martinez de Haro LF, Molina J, Parrilla P. Ineffective oesophageal motility does not affect the clinical outcome of open Nissen fundoplication. Br J Surg. 2004;91(8):1010–4.
60. Ravi N, Al-Sarraf N, Moran T, O'Riordan J, Rowley S, Byrne PJ, et al. Acid normalization and improved esophageal motility after Nissen fundoplication: equivalent outcomes in patients with normal and ineffective esophageal motility. Am J Surg. 2005;190(3):445–50.
61. Simić AP, Skrobić OM, Gurski RR, Šljukić VM, Ivanović NR, Peško PM. Can different subsets of ineffective esophageal motility influence the outcome of nissen fundoplication? J Gastrointest Surg. 2014;18(10):1723–9.
62. Smout A, Fox M. Weak and absent peristalsis. Neurogastroenterol Motil. 2012;24(Suppl 1):40–7.
63. Pouderoux P, Shi G, Tatum RP, Kahrilas PJ. Esophageal solid bolus transit: studies using concurrent videofluoroscopy and manometry. Am J Gastroenterol. 1999;94(6):1457–63.
64. Gonzalez R, Dunkel R, Koletzko B, Schusdziarra V, Allescher HD. Effect of capsaicin-containing red pepper sauce suspension on upper gastrointestinal motility in healthy volunteers. Dig Dis Sci. 1998;43(6):1165–71.
65. Grossi L, Cappello G, Marzio L. Effect of an acute intraluminal administration of capsaicin on oesophageal motor pattern in GORD patients with ineffective oesophageal motility. Neurogastroenterol Motil. 2006;18(8):632–6.
66. Vigneri S, Bonventre S, Inviati A, Schifano D, Cosentino G, Puma A, et al. Effects of transcranial direct current stimulation on esophageal motility in patients with gastroesophageal reflux disease. Clin Neurophysiol. 2014;125(9):1840–6.
67. Maddern GJ, Kiroff GK, Leppard PI, Jamieson GG. Domperidone, metoclopramide, and placebo. All give symptomatic improvement in gastroesophageal reflux. J Clin Gastroenterol. 1986;8(2):135–40.
68. Maddern GJ, Horowitz M, Jamieson GG. The effect of domperidone on oesophageal emptying in diabetic autonomic neuropathy. Br J Clin Pharmacol. 1985;19(4):441–4.
69. Ruth M, Finizia C, Cange L, Lundell L. The effect of mosapride on oesophageal motor function and acid reflux in patients with gastro-oesophageal reflux disease. Eur J Gastroenterol Hepatol. 2003;15(10):1115–21.

70. Chen CL, Yi CH, Liu TT, Orr WC. Effects of mosapride on secondary peristalsis in patients with ineffective esophageal motility. Scand J Gastroenterol. 2013;48(12):1363–70.
71. Lee JY, Kim SK, Cho KB, Park KS, Kwon JG, Jung JT, et al. A double-blind, randomized, multicenter clinical trial investigating the efficacy and safety of esomeprazole single therapy versus mosapride and esomeprazole combined therapy in patients with esophageal reflux disease. J Neurogastroenterol Motil. 2017;23(2):218–28.
72. Kessing BF, Smout AJ, Bennink RJ, Kraaijpoel N, Oors JM, Bredenoord AJ. Prucalopride decreases esophageal acid exposure and accelerates gastric emptying in healthy subjects. Neurogastroenterol Motil. 2014;26(8):1079–86.
73. Lei WY, Hung JS, Liu TT, Yi CH, Chen CL. Influence of prucalopride on esophageal secondary peristalsis in reflux patients with ineffective motility. J Gastroenterol Hepatol. 2018;33(3):650–5.
74. Chrysos E, Tzovaras G, Epanomeritakis E, Tsiaoussis J, Vrachasotakis N, Vassilakis JS, et al. Erythromycin enhances oesophageal motility in patients with gastro-oesophageal reflux. ANZ J Surg. 2001;71(2):98–102.
75. Mertens V, Blondeau K, Pauwels A, Farre R, Vanaudenaerde B, Vos R, et al. Azithromycin reduces gastroesophageal reflux and aspiration in lung transplant recipients. Dig Dis Sci. 2009;54(5):972–9.
76. Di Stefano M, Papathanasopoulos A, Blondeau K, Vos R, Boecxstaens V, Farré R, et al. Effect of buspirone, a 5-HT1A receptor agonist, on esophageal motility in healthy volunteers. Dis Esophagus. 2012;25(5):470–6.
77. Blonski W, Vela MF, Freeman J, Sharma N, Castell DO. The effect of oral buspirone, pyridostigmine, and bethanechol on esophageal function evaluated with combined multichannel esophageal impedance-manometry in healthy volunteers. J Clin Gastroenterol. 2009;43(3):253–60.
78. Aggarwal N, Thota PN, Lopez R, Gabbard S. A randomized double-blind placebo-controlled crossover-style trial of buspirone in functional dysphagia and ineffective esophageal motility. Neurogastroenterol Motil. 2018;30(2):e13213.
79. Karamanolis GP, Panopoulos S, Karlaftis A, Denaxas K, Kamberoglou D, Sfikakis PP, et al. Beneficial effect of the 5-HT1A receptor agonist buspirone on esophageal dysfunction associated with systemic sclerosis: a pilot study. United European Gastroenterol J. 2015;3(3):266–71.
80. Karamanolis GP, Panopoulos S, Denaxas K, Karlaftis A, Zorbala A, Kamberoglou D, et al. The 5-HT1A receptor agonist buspirone improves esophageal motor function and symptoms in systemic sclerosis: a 4-week, open-label trial. Arthritis Res Ther. 2016;18:195.

Chapter 10
Functional Dysphagia

Ofer Z. Fass and Ronnie Fass

Introduction

Functional dysphagia, also known in the literature as nonobstructive dysphagia, is one of the five functional esophageal disorders recognized by the Rome IV committee for functional esophageal disorders [1]. It is an infrequent cause of dysphagia symptoms and the least common functional esophageal disorder [2]. Thus, much is still unknown about disease epidemiology, pathophysiology, and treatment. Functional dysphagia remains a significant source of functional impairment and emotional distress in affected patients. In addition, it poses a diagnostic and therapeutic challenge to clinicians in their everyday practice. Although there is limited clinical information about its management, evidence regarding treatment of other functional esophageal disorders is often applied to functional dysphagia, which includes a multimodal approach of neuromodulators and management of psychological comorbidities. In refractory cases, empiric esophageal dilation and botulinum toxin injections into the distal esophagus are commonly considered.

In this chapter, functional dysphagia will be reviewed in detail as well as areas requiring further investigation. All provided recommendations are accompanied by a grade, which reflects the quality of available evidence in the current literature (Table 10.1).

O. Z. Fass
Department of Medicine, New York University Langone Health, New York University, New York, NY, USA

R. Fass (✉)
Case Western Reserve University, Digestive Health Center, Division of Gastroenterology and Hepatology, MetroHealth Medical Center, Cleveland, OH, USA

© Springer Nature Switzerland AG 2020
D. A. Patel et al. (eds.), *Evaluation and Management of Dysphagia*,
https://doi.org/10.1007/978-3-030-26554-0_10

Table 10.1 Levels of evidence

Level 1A	Large randomized control trials, systematic reviews/meta-analyses
Level 1B	High-quality cohort study
Level 1C	Moderate-sized randomized control trial or meta-analysis of small trials
Level 1D	At least one randomized control trial
Level 2	One high-quality, non-randomized cohort study
Level 3	At least one high-quality case-control study
Level 4	High-quality case series
Level 5	Opinions from experts

Definition

Functional dysphagia is defined as the sensation of abnormal bolus transit through the esophagus in the absence of structural, mucosal, or motor abnormalities [1]. Patients may report a sensation of solid or liquid foods sticking, lodging, or passing abnormally when swallowing. The definition of functional dysphagia requires the exclusion of alternative etiologies for esophageal dysphagia, including mucosal, structural, and motility disorders. Rome IV emphasized the need to exclude esophageal disorders that may present with dysphagia but without clear mucosal abnormalities, such as gastroesophageal reflux disease (GERD) and eosinophilic esophagitis (EoE). In addition, major esophageal motor disorders should be excluded as they commonly present with normal endoscopy. Therefore, it is important to obtain ancillary testing, such as reflux testing, high-resolution esophageal manometry (HREM), and mucosal biopsies, prior to establishing the diagnosis of functional dysphagia.

Rome IV outlines specific criteria for the diagnosis of functional dysphagia, all of which must be present [1].

- Sense of solid and/or liquid food sticking, lodging, or passing abnormally through the esophagus.
- Absence of evidence that esophageal mucosal or structural abnormality is the cause of the symptom.
- Absence of evidence that GERD or EoE is the cause of the symptom.
- Absence of major esophageal disorders (achalasia, esophagogastric junction outflow obstruction, distal esophageal spasm, jackhammer esophagus, and absent peristalsis).

Criteria must be fulfilled for the past 3 months with symptom onset at least 6 months before diagnosis with a frequency of at least once a week. Importantly, the presence of minor esophageal motor disorders, such as ineffective esophageal motility and fragmented peristalsis, does not exclude the diagnosis of functional dysphagia.

Ruling out EoE and major esophageal motility disorders as a prerequisite for diagnosing functional dysphagia is new to Rome IV as compared with previous Rome criteria. Similarly, the required symptom frequency of once per week is also new. EoE may cause dysphagia without any visible structural abnormalities on upper endoscopy. Consequently, esophageal mucosal biopsies are needed to exclude or make the diagnosis of eosinophilic esophagitis in these patients. Major esophageal motility disorders may cause a variety of symptoms, including dysphagia, chest pain, and heartburn. In Rome III, only pathology-based esophageal motor disorders were excluded. This meant only achalasia, ignoring the importance of excluding the other major esophageal motor disorders. Rome IV assumed that minor esophageal motility disorders, such as ineffective esophageal motility and fragmented peristalsis, are unlikely to be an important cause for dysphagia, and thus their presence does not exclude the diagnosis of functional dysphagia.

Rome IV recognized that functional dysphagia is an evolving concept, which is dependent on the diagnostic accuracy of the currently available technology. Thus, the definition of functional dysphagia will continue to change overtime as new and more refined equipment are introduced into our clinical practice, possibly shrinking the pool of patients with an unknown etiology for their dysphagia. Furthermore, while Rome IV allows the inclusion of dysphagia patients with minor esophageal motor disorders under the definition of functional dysphagia, future Rome committees may decide to exclude all or subset of these patients from the diagnosis.

Epidemiology

Epidemiological data for functional dysphagia are limited due to its complex diagnosis. Several esophageal tests are required prior to establishing the diagnosis, and consequently many clinicians outside the field of neurogastroenterology and motility remain unacquainted with the disorder. Furthermore, studies addressing disease prevalence often fail to meet all of the exclusionary criteria outlined by Rome IV.

In one of the first studies attempting to estimate the prevalence of swallowing disorders in the general population, the investigators surveyed 600 individuals aged 50–79 years old regarding swallowing and esophageal complaints. Of the 556 respondents, approximately 3% reported dysphagia symptoms. However, the number of persons with functional dysphagia was not determined in this study [3]. A mailed questionnaire study performed in Olmsted County, Minnesota, found similar results [4]. Investigators surveyed 3669 patients about dysphagia symptoms, and the medical records of patients reporting positive symptoms were examined for organic causes of dysphagia. The prevalence of dysphagia symptoms was shown to be 3% in both men and women. Approximately 2.5% of all respondents were noted to have dysphagia without an identifiable etiology. Of the 168 patients reporting frequent symptoms (at least weekly), approximately 50% had no clear etiology, suggesting a diagnosis of functional dysphagia. Another study also utilizing mailed questionnaires estimated the prevalence of functional dysphagia to be between 7 and 8% [2]. However, it was limited by the use of the old Rome I diagnostic criteria. A different study assessed the prevalence of functional gastrointestinal disorders in nine Asian countries [5]. Among the 1012 patients identified with functional gastrointestinal disorders, 0.6% reported symptoms of functional dysphagia. Of the five functional esophageal disorders, functional dysphagia had the lowest prevalence. Similar to the aforementioned studies, assessment of dysphagia prevalence was limited by the use of the Rome II criteria and lack of clinical confirmation.

A notable limitation of survey studies is the inability to perform exclusionary testing in patients reporting dysphagia, suggesting that the actual prevalence of functional dysphagia may be much lower than reported. In nearly 80% of patients presenting with dysphagia, an organic cause can be identified by taking a careful history. In patients undergoing endoscopic evaluation of dysphagia, a structural or mucosal etiology is identified in 75% of the cases [6, 7].

Advances in esophageal manometry have improved diagnostic accuracy of swallowing and motility disorders. A recent study evaluated 236 patients with esophageal dysphagia using high-resolution esophageal manometry (HREM) [8]. Only 32 (13.6%) patients demonstrated normal testing, suggesting that the prevalence of functional dysphagia may be lower in different populations and ethnic backgrounds.

Advances in manometric and impedance testing have enabled the detection of organic etiologies in patients previously thought to have a functional disorder. It is anticipated that with continued improvements in diagnostic testing, many patients with functional dysphagia will be reclassified as having an organic disorder resulting in further decrease in disease prevalence.

Pathophysiology

The pathophysiology of functional dysphagia is incompletely understood and remains an area of intense research. As with all functional esophageal disorders, symptoms are thought to arise in part from a complex interaction between esophageal hypersensitivity, abnormal central processing of esophageal stimuli, and psychological comorbidity. Evidence also suggests that intermittent peristaltic dysfunction may contribute to symptom generation. Thus, functional dysphagia is likely driven by multiple mechanisms which may differ among patients.

Key etiological principles of functional esophageal disorders are esophageal hypersensitivity and altered central perception of intraesophageal stimuli. Intraesophageal acid perfusion and balloon distension have both been shown to reproduce symptoms in patients with functional dysphagia [9].

Several mechanisms have been proposed as part of the intermittent abnormal esophageal motility theory. In 1 study, 30 patients with endoscopy-negative heartburn symptoms underwent acidic swallows with pomegranate juice while simultaneously being evaluated by HREM [10]. Patients were noted to have hypercontractile responses of the distal esophageal smooth muscle during perfusion of the acidic juice. Another study evaluated manometric recordings in 30 patients with functional dysphagia who underwent intraesophageal graded balloon distension. Distal esophageal contractions were demonstrated in 70% of the patients compared to 0% in healthy controls [11]. It should be noted that 30% of the functional dysphagia patients in this study did not show any peristaltic abnormalities in response to balloon distension. Other studies that support the esophageal dysmotility theory offer an alternative explanation for symptom generation in patients with functional dysphagia. Rather than hypercontractile responses induced by intraesophageal stimulation, they suggest hypocontractility, or peristaltic dysfunction, as the primary mechanism [12]. A study using barium boluses concomitantly with esophageal manometry in patients with nonobstructive dysphagia has shown that impaired or absent peristaltic waves resulted in incomplete bolus clearance [9]. As peristaltic wave amplitudes become weaker, esophageal clearance becomes progressively more ineffective [13]. A study investigating esophageal motility patterns in dysphagia patients during feeding demonstrated markedly reduced peristalsis, which could be provoked or exacerbated by increasing swallow frequency [14]. One hypothesis was that impaired peristalsis may be driven in part by esophageal acid exposure. A study in patients with endoscopy-negative reflux disease demonstrated decreased effective peristaltic contractions with increasing esophageal acid exposure ($r = 0.52$ for liquid boluses, $r = 0.27$ for solid boluses), which might also be applied to patients with functional dysphagia [15].

While Rome IV requires the exclusion of major esophageal motor disorders, it allows for the presence of minor disorders, such as ineffective esophageal motility and fragmented peristalsis. However, "minor esophageal motility disorders" is a broad category encompassing some conditions that have yet to be labeled by the Chicago classification. Future Rome guidelines may choose to exclude all motility disorders, both major and minor, further reducing the prevalence of functional dysphagia and altering our current understanding of its pathophysiology.

Despite the proposed role of disordered peristalsis in functional dysphagia, recent studies utilizing HREM have shown poor correlation between esophageal peristaltic patterns and patient-reported symptoms [16]. It appears that even with successful clearance of the food bolus, dysphagia symptoms may continue to persist [17]. Furthermore, stasis of liquid and solid boluses is observed in both functional dysphagia patients and healthy controls, suggesting that esophageal hypersensitivity, rather than disordered peristalsis, is the likely primary trigger of symptoms [18].

Another mechanism for symptom generation in patients with functional dysphagia has been established by using high-frequency intraesophageal ultrasonography, which examines simultaneous longitudinal and circular muscle contractions within the esophageal wall. A study in patients with nutcracker esophagus demonstrated asynchrony between longitudinal and circular muscle contractions during swallowing as compared to healthy controls. This abnormality could be extrapolated to patients with functional dysphagia [19, 20].

The mechanism by which esophageal hypersensitivity develops in some patients continues to be an important area of investigation. Studies in patients with functional esophageal disorders suggest that peripheral mucosal afferents are sensitized by repeated esophageal acid exposure, resulting in dilation of intraepithelial spaces and increased mucosal permeability [21]. The role of esophageal hypersensitivity in functional dysphagia was further supported by the observation that patients with abnormal sensory perception thresholds for balloon distension also demonstrate a significant association with dysphagia as their primary presenting symptom [22].

As with all other functional esophageal disorders, psychological comorbidities have also been observed in patients with functional dysphagia, suggesting a potential role in disease presentation. Patients with dysphagia without a clear structural etiology have been shown to have higher rates of anxiety, depression, and somatization disorders [23]. One study reported an association between emotional distress and anxiety with functional dysphagia [24]. Another study demonstrated a relationship between emotional stress and altered esophageal motility. Both patients who were reporting unpleasant memories, and those who were subjected to stressful interviews, demonstrated altered barium transit [23]. Challenging cognitive tasks have similarly been shown to induce altered esophageal manometry findings. Psychological comorbidity contributes to altered perception of intraesophageal stimuli and may drive symptom severity in patients with functional esophageal disorders. However, whether altered motility observed in patients under psychological stress contributes to dysphagia symptoms is uncertain. Alternatively, patients with psychological comorbidities may experience greater distress from their symptoms and be more likely to pursue medical attention.

Clinical Presentation

The characteristic symptom of functional dysphagia is the sensation of sticking, lodging, abnormal passage, or incomplete passage of solid or liquid boluses [1]. The symptoms of functional dysphagia are indistinguishable from those of dysphagia due to organic etiologies. Thus, a patient presenting with suspected functional dysphagia must undergo detailed diagnostic testing to rule out structural, mucosal, and major motor abnormalities.

New to the Rome IV criteria is the addition of EoE as an exclusion criterion. Biopsies of the esophageal mucosa are routinely obtained during endoscopic evaluation of dysphagia to assess for the presence of eosinophils. Additionally, the presence of GERD is similarly specified as an exclusion criterion. Therefore, the presence of typical heartburn symptoms in addition to dysphagia suggests an alternative diagnosis.

Psychological comorbidities are associated with functional dysphagia, specifically anxiety, depression, somatization, and stress [24]. Although not diagnostic, the presence of clinically significant anxiety in a patient with dysphagia and no obvious organic etiology should heighten the suspicion for functional dysphagia.

Diagnosis

Diagnostic workup of dysphagia begins with a thorough history to exclude other conditions that can mimic dysphagia, such as xerostomia, globus sensation, odynophagia, and choking sensation. Thereafter, oropharyngeal dysphagia is excluded by the presence of the following symptoms: sialorrhea, food sticking immediately in the throat, inability to chew, difficulty initiating a swallow, nasopharyngeal regurgitation, inability or delay in initiating a swallow, the need for repetitive swallows to clear the hypopharynx, aspiration, coughing, or choking [25]. The patient may also report various neuromuscular symptoms, such as dysarthria, diplopia, muscle weakness, vertigo, nausea, vomiting, tremor, and ataxia. Importantly, dysphagia can be the initial symptom of a neurologic disease.

In general, intrinsic and extrinsic mechanical causes commonly lead to dysphagia for solid foods, whereas patients with motility disorders tend to complain of progressive or nonprogressive dysphagia for both liquids and solids from the onset.

Useful information can be obtained from the reported course of the dysphagia. Acute onset of dysphagia due to food impaction is usually indicative of mechanical obstruction. Additionally, a sudden onset of dysphagia in association with other neurologic symptoms may indicate an acute cerebrovascular accident. Patients who have lower esophageal mucosal rings typically complain of dysphagia that is intermittent and nonprogressive. In contrast, esophageal strictures or malignancies commonly cause progressive dysphagia.

The duration of the dysphagia is often an important sign as to whether the underlying cause is benign or malignant. Malignant dysphagia, for example, presents with relatively short progressive history and is frequently associated with significant weight loss.

Commonly, patients with oropharyngeal dysphagia can accurately localize the swallow dysfunction to the oropharynx. In contrast, patients with esophageal dysphagia symptoms may not be able to localize the level of the disease. The patient pointing to the jugular notch may reflect a referral of sensation from the distal esophagus. Pointing to the xiphoid bone is more sensitive for the location of the swallowing dysfunction.

Associated symptoms, such as heartburn, regurgitation, aspiration, weight loss, and chest or abdominal pain, may help to narrow the differential diagnosis. History of chronic heartburn may suggest that the dysphagia is caused by an esophageal peptic stricture or erosive esophagitis. The symptoms of chest pain, wheezing, chronic cough, hoarseness, and sleep disruption may be atypical, or extraesophageal manifestations of gastroesophageal reflux disease. History of chest pain may also suggest the possibility of spastic motility disorders of the esophagus as a cause for the dysphagia.

Pain during swallowing or persistent sore throat may indicate malignancy, infection, or inflammation from corrosive agents or ionizing radiation. In some patients, change in voice quality is the first symptom suggestive of a swallowing disorder. In contrast, patients with mechanical obstruction or achalasia may present with weight loss.

As mentioned above, difficulties in swallowing may be the presenting symptom of a much more generalized neuromuscular disorder or systemic disease [26]. For example, dysphagia could be the presenting symptom of collagen vascular disorders such as scleroderma or systemic lupus erythematosus.

Dysphagia in patients on chronic immunosuppressive treatment may suggest infectious esophagitis (fungal or viral). Although the predominant symptom for these patients is usually odynophagia, most patients experience dysphagia as well.

A detailed history of medication consumption is also important, as a number of centrally acting drugs can impair oropharyngeal function and cause tardive dyskinesia with masticatory and swallowing difficulties, as well as toxic or inflammatory myopathy or dysfunction in neuromuscular transmission. In addition, medications such as nonsteroidal anti-inflammatory drugs, tetracyclines, potassium, iron, and vitamin C tablets can cause pill-induced esophagitis that presents as acute esophageal dysphagia. These types of medications can cause mid- or distal esophageal ulceration and even a stricture [27].

Physical examination in patients with dysphagia may reveal clues for diagnosis and the patient's nutritional status. Unfortunately, physical examination is commonly skipped in patients with dysphagia, depriving physicians from obtaining additional important clinical information. Careful examination of the head and neck for masses, lymph nodes, or enlarged thyroid is pivotal. Signs of prior surgery and radiotherapy should be noted. The oral cavity, including dentition or dentures, tongue, and oropharynx, should be inspected. Eye signs, sweating, tremor, and tachycardia may be present in patients with thyrotoxic myopathy. Examination of the chest may reveal signs of pneumonia due to aspiration, particularly in patients with oropharyngeal dysphagia. A neurologic examination is mandatory when evaluating patients with oropharyngeal dysphagia. Physical findings may indicate cranial nerve dysfunction, neuromuscular disease, cerebellar dysfunction, or a movement disorder [28]. For patients with dysphagia caused by a collagen vascular disease, physical examination may detect joint abnormalities, calcinosis, sclerodactyly, telangiectasia, and other findings.

It has been demonstrated that a careful and detailed physical examination with a good history of the medical problem should lead a physician to the correct diagnosis in 80–85% of dysphagia cases [29]. However, some patients may present with atypical symptoms and signs. In these cases, the physician must rely on other diagnostic studies to establish the correct diagnosis.

If esophageal dysphagia is suspected, an upper endoscopy should be performed first to assess for structural and mucosal etiologies. If the test is unremarkable, esophageal biopsies are obtained to assess for EoE, a new exclusion criterion offered by Rome IV [1]. Although an upper endoscopy is typically sufficient to identify structural causes of dysphagia, a barium swallow using solid boluses, like a tablet or marshmallow, may be employed to identify subtle structural irregularities, such as rings or extrinsic compression of the esophagus [30]. Some clinicians may use timed barium esophagram to obtain a physiological assessment of patient's capacity to empty their esophagus.

While erosive esophagitis and Barrett's esophagus can be excluded during upper endoscopy, patients with nonerosive reflux disease (NERD), and thus negative upper endoscopy, can present with dysphagia symptoms and should be excluded as part of the diagnostic workup. This is in particular important in those with both dysphagia and heartburn symptoms who should undergo empiric treatment with a

PPI and subsequently assessed for improvement in their dysphagia. Ambulatory pH monitoring or impedance plus pH is not considered part of the routine diagnostic algorithm for functional dysphagia but can be considered in patients with associated persistent heartburn and/or regurgitation symptoms who are not responsive to aggressive anti-reflux treatment.

In the absence of structural etiologies and heartburn symptoms, the next diagnostic step is the exclusion of major esophageal motor disorders. This is accomplished by using HREM which assesses esophagogastric function and esophageal body peristalsis that can impede bolus transit [31]. As previously mentioned, Rome IV allows for minor esophageal motor abnormalities to be present, such as ineffective esophageal motility and fragmented peristalsis, in patients with the diagnosis of functional dysphagia. This is because low-amplitude esophageal contractions and liquid/solid bolus stasis requiring multiple swallows to clear the esophagus have been observed in both patients and healthy controls [16, 32]. Certain maneuvers, such as rapid swallowing or ingestion of solid food during esophageal manometry, can enhance the detection of esophageal motor abnormalities that may explain dysphagia symptoms [20, 33].

The exclusion of intrinsic structural esophageal abnormalities, extrinsic compression, EoE, NERD, and major esophageal motor disorders supports the diagnosis of functional dysphagia (Fig. 10.1). Other experimental modalities may have a role in functional dysphagia, although most have not been studied in this area. High-frequency intraesophageal ultrasonography has been used to demonstrate lack of coordination between the longitudinal and circular esophageal muscle contractions in patients with dysphagia and nutcracker esophagus [19]. Endoscopic functional luminal imaging probe (EndoFLIP) is a new technology that is able to measure esophagogastric junction distensibility [34]. Studies using EndoFLIP in patients with EoE, achalasia, or those who are pre- or postsurgical intervention in the esophagus demonstrated a correlation between the degrees of distensibility and the risk for reporting dysphagia [35]. While the EndoFLIP technique requires further validation, it may be used in patients with functional dysphagia to identify distensibility abnormalities and thus further classify them. High-resolution impedance manometry (HRIM) has been used to evaluate esophageal bolus flow and retention, simultaneously with esophageal peristalsis and esophagogastric function [36]. This technique may further help to investigate patients with dysphagia, but its value in functional dysphagia remains to be determined.

Future developments in technology that assess esophageal function will continue to challenge our definition of functional dysphagia. In addition, currently available diagnostic techniques demonstrate that ineffective esophageal motility is the most commonly diagnosed esophageal motor disorder in clinical practice. This is primarily due to the wide range of peristaltic abnormalities that are encompassed under this category, all the way from 50% weak swallows to 90% failed swallows. Future changes to the definition of ineffective esophageal motility may alter the definition of functional dysphagia. Table 10.2 summarizes all recommendations for the diagnosis of functional dysphagia.

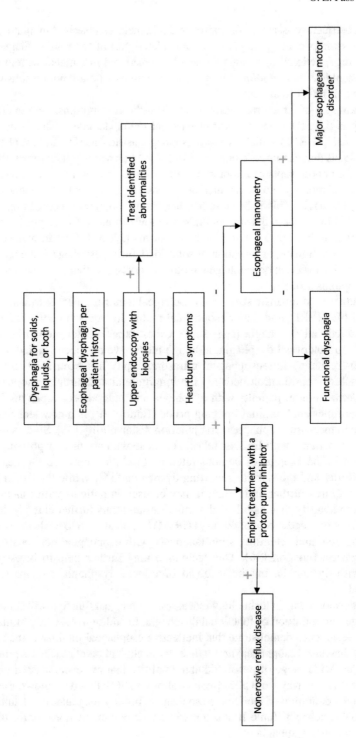

Fig. 10.1 Diagnostic algorithm for functional dysphagia

Table 10.2 Diagnostic recommendations for functional dysphagia

Recommendation	Level of evidence
1. A thorough history and physical examination should be obtained to exclude esophageal dysphagia due to structural, mucosal, and motor abnormalities	Level 2
2. Upper endoscopy should be performed to assess for structural and mucosal etiologies	Level 1a
3. Mucosal biopsies during upper endoscopy should be obtained to assess for EoE and other mucosal abnormalities	Level 1a
4. Barium swallow with tablet or marshmallow should be considered in dysphagia patients with normal endoscopy	Level 5
5. Patients with heartburn symptoms should be initially treated with empiric PPI therapy	Level 1C
6. High-resolution esophageal manometry should be performed to rule out major motility disorders after structural and mucosal abnormalities are excluded	Level 3
7. Provocative maneuvers, such as rapid swallowing or ingestion of food during manometry, may be used to enhance the detection of esophageal motor abnormalities	Level 3

EoE eosinophilic esophagitis, *PPI* proton pump inhibitor

Treatment

There is limited evidence to guide the management of functional dysphagia, and recommendations are primarily empiric. Furthermore, dysphagia symptoms may resolve over time and occasionally not require aggressive treatment [1]. Thus, initial management is commonly conservative and entails lifestyle modifications, such as sitting upright when eating, avoiding food triggers, swallowing smaller food boluses, and using water, sauce, or gravy as food lubricants [37].

If symptoms persist despite conservative management, the next best course of treatment remains unclear. Some experts advocate for a trial of PPI therapy over a period of 4–8 weeks, especially in patients with associated heartburn symptoms. If the patient remains symptomatic, then anti-reflux treatment should be discontinued [38]. Subsequent medical therapy may include neuromodulators (Table 10.3). These medications have proven to be beneficial in other functional esophageal disorders because of their effect on reducing esophageal hypersensitivity [39]. The main esophageal neuromodulators include tricyclic antidepressants, selective serotonin reuptake inhibitors, and selective norepinephrine reuptake inhibitors. Other esophageal neuromodulators include trazadone, pregabalin, and gabapentin. However, no randomized controlled trials are available in functional dysphagia, and thus the use of neuromodulators in this disorder remains empiric.

Prokinetics and parasympathomimetic drugs have been proposed as novel therapeutic modalities in functional dysphagia; however, data to support their routine use in practice is still lacking. Furthermore, the few trials investigating their efficacy in patients with esophageal peristaltic dysfunction have yielded disappointing results

Table 10.3 Neuromodulators studied in randomized controlled trials of patients with functional or nonfunctional esophageal disorders

Name	Class of drugs	Disorder	Dose	Response rate	Side effects
Imipramine	TCAs	NCCP	50 mg/day	52%	QT prolongation
Imipramine	TCAs	NCCP	50 mg/day	Significant	Dry mouth, dizziness
Imipramine	TCAs	FH, RH	25 mg/day	37.2%	Constipation
Amitriptyline	TCAs	NCCP, globus	10.25 mg/day	52%, significant	Excessive sleeping, dizziness
Sertraline	SSRIs	NCCP	50–200 mg/day	57%	Nausea, restlessness
Sertraline	SSRIs	NCCP	50–200 mg/day	Modest	Dry mouth, diarrhea
Paroxetine	SSRIs	NCCP	10–50 mg/day	Modest	Fatigue, dizziness
Paroxetine	SSRIs	NCCP	10–50 mg/day	21.70%	None
Citalopram	SSRIs	RH	20 mg/day	Significant	None
Fluoxetine	SSRIs	FH/RH	20 mg/day	Significant	Headache, dry mouth
Trazodone	SRIs	Dysmotility	100–150 mg/day	29–41%	Dry mouth, dizziness
Venlafaxine	SNRIs	NCCP	75 mg/day	52%	Sleep disturbances
Ranitidine	H2RAs	FH	300 mg/day	Significant	None
Theophylline	Adenosine antagonists	NCCP	200 mg twice per day	58%	Nausea, insomnia, tremor
Gabapentin	GABA analog	Globus	300 mg 3 times per day	66%	None

With permission from Ref. [44]
FH functional heartburn, *GABA* gamma-aminobutyric acid, *NCCP* noncardiac chest pain, *RH* reflux hypersensitivity, *SNRIs* serotonin-norepinephrine reuptake inhibitors, *SRIs* serotonin reuptake inhibitors, *SSRIs* selective serotonin reuptake inhibitors, *TCAs* tricyclic antidepressants

in addition to concerns about their safety profile [37]. Future studies in functional dysphagia patients may be needed before definitive recommendations can be made regarding the value of prokinetics.

A number of studies have evaluated the role of empiric esophageal dilation in the management of functional dysphagia. One study by Naini et al. compared esophageal dilation using a 54- or 57-Fr bougie to medical therapy with a PPI or histamine-2 receptor antagonist in patients with functional dysphagia. Complete resolution of symptoms was reported in 68.3% of patients treated with esophageal dilation compared to 59.5% of those treated with medical therapy, although the difference was not statistically significant [40]. Another study by Colon et al. compared the efficacy of different bougie sizes on symptom response of patients with nonobstructive dysphagia [41]. Patients were randomized to receive dilation with a 50-Fr bougie ($n = 13$) or a 26-Fr bougie ($n = 10$). Patients undergoing dilation with the 50-Fr bougie had a significantly greater symptomatic response compared to those undergoing dilation with the 26-Fr bougie (84.6 vs 40%, $P = 0.03$), (Fig. 10.2). At 2-year follow-up, 80% of the patients initially respond-

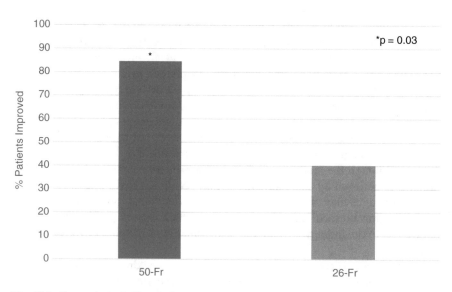

Fig. 10.2 Comparison of efficacy of esophageal dilation with 50-Fr bougie versus 26-Fr bougie in patients with functional dysphagia immediately after dilation. (With permission from Ref. [41])

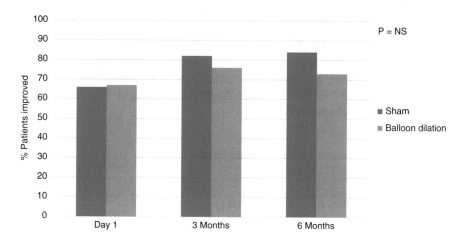

Fig. 10.3 Comparison of through-the-endoscope balloon dilation versus sham dilation in patients with dysphagia but without endoscopic evidence of disease. (With permission from Ref. [42])

ing to the 50-Fr bougie had a sustained response. It is thought that the response to dilation with a 50–54-Fr bougie may be due to interruption of subtle structural abnormalities such as rings, which may not be identified during endoscopy or barium swallows. In contrast, dilation with through-the-endoscope balloons has not been shown to benefit patients with functional dysphagia. A trial comparing endoscopic balloon dilation to sham dilation did not demonstrate a significant difference in dysphagia symptoms at day 1, 3 months, or 6 months posttreatment (Fig. 10.3) [42].

Botulinum toxin injections, which are commonly used for esophageal hyper-contractile disorders, have been considered for the treatment of refractory cases of functional dysphagia. A study by Vanuytsel et al. investigated the role of botulinum toxin injections into the distal esophagus in patients with diffuse esophageal spasm and nutcracker esophagus [43]. As compared with patients who had received sham saline injections, botulinum toxin injections were associated with a significant reduction in symptom scores and esophagogastric junction pressures. However, response to treatment does not appear to be durable. Only 50% of the patients reported response to treatment at 1 month and 30% at 1 year. Although the study population had a primary esophageal motility disorder, it is believed by some authorities that botulinum toxin injection into the lower esophagus may also benefit patients with functional dysphagia. However, what injection protocol should be used and which factors predict response to botulinum toxin therapy in patients with functional dysphagia remain to be determined.

As with all functional esophageal disorders, addressing psychological comorbidities is essential for any therapeutic intervention in patients with functional dysphagia. While none has been studied in functional dysphagia patients, psychological interventions, such as cognitive behavioral therapy, muscle relaxation techniques, hypnotherapy, mindfulness, dynamic psychotherapy, and multicomponent psychosocial therapy, have been used successfully in other functional esophageal disorders and noncardiac chest pain. It is evident from other functional esophageal disorders that addressing psychological comorbidity is pivotal for treatment success. Table 10.4 summarizes recommendations for medical management, and Table 10.5 summarizes recommendations for nonmedical management of patients with functional dysphagia. Figure 10.4 provides a suggested treatment algorithm.

Table 10.4 Medical management of functional dysphagia

Recommendation	Level of evidence
1. Lifestyle modifications should be the first line of management	Level 5
2. PPI therapy for 4–8 weeks should be considered for patients with associated heartburn or regurgitation symptoms	Level 5
3. Neuromodulators (SSRIs, SNRIs, TCAs) should be considered early in patient management	Level 5
4. Prokinetics and parasympathomimetic medications should not be considered as part of medical management	Level 5

PPI proton pump inhibitor, *SNRI* selective norepinephrine reuptake inhibitors, *SSRI* selective serotonin reuptake inhibitors, *TCA* tricyclic antidepressant

Table 10.5 Nonmedical management of functional dysphagia

Recommendation	Level of evidence
1. All patients with psychological comorbidities should be evaluated by a psychiatrist or psychologist. Treatment may include cognitive behavioral therapy, biofeedback, and stress reduction techniques	Level 5
2. Patients failing medical management should undergo esophageal dilation with a 50–54-Fr bougie	Level 1D
3. Through-the-endoscope balloon dilation should not be used as treatment and is not equivalent to dilation with a bougie	Level 1D
4. Botulinum toxin injections should be offered if dilation failed	Level 5

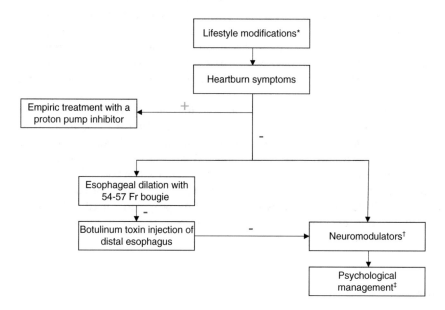

*Lifestyle modifications entail sitting upright when eating, avoiding food triggers, swallowing smaller food boluses, and using water, sauce, or gravy as food lubricants.

†Neuromodulators include selective serotonin reuptake inhibitors, selective norepinephrine reuptake inhibitors, and tricyclic antidepressants, and GABA analogs.

‡Psychological management involves cognitive behavioral therapy, biofeedback, and stress-reduction techniques.

Fig. 10.4 Treatment algorithm for functional dysphagia

Summary

Functional dysphagia is an uncommon cause of dysphagia symptoms and presents a diagnostic and therapeutic challenge. It is defined as a sensation of solid and/ or liquid food sticking, lodging, or passing abnormally through the esophagus in the absence of any mucosal, structural, or major functional abnormalities of the esophagus.

Functional dysphagia accounts for 7–8% of the patients presenting with dysphagia [2]. Etiology is presumed to be secondary to esophageal hypersensitivity, abnormal central processing of esophageal stimuli, intermittent abnormal esophageal motor disorder, and psychological comorbidities.

Diagnosis begins with a careful history and physical examination. Upper endoscopy with mucosal biopsies should be performed in all patients presenting with dysphagia. If endoscopy is unremarkable and the patient reports heartburn or regurgitation symptoms, an empiric PPI trial should be considered. If there is no improvement, subsequent testing with HREM can help to exclude major esophageal motor disorders.

Treatment of functional dysphagia includes lifestyle changes and avoidance of triggers, neuromodulators (tricyclic antidepressants, selective serotonin reuptake inhibitors, selective norepinephrine reuptake inhibitors, trazadone, pregabalin, and gabapentin), and psychological interventions if needed. Nonpharmacologic management can also be employed, which includes dilation with a 50–54-Fr bougie and in carefully selected patients botulinum toxin injections into the distal esophagus. Regardless, there are many areas in functional dysphagia that need to be further studied, and thus definition, epidemiology, diagnosis, and treatment of functional dysphagia are likely to further evolve in the future.

References

1. Aziz Q, et al. Esophageal disorders. Gastroenterology. 2016;150(6):1368–79.
2. Drossman DA, et al. U. S. householder survey of functional gastrointestinal disorders. Dig Dis Sci. 1993;38(9):1569–80.
3. Lindgren S, Janzon L. Prevalence of swallowing complaints and clinical findings among 50–79-year-old men and women in an urban population. Dysphagia. 1991;6(4):187–92.
4. Cho SY, et al. Prevalence and risk factors for dysphagia: a USA community study. Neurogastroenterol Motil. 2015;27(2):212–9.
5. Kwan AC-P, et al. Validation of Rome II criteria for functional gastrointestinal disorders by factor analysis of symptoms in Asian patient sample. J Gastroenterol Hepatol. 2003;18(7):796–802.
6. Lind CD. Dysphagia: evaluation and treatment. Gastroenterol Clin North Am. 2003;32(2):553–75.
7. Rosenstock AS, et al. Su1509 diagnostic yield in the evaluation of dysphagia. Gastrointest Endosc. 2011;73(4):AB287.
8. Wang D, et al. Assessment of esophageal motor disorders using high-resolution manometry in esophageal dysphagia with normal endoscopy. J Neurogastroenterol Motil. 2019;25(1):61–7.
9. Kahrilas PJ, Dodds WJ, Hogan WJ. Effect of peristaltic dysfunction on esophageal volume clearance. Gastroenterology. 1988;94(1):73–80.

10. Lee H, et al. Effect of acid swallowing on esophageal contraction in patients with heartburn related to hypersensitivity. J Gastroenterol Hepatol. 2013;28(1):84–9.
11. Deschner WK, et al. Manometric responses to balloon distention in patients with nonobstructive dysphagia. Gastroenterology. 1989;97(5):1181–5.
12. Roman S, et al. Weak peristalsis in esophageal pressure topography: classification and association with dysphagia. Am J Gastroenterol. 2011;106(2):349–56.
13. Tutuian R, Castell DO. Clarification of the esophageal function defect in patients with manometric ineffective esophageal motility: studies using combined impedance-manometry. Clin Gastroenterol Hepatol. 2004;2(3):230–6.
14. Howard PJ, et al. Esophageal motor patterns during episodes of dysphagia for solids. Neurogastroenterol Motil. 1991;3(3):123–30.
15. Daum C, et al. Failure to respond to physiologic challenge characterizes esophageal motility in erosive gastro-esophageal reflux disease. Neurogastroenterol Motil. 2011;23(6):517–e200.
16. Bogte A, et al. Relationship between esophageal contraction patterns and clearance of swallowed liquid and solid boluses in healthy controls and patients with dysphagia. Neurogastroenterol Motil. 2012;24(8):e364–72.
17. Bogte A, et al. Sensation of stasis is poorly correlated with impaired esophageal bolus transport. Neurogastroenterol Motil. 2014;26(4):538–45.
18. Pouderoux P, et al. Esophageal solid bolus transit: studies using concurrent videofluoroscopy and manometry. Am J Gastroenterol. 1999;94(6):1457.
19. Jung H-Y, et al. Asynchrony between the circular and the longitudinal muscle contraction in patients with nutcracker esophagus. Gastroenterology. 2005;128(5):1179–86.
20. Fox M, Sweis R. Future directions in esophageal motility and function – new technology and methodology. Neurogastroenterol Motil. 2012;24(s1):48–56.
21. Szczesniak MM, Fuentealba SE, Cook IJ. Acid sensitization of esophageal mucosal afferents: implication for symptom perception in patients across the gastroesophageal reflux disease spectrum. Clin J Pain. 2013;29(1):70–7.
22. Clouse RE, et al. Clinical correlates of abnormal sensitivity to intraesophageal balloon distension. Dig Dis Sci. 1991;36(8):1040–5.
23. Galmiche JP, et al. Functional esophageal disorders. Gastroenterology. 2006;130(5):1459–65.
24. Barofsky I, Fontaine KR. Do psychogenic dysphagia patients have an eating disorder? Dysphagia. 1998;13(1):24–7.
25. Gasiorowska A, Fass R. Current approach to dysphagia. Gastroenterol Hepatol. 2009;5(4):269–79.
26. Jones B, Donner MW. Examination of the patient with dysphagia. Radiology. 1988;167(2):319–26.
27. Abid S, et al. Pill-induced esophageal injury: endoscopic features and clinical outcomes. Endoscopy. 2005;37(08):740–4.
28. Achem SR, Devault KR. Dysphagia in aging. J Clin Gastroenterol. 2005;39(5):357–71.
29. Castell DO, Donner MW. Evaluation of dysphagia: a careful history is crucial. Dysphagia. 1987;2(2):65–71.
30. van Westen D, Ekberg O. Solid bolus swallowing in the radiologic evaluation of dysphagia. Acta Radiol. 1993;34(4):372–5.
31. Gyawali CP, et al. Evaluation of esophageal motor function in clinical practice. Neurogastroenterol Motil. 2013;25(2):99–133.
32. Kahrilas PJ, et al. The Chicago classification of esophageal motility disorders, v3.0. Neurogastroenterol Motil. 2015;27(2):160–74.
33. Shaker A, et al. Multiple rapid swallow responses during esophageal high-resolution manometry reflect esophageal body peristaltic reserve. Am J Gastroenterol. 2013;108:1706.
34. Hirano I, Pandolfino JE, Boeckxstaens GE. Functional lumen imaging probe for the management of esophageal disorders: expert review from the clinical practice updates committee of the AGA Institute. Clin Gastroenterol Hepatol. 2017;15(3):325–34.
35. Nicodème F, et al. Esophageal distensibility as a measure of disease severity in patients with eosinophilic esophagitis. Clin Gastroenterol Hepatol. 2013;11(9):1101–1107.e1.

36. Singendonk MJ, et al. High-resolution impedance manometry parameters in the evaluation of esophageal function of non-obstructive dysphagia patients. Neurogastroenterol Motil. 2019;31(2):e13505.
37. Smout A, Fox M. Weak and absent peristalsis. Neurogastroenterol Motil. 2012;24(s1):40–7.
38. Vakil NB, Traxler B, Levine D. Dysphagia in patients with erosive esophagitis: prevalence, severity, and response to proton pump inhibitor treatment. Clin Gastroenterol Hepatol. 2004;2(8):665–8.
39. Dickman R, Maradey-Romero C, Fass R. The role of pain modulators in esophageal disorders – no pain no gain. Neurogastroenterol Motil. 2014;26(5):603–10.
40. Naini P, et al. Critical evaluation of esophageal dilation in nonobstructive dysphagia with and without esophageal rings. J Clin Gastroenterol. 2007;41(4):362–5.
41. Colon VJ, Young MA, Ramirez FC. The short- and long-term efficacy of empirical esophageal dilation in patients with nonobstructive dysphagia: a prospective, randomized study. Am J Gastroenterol. 2000;95(4):910–3.
42. Scolapio JS, et al. Dysphagia without endoscopically evident disease: to dilate or not? Am J Gastroenterol. 2001;96(2):327–30.
43. Vanuytsel T, et al. Botulinum toxin reduces dysphagia in patients with nonachalasia primary esophageal motility disorders. Clin Gastroenterol Hepatol. 2013;11(9):1115–1121.e2.
44. Gyawali CP, Fass R. Management of gastroesophageal reflux disease. Gastroenterology. 2018;154(2):302–18.

Index

© Springer Nature Switzerland AG 2020
D. A. Patel et al. (eds.), *Evaluation and Management of Dysphagia*,
https://doi.org/10.1007/978-3-030-26554-0